Controversies in Clinical Thyroidology

Controversies in
Clinical Thyroidology

Edited by
Joel I. Hamburger
J. Martin Miller

With 56 Figures

Springer-Verlag
New York   Heidelberg   Berlin

Joel I. Hamburger
Associated Endocrinologists
4400 Prudential Town Center
Southfield
Michigan 48075 U.S.A.

J. Martin Miller
Division of Endocrinology
Henry Ford Hospital
Detroit
Michigan 48202 U.S.A.

Library of Congress Cataloging in Publication Data
Main entry under title:
Controversies in clinical thyroidology.
  Includes index.
  1. Thyroid gland—Diseases.   I. Hamburger, Joel I.
II. Miller, J. Martin.   [DNLM: 1. Thyroid
diseases.   WK 200 C764]
RC655.C64   616.4′4   81-5270
                              AACR2

© 1981 by Springer-Verlag New York Inc.
Softcover reprint of the hardcover 1st edition 1981

9 8 7 6 5 4 3 2 1

ISBN-13:978-1-4612-5918-3   e-ISBN-13:978-1-4612-5916-9
DOI: 10.1007/978-1-4612-5916-9

Preface

"Man's natural instinct, in fact, is never toward what is sound and true. It is toward what is specious and false . . .

The ideas that conquer the race most rapidly and arouse the wildest enthusiasm and are held most tenaciously are precisely the ideas that are most insane. This has been true since the first 'advanced' gorilla put on underwear, cultivated a frown and began his first lecture tour, . . ."

H. L. Mencken, from
Meditation On Meditation
in the Smart Set, June, 1920
pp 45–46

In our opinion there is no field of clinical medicine in such a state of dynamic disequilibrium as clinical thyroidology. Thyroid diseases are very common. The moderately complex but easily understandable physiological interrelationships between the thyroid, pituitary and hypothalamus have provided stimuli for the application of modern technology in the development of an array of diagnostic procedures. Although therapeutic methods have been more stable, and recent advances more limited, their application by physicians representing different disciplines has provided an ample basis for the expression of differing viewpoints.

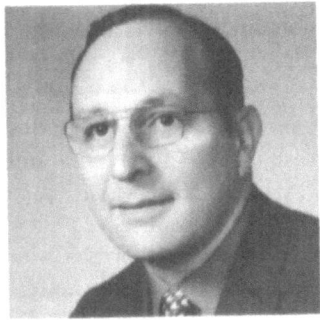

Joel I. Hamburger, M.D.

Unfortunately there are few opportunities for in-depth exploration of different attitudes and experience relevant to issues of current interest. The review process employed by medical journals often seems to stifle the expression of controversial viewpoints. The discussions afforded by "Letters to the Editor" are limited and suffer from an interval of several months between the original presentation and the controversy it provoked. At

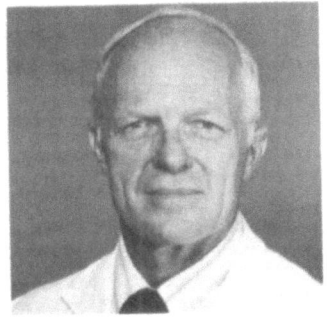

J. Martin Miller, M.D.

medical meetings discussions almost invariably are closed for lack of time before
the issues can be resolved. Finally, it is seldom possible to bring together in one
location at the same time experts from around the world.

The objective of this volume is to provide a forum for thorough discussions of
controversial issues which the editors believe will be of interest to physicians who
care for thyroid patients. The editors and their colleagues have provided the
framework for each discussion by listing the issues, reporting their experience and
offering their opinions, based upon that experience. The editors have been in close
contact and have worked together on projects for the past twenty years. During
this time they have been engaged primarily in patient care. Therefore they believe
they know the answers. Curiously, however, they do not always agree with each
other's answers. Be that as it may, after the initial presentations we come to the
heart of the volume, the invited commentaries from authorities from around the
world. These physicians were asked to present their experience and opinion on the
issues because of their demonstrated interest and expertise, and previous contributions to the thyroid literature. Special effort has been made to obtain input from
physicians holding opinions contrary to those of the editors. The contributors were
given the opportunity to review the material prepared by the editors so that they
could focus their remarks on the issues which were raised. They have been given
free rein to express themselves at whatever length they deemed appropriate, and
their remarks, in agreement or otherwise, have been printed as submitted.
Although the inclusion of supporting data has been encouraged, since the contributors are all physicians who have published papers on the subject, we were mostly
interested in their opinions.

The final summations by the editors may be of assistance to some, but may be
ignored by others who prefer to arrive at their own conclusions. Regardless of this,
we hope that the reader will find that this form of presentation provides an easy
way to reach decisions on controversial issues in clinical thyroidology.

Before closing these remarks we feel obliged to beg the indulgence of the many
outstanding authorities who were not invited to participate. We sincerely hope
that they will submit material for consideration for the next volume. We plan to
produce new editions on different issues at about two year intervals. Such submissions may be of two types:

1. A suggestion of a controversial issue which a physician would like to have
presented in the format of this volume.

2. An in-depth presentation of experience on an issue which can be discussed
by other authorities.

Instructions for authors are included at the end of the book.

Joel I. Hamburger, M.D.
J. Martin Miller, M.D.

Contents

Some Contributors to This Volume

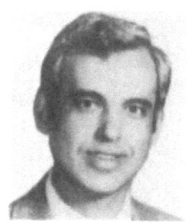

Michael Garcia, M.D.

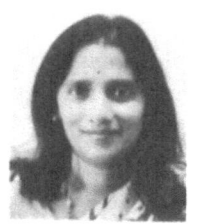

Sudha R. Kini, M.D.

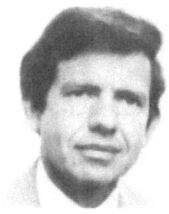

Donald A. Meier, M.D.

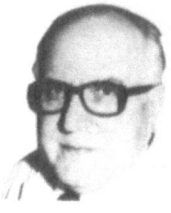

John Rebuck, M.D.

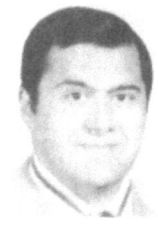

Sheldon S. Stoffer, M.D.

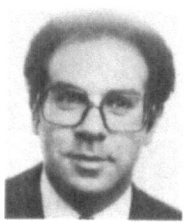

Charles I. Taylor, M.D.

List of Contributors

Nobuyuke Amino, M.D. Assistant Professor of Medicine, The Central Laboratory for Clinical Investigation, Osaka University Hospital, Osaka, Japan

David Barzilai, M.D. Professor of Medicine and Endocrinology; Dean, Faculty of Medicine, Technion-Israel Institute of Technology, Haifa, Israel

David V. Becker, M.D. Professor of Medicine and Radiology; Director, Division of Nuclear Medicine, New York Hospital–Cornell Medical Center, New York, New York, U.S.A.

William H. Beierwaltes, M.D. Professor of Medicine; Director, Division of Nuclear Medicine, University of Michigan Hospital, Ann Arbor, Michigan, U.S.A.

Manfred Blum, M.D. Associate Professor of Clinical Medicine; Director, Nuclear Endocrine Division, New York University School of Medicine, New York, New York, U.S.A.

Lewis E. Braverman, M.D. Professor of Medicine and Physiology; Director, Endocrinology and Metabolism, University of Massachusetts Medical School, Worcester, Massachusetts, U.S.A.

John J. Canary, M.D. Professor of Medicine; Director, Division of Endocrinology and Metabolism, Georgetown University School of Medicine, Washington, D.C., U.S.A.

Angelo Carpi, M.D. Center of Nuclear Medicine, University of Pisa, Pisa, Italy

Robert G. Carroll, M.D.   Associate Professor of Radiology, University of Florida, Gainesville, Florida, U.S.A.

N. David Charkes, M.D.   Research Professor of Nuclear Medicine and Professor of Medicine, Temple University Medical School and Hospital, Philadelphia, Pennsylvania, U.S.A.

Orlo H. Clark, M.D.   Associate Professor of Surgery, Veterans Administration Medical Center and University of California Medical Center, San Francisco, California, U.S.A.

George Crile, Jr., M.D.   Emeritus Consultant, Department of General Surgery, Cleveland Clinic Foundation, Cleveland, Ohio, U.S.A.

Nelly Demeester-Mirkine, M.D.   Department of Medicine, Brugmann Hospital, Free University of Brussels, Brussels, Belgium

Israel Doniach, M.D.   Emeritus Professor of Pathology, The University of London; Honorary Lecturer, Department of Histopathology, St. Bartholomew's Hospital, London, England

Michael Garcia, M.D.   Associated Endocrinologists, 4400 Prudential Town Center, Southfield, Michigan, U.S.A.

Colum A. Gorman, M.B., B.Ch., Ph.D.   Assistant Professor of Medicine, Mayo Clinic, Rochester, Minnesota, U.S.A.

Francis S. Greenspan, M.D.   Clinical Professor of Medicine; Chief, Thyroid Clinic, University of California Medical Center, San Francisco, California, U.S.A.

Monte A. Greer, M.D.   Professor of Medicine; Head, Division of Endocrinology, University of Oregon Health Sciences Center, Portland, Oregon, U.S.A.

Ian B. Hales, M.D.   Director of Nuclear Medicine and Endocrinology, Royal North Shore Hospital, Sydney, Australia

William A. Hawk, M.D.   Senior Pathologist, Cleveland Clinic Foundation, Cleveland, Ohio, U.S.A.

C. Stratton Hill, Jr., M.D.   Associate Professor of Medicine, University of Texas–M.D. Anderson Hospital, Houston, Texas, U.S.A.

Mitsuo Inada, M.D.   Second Division, Department of Internal Medicine, Kyoto University School of Medicine, Kyoto, Japan

Flemming Jensen, M.D.   Chief Resident, Ultrasonic Laboratory, Gentöfte Hospital, University of Copenhagen, Copenhagen, Denmark

Edwin L. Kaplan, M.D.   Professor of Surgery, Vice-Chairman for General Surgery, The University of Chicago, Chicago, Illinois, U.S.A.

Sudha R. Kini, M.D.   Department of Pathology, Henry Ford Hospital, Detroit, Michigan, U.S.A.

Demetrios A. Koutras, M.D.   Associate Professor, "Alexandra" Hospital, Athens, Greece

Robert D. Leeper, M.D.   Attending Physician, Memorial Hospital, New York, New York; Associate Member, Sloan Kettering Institute, New York, New York, U.S.A.

Farahe Maloof, M.D.   Associate Professor in Medicine, Harvard Medical School; Physician, Massachusetts General Hospital, Boston, Massachusetts, U.S.A.

William M. McConahey, M.D.   Professor of Medicine, Mayo Medical School; Senior Consultant, Endocrinology and Internal Medicine, Mayo Clinic, Rochester, Minnesota, U.S.A.

Donald A. Meier, M.D.   Associated Endocrinologists, 4400 Prudential Town Center, Southfield, Michigan, U.S.A.

Shigenobu Nagataki, M.D.   Third Department of Internal Medicine, Faculty of Medicine, University of Tokyo, Tokyo, Japan

Thomas F. Nikolai, M.D.   Staff Physician, Section of Endocrinology, Department of Internal Medicine, Marshfield Clinic, Marshfield, Wisconsin, U.S.A.

Sten Nørby Rasmussen, M.D.   Chief Resident, Department of Medical Gastroenterology, Rigshospitalet, University of Copenhagen, Copenhagen, Denmark

John W. Rebuck, M.D.   Senior Hematopathologist, Department of Pathology, Henry Ford Hospital, Detroit, Michigan, U.S.A.

Thomas S. Reeve, M.B.   Professor of Surgery, The University of Sydney (at Royal North Shore Hospital), Sydney, Australia

Horst P. Schleusener,   Professor, Freie Universität Berlin, Berlin, Federal Republic of Germany

O. Peter Schumacher, M.D., Ph.D.   Consultant in Endocrinology, Cleveland Clinic Foundation, Cleveland, Ohio, U.S.A.

James C. Sisson, M.D.   Professor of Internal Medicine, University of Michigan Medical Center, Ann Arbor, Michigan, U.S.A.

D. Ward Slingerland, M.D.   Associate Chief, Nuclear Medicine; Associate Research Professor of Medicine, VA Medical Center, Boston University School of Medicine, Boston, Massachusetts, U.S.A.

Kenneth Sterling, M.D.   Clinical Professor of Medicine, Columbia University College of Physicians and Surgeons; Director, Protein Research Laboratory, Va Medical Center, New York, New York, U.S.A.

Sheldon S. Stoffer, M.D.   Associated Endocrinologists, 4400 Prudential Town Center, Southfield, Michigan, U.S.A.

Charles I. Taylor, M.D.   Associated Endocrinologists, 4400 Prudential Town Center, Southfield, Michigan, U.S.A.

Robert D. Utiger, M.D.   Professor of Medicine, University of North Carolina School of Medicine, Chapel Hill, North Carolina, U.S.A.

Robert Volpé, M.D.   Professor, Department of Medicine, University of Toronto School of Medicine, Toronto, Ontario, Canada

Paul G. Walfish, M.D.   Associate Professor, Department of Medicine, University of Toronto School of Medicine; Director, Thyroid Research Laboratory and Endocrine Division, Mount Sinai Hospital, Toronto, Ontario, Canada

Jan D. Wiener, Ph.D   Academisch Ziekenhuis der Vrije Universiteit, Amsterdam, The Netherlands

Lawrence C. Wood, M.D.   Instructor in Medicine, Harvard Medical School; Assistant Physician, Massachusetts General Hospital, Boston, Massachusetts, U.S.A.

Chapter 1

Is Thyroid Imaging an Overutilized Diagnostic Procedure?

Joel I. Hamburger, M.D.
J. Martin Miller, M.D.
Michael Garcia, M.D.
Donald A. Meier, M.D.
Sheldon S. Stoffer, M.D.
Charles I. Taylor, M.D.

INTRODUCTION

The technique for thyroid imaging has improved dramatically over the past 30 years so that modern images are remarkably clear and may provide striking pictures of abnormal thyroid structure. Also the patient radiation burden has been reduced by a factor of 100. However, advanced technology carries a correspondingly advanced price tag. As physicians are being held increasingly accountable for the rising cost of health care it becomes incumbent upon us to consider the cost effectiveness of thyroid imaging in relation to the indications for its use. This issue is particularly pertinent now because of improvement in the sensitivity and reliability of in vitro thyroid function testing. Also, needle biopsy is gaining favor as the procedure of choice for the diagnosis of the thyroid nodule.[1]

Two recent experiences provoked consideration of this issue. First, at a local medical meeting a nuclear medicine specialist presented a family with Hashimoto's thyroiditis. All members had been imaged. When asked why imaging was ordered he responded: "It's part of the routine workup." Second, a 26-year-old woman came to our clinic for a second opinion to determine whether she needed an annual thyroid scan. One had been done by her physician every year since age 16. The tracer employed was [131]I.

It is the objective of this report to assess retrospectively the medical value of thyroid images performed on 2000 consecutive patients. Half the images were performed in a private fee-for-service referral clinic, Northland Thyroid Laboratory (NTL) in which imaging was performed (with few exceptions) only when considered necessary by the staff endocrinologists. The other half were performed in a large multispecialty group practice, Henry Ford Hospital (HFH), in which images were performed whenever ordered by the attending salaried physicians, in the majority of instances not endocrinologists. The experiences of the two clinics will be compared in an effort at addressing the following controversial issues:

(1) Is thyroid imaging overutilized?

(2) If so, what are the relative contributions of economic self-interest and inexperience to this overutilization?

(3) What are the principal indications for thyroid imaging at this time, and for which of these indications are the data obtained likely to be of importance in the management of the patient's problem?

EXPERIENCE OF THE TWO CLINICS: INDICATIONS FOR IMAGING

Each record was assessed to determine the reason for imaging and the final diagnosis. After the records were reviewed the authors evaluated each indication in terms of its importance to patient management and with respect to cost-benefit considerations. Agreement was reached on the following grading scale:

Necessity Category I: Justified

Necessity Category II: Limited value

Necessity Category III: Not justified

The bases for these judgments will be presented, and the performance of the two clinics in terms of cost effectiveness will be compared.

Table 1-1 presents the indications for imaging in the two institutions and the number of images performed for each. The necessity category is also shown, as is the percentage (in parentheses) of images performed for necessity category III indications.

Discrete Solitary or Dominant Thyroid Nodules

Twenty-six percent of the images were for the evaluation of a solitary or discrete dominant nodule. In the NTL series 22% of these lesions were autonomously functioning thyroid nodules (AFTN). This was the case only for 10% of the HFH series, but HFH patients did not in all instances have the necessary confirmatory studies performed. AFTN diagnoses were of value in excluding thyroid cancer. A finding of reduced nodular function was less helpful, because most of these nodules are benign. Nevertheless the information had limited usefulness for two reasons. First, for those patients who have surgery for what proves to be carcinoma, it is helpful to know the preoperative relationship of the nodule to the remaining thyroid tissue and other anatomic structures of the neck. These data may be critical for comparison with postoperative imaging data. Second, for many patients who do not have surgical treatment, thyroid hormone will be given. Demonstra-

Table 1-1. Indications for thyroid imaging at Northland Thyroid Laboratory and Henry Ford Hospital, and the necessity category assigned to each.

Indications	Northland Thyroid Laboratory	Henry Ford Hospital	Necessity category
1. Discrete solitary or dominant thyroid nodule	215	306	I
2. To assess function of thyroid remnants after thyroidectomy for benign disease	34	40	I
3. Cancer follow-up	17	39	I
4. Post-TSH in assessment of further need for exogenous thyroid hormone	125	0	II
5. Suspected subacute thyroiditis	64	21	II
6. Suspected thyroglossal duct cyst, or to determine whether there is thyroid in the normal position when a midline mass consistent with a thyroglossal duct cyst is found	1	21	II
7. To determine if retromanubrial mass is thyroid	0	42	II
8. Assessment of uniformity of function in diffuse or multinodular goiter, no dominant nodule	282 (28%)	234 (23%)	III
9. Graves' disease with goiter	99 (10%)	79 (8%)	III
10. To assess function of thyroid remnants after radioactive iodine therapy	72 (7%)	29 (3%)	III
11. Searching for impalpable nodules (history radiation therapy)	41 (4%)	71 (7%)	III
12. To assess thyroid function in nongoitrous individuals	36 (4%)	81 (8%)	III
13. To assess thyroid size	9 (1%)	18 (2%)	III
14. Miscellaneous	5	19	
Total	1000	1000	

tion of reduced nodular function excludes autonomous function, which would contraindicate the use of thyroid hormone. We do not agree that needle biopsy makes imaging unnecessary,[2] nor that all nodules should be biopsied. Because imaging of thyroid nodules may exclude a diagnosis of cancer for 10–20% of patients, and provides information of limited value for the rest, this indication was graded category I.

Following Thyroidectomy for Benign Disease

Four percent of the images were performed to assess thyroid tissue remaining after thyroidectomy for benign disease. Many of these remnants had undergone nodular hyperplasia because of failure to administer thyroid hormone postoperatively. Most of these nodules were functional, but 1 of 40 in the HFH series and 2 of 34 from the NTL series were functionless. This information is useful. Demonstration of function provides an explanation for the development of the lesion (compensatory hyperplasia) and permits a prediction that the nodule might regress in response to thyroid hormone. Of course, if the operation is for Graves' disease the persistent tissue may not be suppressible. Hypofunctional nodules might be neoplasms or degenerated hyperplastic remnants. This indication for imaging was graded category I.

Cancer Follow-up

Three percent of the images were performed for follow-up of thyroid cancer. These studies were helpful in either a negative or positive sense. Therefore, this indication for imaging was graded category I.

To Assess Necessity for Continued Treatment with Thyroid Hormone

Six percent of the images were done after thyroid-stimulating hormone (TSH) administration to assess the need for continued treatment with thyroid hormone for patients who were receiving this medication without substantial evidence that it was necessary. If the thyroid gland seemed normal, thyroid hormone was discontinued. Although withdrawal from thyroid hormone was successful most of the time, for some patients the thyroid was unable to produce enough hormone to maintain the euthyroid state. Thyroid hormone was continued for those who failed to respond to TSH administration or whose thyroid images were grossly abnormal. These imaging procedures were employed primarily to avoid a trial of thyroid hormone withdrawal in patients (30% of those studied) for whom an episode of myxedema could be predicted on the basis of poor response to TSH administration. This indication for thyroid imaging would be eliminated in a "bare bones" health care system in which all patients for whom the necessity for continued treatment is questioned would be asked to discontinue treatment for a suitable period of time. As a compromise one could use some value for the 24-h radioactive iodine uptake after TSH administration as the basis for continuing or discontinuing treatment. Unfortunately the increased iodine intake by the public makes it difficult to decide what an appropriate cut-off value might be. Since these studies had limited clinical value this indication for imaging was graded category II.

Suspected Subacute Thyroiditis

Four percent of the images were performed in patients with suspected subacute thyroiditis. The presenting complaint was usually neck pain, but sometimes the diagnosis was considered because of mild hyperthyroidism with an unusually firm goiter and a low radioactive iodine uptake. In a patient with clinical and biochemical evidence of hyperthyroidism, failure to obtain a very sharply defined thyroid image is suggestive of the painless thyroiditis syndrome or subacute thyroiditis. This information is of no greater value than that which a low radioactive iodine uptake provides. Occasionally imaging may reveal a moth-eaten appearance with better visualization of areas of lesser involvement. Imaging can be performed without requiring the second patient visit which is necessary for a radioactive iodine uptake. If a very poor image is obtained the radioactive iodine uptake will be low, and the additional visit can be avoided. This advantage is offset by the higher cost of imaging. Nevertheless we consider these images of limited clinical utility and grade this indication category II.

Midline Neck Masses

One percent of the images were performed to determine whether a midline neck mass (suspected thyroglossal duct cyst) contained any functioning thyroid tissue. Most patients were seen preoperatively to exclude the possibility that the mass was the only functioning thyroid tissue, i.e., an ectopic thyroid. Since ectopic functioning thyroid tissue masses often regress in response to thyroid hormone treatment (Figs. 1-1 and 1-2), operation is avoidable. However, only one patient had any functional tissue, and this was a mass on the right side of the thyroid cartilage, part of a pyramidal lobe. No function was observed in any mass superior to the thyroid cartilage in this series of images (although occasional examples of lingual

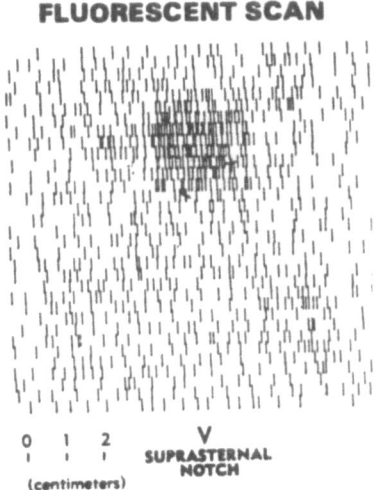

FLUORESCENT SCAN

0 1 2   V
        SUPRASTERNAL
          NOTCH
(centimeters)

Figure 1-1. A fluorescent thyroid image reveals thyroid tissue in the midline high in the neck and no thyroid tissue in the normal position.

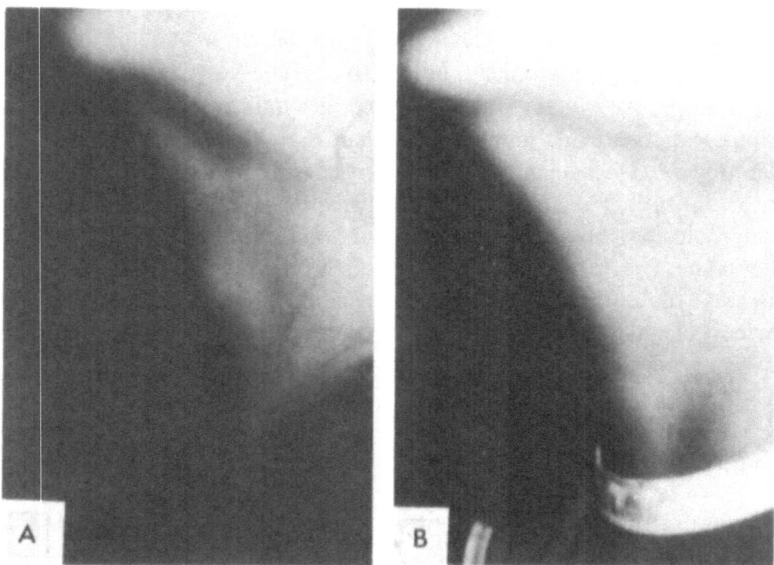

Figure 1-2. **A** Visible mass of ectopic thyroid tissue protruding from the anterior neck. **B** Regression of mass after treatment with levothyroxine, 0.15 mg daily for 6 months.

or high cervical ectopic thyroid remnants have been detected by images at both institutions on other occasions). Usually the exclusion of ectopic thyroid tissue can be made by palpation of thyroid tissue in the normal location. Otherwise, imaging a midline mass would be useful. Therefore we graded imaging for this indication category II.

Retromanubrial Masses

Two percent of the images were performed to determine whether retromanubrial masses were thyroidal in origin. Half these procedures could have been avoided because a normal thyroid gland had been identified in the usual cervical location. Retromanubrial thyroid tissue is almost always associated with cervical goiter. Since these images provided information of limited usefulness, this indication was graded category II.

Diffuse or Multinodular Goiter

Twenty-six percent of the images were performed for diffuse, lobulated, or multinodular goiters without a single dominant nodule suggesting malignancy. The physicians were looking for uniformity of thyroid function and particularly for any areas of reduced function (possible malignancy) or "hot" areas (possible autonomous function). Without a dominant discrete nodule, areas of reduced function, when discovered, did not differentiate malignancy from degeneration or atrophic changes. Also, the absence of discrete areas of increased function did not rule out autonomous function. Therefore this indication for imaging was graded category III.

Graves' Disease

Nine percent of the images were performed to establish goiter size prior to treatment of Graves' disease. Imaging may be of limited value for this purpose in patients with short necks and goiters which are relatively small and low lying. However, radioactive iodine dosage was based primarily upon estimates of goiter size made by palpation and the magnitude of the 24-h radioactive iodine uptake. Therefore these images contributed negligibly to the management of the patients and this indication was graded category III. Imaging might be of some medicolegal value to document the presence of a goiter prior to destructive therapy, in the event that the patient or a subsequent physician questions the diagnosis at a later date.

Following Radioactive Iodine Therapy

Five percent of the images were performed to assess thyroid status following radioactive iodine therapy. Most of the time these were performed because of persistent goiter or a persistent nodule if the patient had been treated for a toxic AFTN. The decision to retreat with radioactive iodine, or to treat for hypothyroidism, was based upon assessments of thyroid function. The image played a negligible part in the decision relative to dosage. Demonstration of reactivation of suppressed extranodular tissue after ablation of a toxic AFTN may be satisfying, but did not contribute to the management. If the AFTN was still palpable, imaging was not needed if the patient was euthyroid. If the patient was still hyperthyroid, obviously the treatment had been inadequate and a repeat dose of ^{131}I was needed. This dose should be based upon the size of the nodule, estimated by palpation, and the 24-h radioactive iodine uptake. Therefore images for this indication were graded category III.

Searching for Impalpable Nodules

Six percent of the images were performed to search for impalpable nodules after a history of prior radiation therapy to the upper body, or less often, in a search for a primary lesion after discovery of a metastatic malignancy elsewhere. In these cases no hypofunctional defects were detected. Regardless of the findings these studies, in our opinion, are worthless in the absence of a palpable lesion. In the irradiated patient finding a zone of reduced function does not mean that this is a malignancy. Most of these image defects represent benign processes. Also, the absence of a defect does not preclude the presence of malignancy. It is well accepted that the diagnosis of thyroid malignancy can be deferred with safety until the lesion is palpable. This assumes that the palpator has reasonable experience in the evaluation of thyroid patients. Essentially the same argument holds in the case of a search for a primary in a patient with known metastatic thyroid malignancy and no palpable thyroid abnormality. Therefore this indication for imaging was graded category III.

To Assess Thyroid Function in Nongoitrous Individuals

Six percent of the images were performed in patients without thyroid enlargement in the diagnosis of thyroid function. Thyroid imaging data add no important information to standard in vitro studies. In fact, patients with Hashimoto's thyroiditis often concentrate the tracer well but are unable to complete the additional steps essential for the synthesis of thyroid hormone. A normal-appearing image may mislead the unwary physician to diagnose normal thyroid function, when the patient is severely hypothyroid. Some patients with Hashimoto's thyroiditis even have images suggesting hyperthyroidism. Since these images are not only useless, but may be misleading, this indication was graded category III.

To Assess Thyroid Size

For 1.4% of the patients imaging was performed to assess thyroid size in the absence of goiter. These studies were requested by physicians without expertise in thyroidology and images were uniformly normal and useless. This indication was graded category III.

Differences Between the Two Clinics

Although more cancers are discovered and followed yearly at NTL than at HFH, a greater proportion of images performed at HFH were for follow-up of thyroid cancer patients. This discrepancy was not related to different indications for imaging of thyroid cancer patients. At both clinics additional images after the initial postoperative image are obtained only if ^{131}I therapy is given or clinical recurrences develop. However, it took only 4 months to accumulate 1000 images at NTL, but 15 months to accumulate the same number at HFH, where thyroid patients are seen less often. We believe this explains the differences.

The nonendocrinologists at HFH were almost twice as likely as the endocrinologists at NTL to order images to search for impalpable nodules or to assess thyroid function or goiter size.

The discrepancy in the frequency with which imaging was used to explain retromanubrial masses in the two institutions most likely reflects the contribution of inpatients at HFH, especially patients from the oncology service. Such patients are not seen at NTL. The different patient population also explains the near absence of patients at NTL who were imaged for thyroglossal duct masses.

A larger proportion of patients at NTL were imaged for suspected thyroiditis, especially painless thyroiditis associated with spontaneously resolving hyperthyroidism. This difference probably reflects the greater awareness of the endocrinologists of this syndrome. The images were obtained to preclude inappropriate treatment of the spontaneously resolving hyperthyroidism of thyroiditis. A poor image has essentially the same significance as a low radioactive iodine uptake value. At NTL there is emphasis on one-visit complete patient evaluations, and an image can be done at the initial visit, whereas the patient must return the next day for a radioactive iodine uptake determination.

A greater proportion of patients with Graves' disease were imaged initially and following ^{131}I therapy at NTL. In a private clinic it may be considered more important to document objectively what the ^{131}I treatment has accomplished for medicolegal purposes.

Post-TSH imaging to assess the continued need for thyroid hormone administration was performed only at NTL. This may reflect a greater awareness by the endocrinologists at NTL of the technical usefulness of TSH administration, a difference in the type of referral seen in the outpatient setting of NTL, the impact of economic incentives on the NTL physicians' approach to the solution of this problem, or satisfaction with a radioactive iodine uptake after TSH administration without imaging at HFH.

It is of some interest to note that the proportion of images considered as category III was 54% for NTL and 51% for HFH.

DISCUSSION

There may be differences of opinion as to the clinical importance of various indications for thyroid imaging. Our evaluations are admittedly subjective but based upon our mutual long experience in clinical practice. Neither of us have any reason to denigrate the usefulness of thyroid imaging. However, we share a common concern for the ultimate impact upon the practice of medicine of overutilization of laboratory technology in general, and thyroid imaging in particular. Too often whenever the possibility of thyroid disease is raised thyroid imaging comes to mind almost as an automatic reflex.

The issue of economic interest cannot be ignored. The fee-for-service system in the United States provides an incentive for the provision of services, regardless of necessity. When the patient is not paying personally for these services he and his physician are less concerned about the economic implications of diagnostic decisions. Medical insurance further distorts the relationship between patient and physician by rewarding physicians who perform tests, while ignoring physicians who take histories, perform physical examinations, and offer advice.

Economic interests influence hospital policies as well as those of private physicians. In some physicians' offices and clinics diagnostic laboratory services are performed primarily to maximize profits. Exposés of kickback schemes which promote exploitation of third party payers have jolted patient confidence in their physicians. Even conscientious physicians in private practice may have no compunctions about utilizing a profitable office laboratory whenever the information obtained is of any value, even if it is not essential. Hospitals are no more scrupulous in discouraging unessential laboratory services. Indeed the profits from the laboratories support many other hospital activities.

Inexperience and poor teaching contribute to overutilization of diagnostic laboratory services. Students and house officers early in their careers learn to admire the "complete workup."[3] They are more quickly criticized for overlooking some test of marginal importance than complimented for efforts at discrimination in the use of the laboratory. These habits are not changed when the student reaches the staff level. The seductive simplicity of the "routine battery workup" relieves the physician from considering the cost effectiveness of individual procedures. In some institutions the physician can order the thyroid battery or liver battery, for example, without even knowing which tests are included. The "laboratory" takes care of these minor details. When the results come back the physician can then try to figure out what they mean, or failing in this effort may call in a consultant.

This study suggests that about half the thyroid images performed in clinics staffed by reasonably responsible physicians may be considered unnecessary in retrospect. What the proportion might be in the average private office, clinic, or hospital is unknown. Currently at NTL 49.2% of new thyroid patients referred for evaluation have thyroid imaging as part of the initial workup. About 6000 new patients are seen each year. If 1500 images of questionable importance were not performed (assuming a charge per image of $80), a $120,000 reduction in costs could be realized in one year, in one clinic.

The proportion of patients for whom imaging is performed has been dropping over the past few years at NTL. The data from this study have provided the impetus for a further effort in this direction at both institutions. This can be done more easily in a small private clinic where a limited number of physicians are in close communication. In large institutions where imaging is ordered by many physicians, most of whom are not endocrinologists, and some of whom are house officers in training, the problem is more difficult. Active peer review may be effective sometimes. However, the history of peer review does not give grounds for great optimism in most institutions. Where imaging is viewed as an important source of income, it is unlikely that cost-benefit considerations will have much impact upon practice habits, as long as third parties persist in their generosity. It is beyond the scope of this article to offer solutions to these social and professional dilemmas. Perhaps recognition may serve as a first step toward solutions, but we doubt it.

COMMENTARY

William H. Beierwaltes, M.D.

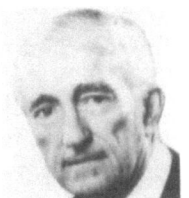

In June, 1980, when I lectured to 1000 surgeons at the University of Minnesota, the question that the Panel Chairman asked was whether every patient with a goiter should have a fine needle aspiration of the thyroid and whether this would significantly take the place of thyroid imaging with either radionuclides or with ultrasound. The point that I emphasized was that when the aspiration is done by experienced persons like Joel Hamburger or Martin Miller, and interpreted by an outstandingly experienced and excellent cytopathologist like Dr. Kini, the fine needle aspiration probably should be done in a very high percentage of patients seen routinely for goiter and it could take the place of a very large number of radionuclide and ultrasound scans being done today.

I also told them that as our experience at the University of Michigan increases and as our cytopathologist becomes more knowledgeable, we are doing fewer scans. On the other hand, I said that I would like to be sure that all 1000 surgeons at the meeting didn't go home to their small local hospitals and expect to start doing needle aspirations and have it contribute significantly to patient care during the first year or two after the introduction of their new procedure. I stressed that not only would the surgeon need experience in doing the aspiration, but most importantly, the pathologist would require 2 to 3 years before he or she could become competent.

I agree with the points regarding "hot nodules." When I see a hot nodule with more radioactivity in it than in the rest of the thyroid gland, or with obvious suppression of the rest of the thyroid gland, it rules out cancer of the thyroid as a cause of the nodule. I see no reason why fine needle aspiration need be done in such patients. In such patients, I then give 25 μg of triiodothyronine four times a day for 8 days to see whether the hot nodule is suppressible. If the radioiodine uptake in the thyroid is decreased by the 8th day to 50% or less of the original values, the serum T_4 falls by greater than 1.5 μg percent, and especially if the uptake in the thyroid nodule is obviously suppressed, then I routinely give the patient a trial of thyroid hormone to see if I can eliminate the nodule.

I do not do a thyroid scan following thyroidectomy for Graves' disease because the findings are frequently bizarre and we know that the usual cause for a recurring nodule is regenerative hyperplasia.

I do use a thyroid scan following thyroidectomy for a nodular goiter when there is a dominant nodule to determine whether it is a hot nodule.

We routinely do a radioiodine scan in follow-up of well-differentiated thyroid cancer treated with radioactive iodine after surgery. We like to do it before surgery so that we can tell whether the "remnant" was actually in the thyroidal bed or outside. We also do it just before radioiodine treatment, off thyroid hormone for 6 weeks, because we never treat with radioactive iodine unless we demonstrate uptake.

If there has been a clear-cut documentation of retrosternal or colloid goiter as the indication for thyroid hormone, I do not take the patients off thyroid hormone because I've not relieved the cause of the goiter by administering thyroid hormone. I ask the patients to continue on it permanently and only see them once a year to be certain the thyroid is shrinking or that it has shrunk to the place where there is nothing by palpation to indicate surgery.

I rarely do thyroid scans anymore for suspected subacute thyroiditis. In a patient with normal or elevated serum T_4 levels, if the uptake is unexpectedly subnormal when there is no other explanation except subacute thyroiditis, that is sufficient.

Yes, I would scan a midline neck mass to be certain that it was functioning.

I have seen patients with retromanubrial goiter whose thyroid glands were apparently normal to palpation, but usually the radioactivity extends from the inferior portion of one lobe down into the chest. I therefore make a great point of telling the technologists that they should continue the scan until the radioactivity related to the thyroid has been followed caudad until it clearly stops.

We do not use radioactive iodine to quantitate goiter size. We do scan when we strongly suspect that the patient has a hot nodule we cannot feel causing T_3 toxicosis, or if the patient has clear-cut thyrotoxicosis and we can't detect a goiter, or if the patient has a short fat neck or inability to dorsiflex his neck, and so on, which might have interfered with our ability to palpate the goiter.

We do not use radionuclide imaging of the thyroid following radioactive iodine therapy of thyrotoxicosis.

We do not do thyroid imaging in the absence of a palpable thyroid lesion, in the evaluation of patients previously exposed to radiation therapy of the head or neck areas.

We do not use thyroid imaging to assess thyroid function in nongoitrous individuals.

There is no doubt in my mind that the number of radionuclide imaging procedures is enhanced in part by profit motive and concern over malpractice suits. However, since at our University Hospital thyroid imaging constitutes only a very small percentage of all procedures, we are in the unique position in our Nuclear Medicine Division of not encouraging thyroid imaging any more than we would encourage any other procedure that seemed to be indicated in the ideal diagnosis and treatment of a patient.

The House Officer most commonly orders a battery of tests on day one because the cost of hospitalization per day has reached almost the cost of any single test he would order. If the first test that comes back is diagnostic, the House Officer very frequently cancels the rest of the tests. If the tests are not diagnostic, the House Officer has then saved the patient several days of hospitalization in order to try to establish a diagnosis and start treatment.

We also have had the experience that the proportion of patients having radio-nuclide imaging has been dropping over the past few years, particularly since the successful use of fine needle aspiration.

COMMENTARY

Angelo Carpi, M.D.

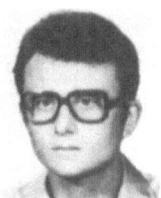

In our clinic 160 thyroid scans are performed monthly. Table 1-2 shows the indications for 944 patients at their first contact with this center. These data do not include repeat images of the same patient. For cancer follow-up an average of 16 whole body scans are performed monthly.

Solitary Thyroid Nodules

In our series, a single thyroid nodule was the indication for imaging in 346 euthyroid subjects (36.6%). An autonomous thyroid nodule inhibiting extranodular tissue was found in 7.5% of these patients. This result is similar to the HFH series. I agree that thyroid scan in this condition confirms a benign disease. When a single thyroid nodule is palpated and the patient is hyperthyroid, thyroid imaging

Table 1-2. Indications for 944 thyroid scans at the Centre of Nuclear Medicine in Pisa.

Indication	No.	%
Solitary thyroid nodule	351	37.2
Multiple thyroid nodules	238	25.2
Postoperative control	22	2.33
To perform complete routine thyroid examinations in absence of clinical findings	87	9.21
To assess thyroid size in euthyroid and toxic goiter	203	21.5
Searching for impalpable nodules	16	1.7
Hypothyroidism	16	1.7
Neck midline mass	3	0.31
Suspected retromanubrial goiter	4	0.42
Suspected subacute thyroiditis	4	0.42

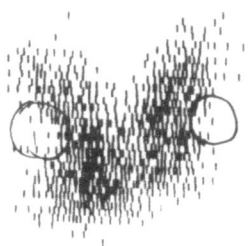

Figure 1-3. Thyroid scan shows that two palpable thyroid nodules are both functionless.

is necessary to show that the nodule is the cause of hyperthyroidism. This was the finding in five patients (6.8% of those hyperthyroid).

Multiple Nodules

Palpation of more than one thyroid nodule, with or without toxicity, was the indication for 238 patients (25.2%). Thyroid scan gave an image of multinodular goiter in 232 of these patients, while in the remaining six subjects (2.52%) thyroid scan showed that all palpable nodules were hyperfunctioning with variable suppression of extranodular tissue. Four of these patients showed mild hyperthyroidism, while two were euthyroid. Therefore thyroid imaging has been useful to identify this condition which likely indicates the presence of multiple benign follicular adenomas (similar to the single hyperfunctioning nodule). Figures 1-3 and 1-4 show thyroid images for two patients each with two palpable nodules of similar size. In one patient (Fig. 1-3) both were functionless; one was a benign follicular adenoma and the other a papillary carcinoma. In the other patient (Fig. 1-4)

Figure 1-4. Thyroid scan shows that two palpable thyroid nodules are both hyperfunctioning. Thyroid scans in basal conditions *(left)* and during T$_3$ suppression test *(right)* are shown.

both were autonomously hyperfunctioning. These data indicate that when more than one thyroid nodule is palpated, thyroid imaging can be useful to differentiate between benign conditions, just as in the case of a single thyroid nodule, although less often. Also, in euthyroid patients with multinodular goiter treated with suppressive doses of thyroid hormone, a thyroid scan can identify autonomously functioning thyroid tissue. This information may suggest the need to withdraw hormone, and in some instances might indicate surgical treatment.

Postoperative Scans

Twenty-two patients in our study (2.33%) had a thyroid scan because they had been operated upon previously for a thyroid disease, and a control postoperative scan was requested. Clinical examination revealed no abnormality in ten patients, palpation of the residual thyroid tissue without nodularity in four patients, and palpation of more than one nodule in the remaining eight patients. Thyroid scans showed functioning nodules in three patients and multiple cold nodules in five patients. Therefore I agree that when a nodule is palpated in the remnant of a thyroid gland after operation a thyroid scan is essential to differentiate compensatory hyperplasia of the remnant from tumor. However, thyroid images gave no useful information when no nodule was palpated. A postoperative thyroid scan is useless for evaluation of thyroid function. Thyroid hormones and TSH circulating levels are the best indexes.

Presently we perform a thyroid scan 1 month after operation of all patients. Nevertheless, the data presented by Hamburger et al. suggest that most of these thyroid scans can be avoided. After thyroidectomy for benign disease, thyroid hormone can be administered without a thyroid scan to prevent or to treat hypothyroidism and to avoid hyperplasia of the remnant. If the operation was for Graves' disease, thyroid hormone should be administered only when in vitro tests show hypothyroidism. For this diagnosis an image of residual thyroid tissue is unnecessary. A thyroid scan after thyroidectomy for benign disease is indicated when the patient, on treatment with thyroid hormone, seems to develop mild hyperthyroidism, and serum thyroid hormone concentrations are at the upper limit of the normal range. Appearance of residual tissue on the scan indicates autonomously functioning tissue and suggests withdrawal of thyroid hormone.

Useless Thyroid Scans

In our series, a thyroid scan did not give any useful information in the following conditions: complete routine thyroid examinations in absence of clinical findings, evaluation of thyroid size in euthyroid and toxic goiter, hypothyroidism, searching for impalpable nodules, study of a midline mass in the neck, and suspected retromanubrial goiter. In some patients thyroid imaging after TSH stimulation was

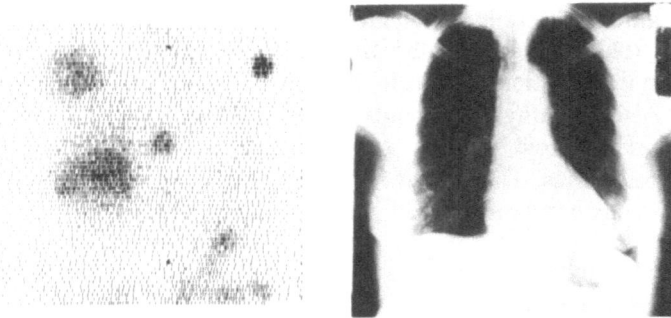

Figure 1-5. Chest ^{131}I scan and radiograph of one patient with differentiated thyroid carcinoma. Scan shows functioning metastases not detected by x ray.

useful to show retromanubrial goiter. When subacute thyroiditis was suspected, a poor quality image or failure to obtain an image were elements in favor of the diagnosis.

Scans in Cancer Follow-up

Whole body ^{131}I scan for differentiated thyroid carcinoma follow-up deserves comment because of the high doses of radioactivity employed and the necessity to make the patient hypothyroid to obtain reliable results. Too frequent repetition of whole body scans after successful ^{131}I treatment is useless. On the other hand, repeating the scan only if there is clinical evidence of recurrent cancer may prevent early diagnosis and treatment of functioning metastases. Large functioning pulmonary metastases of follicular carcinoma, visible on ^{131}I scan, may not be discovered by x ray[4] (Fig. 1-5). Recent data suggest a useful role for serum thyroglobulin, an elevation of which seems to be associated with metastases of differentiated carcinoma.[5] Monitoring with thyroglobulin assays may help to avoid useless whole body scans.

Summary

This retrospective study suggests an overuse of at least 343 thyroid scans (36.3%) in our center. I think that the main reason for this is that physicians have been convinced that scans are necessary for a complete thyroid examination in all thyroid patients.

COMMENTARY

Ian B. Hales, M.D.

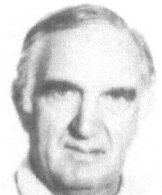

This chapter attempts to critically assess the value of thyroid imaging. My comments will be confined to highlighting areas where differences of opinion might exist. The comments have been based on the three necessity categories described in the introductory section.

Category I

The value of isotope imaging in isolated nodules is generally overrated. For example, in hot nodules, if surgery is to be performed, then scans should not be ordered, but it is still mandatory to assess thyroid function. In the case of cold nodules, these are supposed to suggest a high probability of cancer; however, in our hospital between 1976 and 1979, only 73 of 742 patients having thyroidectomy for single cold nodules had cancer. In assessing the value of scans, one must remember that pertechnetate occasionally fails to show cold areas that will be detected by iodine isotopes. (In our department, 50 consecutive patients having technetium scans also had iodine scans—in two cases this discrepancy resulted and one patient had thyroid cancer.)

The use of tumor-seeking isotopes deserves consideration. The most promising at present is thallium, which could perhaps halve the number of patients being operated on for suspected malignancy.[6] Of 30 of our patients operated upon for cold nodules, only four had cancer and none had cold thallium scans.

There can be no doubt of the usefulness of radioiodine scans in the follow-up of patients whose thyroids have been ablated for thyroid cancer. The demonstration of functioning tissue may be dose-dependent; consequently other parameters, particularly thyroglobulin,[7] should also be measured. This is demonstrated by two patients with suspected spread of malignancy into the esophagus (causing severe dysphagia) and trachea (causing hemoptysis). The scans performed after administering 5 mCi of ^{131}I showed no accumulation of radioiodine in the suspected area, although serum TSH values were greatly elevated.

In both patients, because of the extensiveness of surgery that would have been required to cope with their complications, it was considered worth trying a series of therapeutic doses of [131]I (one received two and one received three, at 3-month intervals). The therapeutic doses were shown to accumulate in the metastatic areas and clinical improvement was also noted. Thyroglobulin levels fell from 2000 to 500 μg/liter and 1000 to 700 μg/liter. Elevated thyroglobulin levels were detected in three additional patients months before the scan became positive. The negative scan result may well be a dose-dependent feature.

Neonatal hypothyroidism should be added to category I. There is excellent evidence to suggest that a scan should be performed before commencing treatment.[8] The identification of functioning tissue raises the possibility of transient hypothyroidism.

Category II

In our experience, post-TSH scans in patients on long-term thyroid replacement have not been helpful. However, in subacute thyroiditis the lack of thyroid uptake (usually using a radioiodine clearance test, which takes 1 h) has been extremely useful in the differential diagnosis of painless thyroiditis. Thyroid imaging in retrosternal extension of goiter is rarely of value in our hands.

Category III

In Graves' disease we have performed a scan prior to ^{131}I therapy to assess the uniformity of uptake, particularly when surgery may be considered an alternative.

I would like to suggest that physicians ask "Will this affect management of the patient?" before ordering any test.

SUMMARY—CHAPTER 1

Just as this volume goes to press another report indicates that physicians, by and large, overutilize laboratory services, without regard to cost-benefit considerations.[9] Yet a second report deals with two strategies to reduce the ordering of laboratory and radiologic tests by medical residents.[10] This objective was fostered in one group of residents by concurrent chart review and discussion sessions. A second group was simply advised that if a reduction in laboratory and radiology procedures were achieved they would be rewarded with cash in an amount up to $375. Interestingly, chart review was more effective than money, but neither method produced a significant reduction in the number of radiology studies.

It is difficult to overcome the seductive simplicity of generations of teaching that objective documentation of all parameters of body function is essential to good medical practice. Yesterday I received a call from an endocrinologist in Cleveland who wanted to know if I could teach him the use of ultrasound evaluation of thyroid nodules. I told him that I considered needle aspiration a simpler, more reliable, and less expensive way to differentiate cystic from solid nodules. However, he asked if ultrasound was not a more precise method than physical examination to document changes in nodule size in response to thyroid hormone treatment. Why he felt the need for such precision was unclear. As Hales put it, "Will this test affect my management of the patient?"

In discussing the subject of this chapter with an outstanding thyroidologist professor from Boston I learned that a baseline thyroid image was considered standard practice for almost any thyroid abnormality. An equally well-known academic colleague agreed with him that patients who have received radiation therapy to the head or neck should have thyroid images, even if the physical examination is negative. Because of reports suggesting that pinhole gamma camera images might detect many impalpable nodules, during the recent period of high concern about radiation-related thyroid cancer we studied 211 consecutive patients with this technique. Only one had defects for which no palpable lesions could be detected. She was an extremely obese woman with a very short neck. However, 15 patients had palpable nodules for which no corresponding defects were demonstrated on the image.[11]

Neither of these physicians would advise operation for imaging abnormalities which did not correspond to palpable nodules. Perhaps they would follow such patients more closely. Neither was much concerned about cost-benefit considerations. Both were concerned about the growing scarcity of funds for medical research.

All of the contributors to this section agree that we can do without much of the thyroid imaging that is currently performed.

One of the principal factors which contribute to overutilization of laboratory services in a fee-for-service system is the income which physicians derive from providing services. Laboratory services are compensated far more generously than those related to examination or counseling. There is more profit from a thyroid image, for which the physician need expend hardly any time, than from a complete history, physical examination, and the subsequent designing of a plan for diagnosis and treatment. This simple fact has created a powerful incentive for the abuses in the provision of laboratory services which have received so much attention in the lay as well as the professional media.

A few years ago the Oakland County (Michigan) Medical Society embarked upon a program to establish ethical guidelines for physicians relative to the provision of laboratory services. Unfortunately the effort was abandoned when it became evident that an outspoken proportion of the membership considered this activity an interference with the free enterprise system.

The failure of physicians, individually and through their professional societies, to control waste, abuse, and outright fraud in the provision of medical care, including unnecessary hospitalization, unnecessary surgery, unnecessarily frequent office examinations, and unnecessary laboratory services, has contributed to the deterioration of the public image of our profession. The consequences of this dereliction are as obvious as they are ominous—for the public as well as for physicians.

Joel I. Hamburger, M.D.

REFERENCES

1. Hamburger JI, Miller JM, Kini SR: Clinical-Pathological Evaluation of Thyroid Nodules. Handbook and Atlas. Southfield, 1979
2. Crile G Jr: Needle biopsy of the thyroid. Clin Nuc Med 2:422, 1977
3. Fitzgerald FT: The clinical examination—a dying art. Forum Med 3:348, 1980
4. Bonte FJ, McConnel RW: Pulmonary metastases from differentiated thyroid carcinoma demonstrable only by nuclear imaging. Radiology 107:585, 1973
5. LoGerfo P, Colacchio T, Colacchio D, Feind C: Thyroglobulin in benign and malignant thyroid disease. JAMA 241:923, 1979
6. Harada T, Ho Y, Shimaoka K, Taniquchi T, Matsudo A, Senoo T: Clinical evaluation of [201] Thallium chloride scan for thyroid nodules. Eur J Nuc Med 5 (2):125, 1980
7. Bridgman MC, Cooper RC, Luttrell BM, Reeve TS, Stiel JN, Wilmshurst EG, Hales IB: Evaluation of serum thyroglobulin levels in the followup of thyroid cancer following ablative therapy. In: Thyroid Research VIII. Canberra, Australian Academy of Science, 1980, pp 483–485
8. Fisher DA: Status of neonatal hypothyroid screening. Report from the Quebec International Conference on Neonatal Thyroid Screening. Thyroid Research VIII. Canberra, Australian Academy of Science, 1980, pp 1–7
9. Herrell JH: Health care expenditures. The approaching crisis. Mayo Clin Proc 55:705, 1980
10. Martin AR, Wolf MA, Thibodeau LA, Dzau V, Braunwald E: A trial of two strategies to modify the test-ordering behavior of medical residents. N Engl J Med 303:1330, 1980
11. Hamburger JI, Stoffer SS: Late thyroid sequellae of radiation therapy to the upper body. In DeGroot LJ (ed): Radiation-Associated Thyroid Carcinoma. New York, Grune & Stratton, 1977, p 20

Chapter 2

Are Silent Thyroiditis and Postpartum Silent Thyroiditis Forms of Chronic Thyroiditis or Different (New) Forms of Viral Thyroiditis?

Joel I. Hamburger, M.D.
Donald A. Meier, M.D.

INTRODUCTION

Subacute (granulomatous) thyroiditis has been regarded as a distinct clinical entity with characteristic histologic findings since the reports of Mygind and De Quervain which appeared near the turn of the century. The 1950 report of Crile and Rumsey[1] is noteworthy because of the clear description of the variable clinical aspects of the disease, from the typical acute presentation to the less clinically overt form, which they designated chronic to indicate the ease with which the diagnosis may be missed. Many patients have hyperthyroidism with low 24-h radioactive iodine uptake (RAIU) which resolves spontaneously in several weeks. This is caused by a discharge of stored thyroid hormone occurring when the inflammatory process produces disruption of the thyroid follicles. As the disease resolves there is commonly a phase of hypothyroidism lasting for about 1 month. Within 3 to 6 months recovery is usually complete. Only a small proportion are left with goiter and even fewer have permanent hypothyrodism. In 10% of the patients the disease is unilateral initially.[2] It may then spread over a few weeks to involve the rest of the gland.[3,4]

Although a painful tender goiter is characteristic of subacute thyroiditis, the severity of these features varies from marked to negligible. Numerous reports between 1950 and 1975 have included patients without pain, but with clinical and laboratory findings otherwise similar to those of the painful patients.[5-14] Indeed the application of the term "subacute" to this disease was surely intended to convey the message that clinical features were often mild. The surgical literature shows that specimens with typical histologic features of subacute thyroiditis were often obtained from patients without pain.[15] These patients came to operation in part because the absence of pain had obscured the diagnosis of subacute thyroiditis.

However, since 1975 several reports have suggested that patients with a painless or silent thyroiditis have a chronic lymphocytic thyroiditis rather than subacute thyroiditis.[16-20] These silent thyroiditis patients usually present with spontaneously resolving hyperthyroidism, pass through a temporary phase of goitrous hypothyroidism, and eventually recover. Many silent thyroiditis patients are seen in the postpartum period.[21-25] These patients often have relapses after successive pregnancies. Silent thyroiditis differs from subacute thyroiditis because of a higher frequency of antithyroid antibodies, often persisting in quite high titer, and the absence of the very high erythrocyte sedimentation rate (ESR). Needle biopsy specimens in silent thyroiditis reveal a consistent pattern of focal lymphocytic infiltration, rather than the giant cell granulomas characteristic of subacute thyroiditis.

It has been suggested that silent thyroiditis is a new form of chronic lymphocytic thyroiditis, or one which is occurring with increasing frequency.[19] Since, in the literature prior to 1975, diagnoses of patients with painless subacute thyroiditis (excluding those from surgical series) were not confirmed histologically, some patients thought to have subacute thyroiditis might have had silent thyroiditis or even postpartum silent thyroiditis.

We shall extract from our experience with thyroiditis clinical and laboratory features which distinguish between subacute (painful) thyroiditis, silent (painless) thyroiditis, and postpartum silent (painless) thyroiditis. The differentiation between subacute thyroiditis and silent thyroiditis is based primarily upon the presence or absence of pain and tenderness, highly subjective phenomena. Hence, it is impossible to guarantee the homogeneity of the three groups. Nevertheless it seems probable that other workers had the same problem.

In the case reports standard methods were employed for in vitro thyroid function tests, and also for RAIU determinations and thyrotropin-releasing hormone (TRH) testing.[26] Antimicrosomal antibody titers were determined by the kit method of the Ames Company (Elkhart, Indiana). Titers of 1/1600 or greater were considered positive. Antithyroglobulin antibody titers were measured by radioimmunoassay.[27] Values of 12% or greater were considered positive. To simplify recording of the data, results of radioimmunoassay were converted to dilution values equivalent to those for antimicrosomal antibody titers.

We shall then review reports dealing with the forms of silent thyroiditis and indicate why we believe (1) that these resemble subacute thyroiditis and (2) that the differences observed may represent slightly different responses to infectious agents (probably viral) which may be more virulent than those which cause subacute thyroiditis.

This review will serve to open the discussion of the following issues:

(1) Do findings of focal lymphocytic infiltration and elevated antithyroid antibody titers mean that silent thyroiditis and postpartum silent thyroiditis are forms of chronic thyroiditis (autoimmune or otherwise)?

(2) Is it coincidence that painful and painless forms of thyroiditis evolve through nearly identical courses from temporary hyperthyroidism to temporary hypothyroidism to more or less complete recovery?

(3) Biopsies in silent forms of thyroiditis (in addition to lymphocytic infiltration) show evidence of marked disruption of follicular architecture with desquamation of follicular epithelium. Essentially identical microscopic findings are seen in subacute thyroiditis. Serial biopsy data indicate that these changes clear as the diseases resolve. Are these parallel microscopic changes coincidental or do they suggest similar acute traumatic events?

(4) Should every hyperthyroid patient have a radioactive iodine uptake to exclude the spontaneously resolving hyperthyroidism of thyroiditis?

(5) Should every patient with spontaneously developing goitrous hypothyroidism be observed for some months before thyroid hormone treatment to exclude a temporary hypothyroidism in the recovery from thyroiditis?

(6) Should patients with repeated episodes of spontaneously resolving hyperthyroidism have thyroid ablation with ^{131}I during recovery, or would thyroid hormone treatment prevent reaccumulation of hormone stores and thus prevent recurrent hormonal discharge?

EXPERIENCE OF NORTHLAND THYROID LABORATORY

In the presentation of our data we shall refer to painful, painless, and postpartum thyroiditis. Table 2-1 gives the age and sex distribution for the three groups. Only 12 of 138 (9%) painful patients were less than 30 years old, compared to 20 of 45 painless (44%) and 54 of 85 (64%) if painless and postpartum patients (who also had no pain) are combined. Although it is unclear why there are fewer young painful patients, this finding provides some support for the concept that the painful and painless diseases are different.

Table 2-2 shows that the frequency of positive antibody titers and the presence

Table 2-1. Comparison of age-sex distribution, painless vs. painful thyroiditis.

	Male		Female		
Age (years)	Painful	Painless	Painful	Painless	Postpartum
<20	0	0	1	7	1
20–29	0	3	11	10	33
30–39	3	4	30	6	6
40–49	9	4	31	4	0
50–59	6	0	32	4	0
60–69	4	1	8	1	0
70+	0	0	3	1	0
Total	22	12	116	33	40

Table 2-2. Positive antibody titers in various types of thyroiditis.

Type of thyroiditis	Frequency	Titer 25,600+
Painful	11/63 (17%)	3/11 (27%)
Painless	16/28 (57%)	8/16 (50%)
Postpartum	35/41 (85%)	19/35 (54%)

Table 2-3. Thyroid function 9 months or longer after acute episode of various types of thyroiditis.

Thyroid function	Painful	Painless	Postpartum
Euthyroid	39 (60%)	10 (33%)	6 (21%)
Euthyroid with goiter	1	2	2
Euthyroid ($\uparrow$ TRH)	13	7	5
Euthyroid ($\uparrow$ TSH)	2	3	3
Hypothyroid	4 (6%)	5 (17%)	13 (39%)
On T_4 for goiter	1	0	3
On T_4 (? indication)	5	3	1
Total	65	30	33

of antibodies in high titer are greater in painless (especially in postpartum) than in painful patients. In some only the antimicrosomal antibody was present in high titer, in others it was the antithyroglobulin antibody, whereas in still others titers for both antibodies were elevated. These findings suggest that not only does the painful disease differ from the painless, but that painless and postpartum also may be different.

Table 2-3 provides further support for this idea. Although frank hypothyroidism developed in only 6% of patients after painful disease, 32% had some persistent abnormality, including goiter, elevated serum TSH level, or an augmented response on TRH test. The following case illustrates this point.

CASE 1:   RECURRENT EPISODES OF SPONTANEOUSLY RESOLVING HYPERTHYROIDISM

A 37-year-old man complained of sweating, hand tremor, and weight loss. Values for the serum T_4 and T_3 resin uptake, were elevated. The RAIU was only 1.5%. A diagnosis of hyperthyroidism was made. The low RAIU was attributed by the radiologist to "an unknown chemical block." Treatment with antithyroid drugs or thyroidectomy was advised. A second opinion was requested. He was then clinically euthyroid. There was no history of the ingestion of iodide or thyroid hormone. The thyroid gland was neither enlarged nor tender. He denied neck pain. A repeat RAIU after TSH stimulation was 9%. Imaging revealed bilateral patchy uptake. The ESR was 21 mm/h. A diagnosis of subsiding "occult" subacute thyroiditis, was made. Three months later he was well.

Three years later he returned with a recurrence of hyperthyroidism with A RAIU of 1%. The thyroid gland was neither enlarged nor tender. The patient was treated with propranolol for a few weeks until he spontaneously recovered.

Two years later he had a third episode of spontaneously resolving hyperthyroidism with low RAIU. Tests for antithyroid antibodies were negative.

Six years after his first episode an enlarged (1.5 times normal) firm thyroid gland was detected. The free thyroxine index (FTI) was 1.5 (NR 1.4–4.0). A TRH test revealed a baseline serum TSH (RIA) level of 6.8 μU/ml and a 20-min post-TRH (100 μg intravenously) value of 51.3 μU/ml, an augmented response. Observation was advised. The patient relocated to another state, and no further data are available.

As we go from painful to painless and then to postpartum patients the proportion of patients who are left with hypothyroidism increases, as does the proportion with lesser functional defects. The following case is an example of a postpartum patient who had persistent hypothyroidism.

CASE 2: POSTPARTUM THYROIDITIS

A 22-year-old woman had an uncomplicated pregnancy which terminated in January 1978 with the delivery of a normal full-term infant. At her 6-week checkup she reported nervousness, a 14-pound weight loss since she was discharged from the hospital, heat intolerance, tremor, and mild palpitation. The thyroid gland was firm and enlarged to about 2.5 times normal. The FTI was 8.0, the serum T_3 (RIA) value 450 ng/dl (NR 80–220), but the RAIU was 1%. The ESR was 22 mm/h. The antimicrosomal antibody titer was positive at 1/25,000. A diagnosis of postpartum thyroiditis was made. Observation was advised. Within 3 months she was hypothyroid. This improved over the succeeding 6 months, but mild symptoms of hypothyroidism persisted, including paresthesias and muscle cramps. The antimicrosomal antibody titer was positive at 1/100,000. The goiter persisted. The FTI was 1.2 and the serum TSH (RIA) was 48 μU/ml. Levothyroxine, 0.15 mg daily, was given.

Most patients with persistent hypothyroidism experienced partial recovery from the more severe hypothyroidism which followed resolution of the hyperthyroidism. The following case illustrates this point.

CASE 3: TRANSIENT HYPOTHYROIDISM AS THE PRESENTING FEATURE IN SILENT THYROIDITIS

A 38-year-old woman was referred for evaluation of a goiter found on routine examination. She reported muscle stiffness, paresthesias, and an abrupt shift from being too warm to being too cold. The heart rate was 68/min. The thyroid gland was 2.5 times normal size, firm, and lobulated. The FTI was 1.2; however, the serum TSH (RIA) value was 2 μU/ml and a repeat assay 20 min after 100 μg of TRH intravenously was 2.2 μU/ml. The antimicrosomal antibody titer was positive at 1/6400. She was questioned in detail and denied any previous neck pain or tenderness. There was a temporary weight loss of 5 to 8 pounds about 1 month earlier. However, she had regained this and an additional 5 pounds as well. Because of the blunted response to the TRH test, and the history compatible with a prior transient hyperthyroidism, the temporary hypothyroid phase in the recovery from silent thyroiditis was suspected. Observation was advised.

One month later she was more overtly hypothyroid. The FTI was 0.4 and the serum TSH (RIA) value was greater than 80. Observation was continued. During the next 3 months she improved progressively. The thyroid gland became normal in size, although somewhat firm and irregular. Thyroid function tests became normal, but the antimicrosomal antibody titer was still positive at 1/6400. One year later the patient was clinically and biochemically euthyroid, but there was an augmented response to TRH, the TSH (RIA) value increasing from 6 to 50 μU/ml, and the antimicrosomal antibody titer was still positive at 1/6400.

Table 2-4. Postpartum thyroiditis: Correlation of thyroid function and elapsed time after parturition.[a]

Elapsed time (months)	Thyroid function						
	Hyperthyroid	Euthyroid (Bl[b] TRH)	Hypothyroid	Euthyroid (↑ TSH)	Euthyroid (↑ TRH)	Goiter	Euthyroid
1	6	—	—	—	—	—	—
2	6	1	1	—	—	2	—
3	7	2	1	—	—	1	—
4	—	2	—	—	1	—	—
5	—	—	1	1	1	2	1
6	—	2	10	3	—	—	1
9	—	—	3	4	1	—	5
12	—	—	—	1	2	—	—
> 12	—	—	2	—	3	1	4

[a]78 examinations were performed in 36 patients.
[b]Bl, blunted response.

The frequency of both painless and postpartum patients seems to have increased in the past few years. Although our clinic has functioned since 1961, 33 of the 45 painless patients and 35 of 40 postpartum patients have been identified in the 3.5-year period from January 1976 to July 1980. About one-half of all painless patients currently are postpartum. Recognition of postpartum thyroiditis requires appreciation that the state of thyroid function which will be observed depends upon the time lapse after delivery. Table 2-4 shows that patients seen soonest after delivery were hyperthyroid or had blunted TRH tests which suggested that hyperthyroidism had been present. If the initial contact with the patient is more delayed, it is more likely that the features of hypothyroidism will predominate. If the patient is seen later than 6 to 9 months postpartum there may have been complete recovery and the diagnosis may be missed.

DISCUSSION

The recent flurry of reports dealing with the silent thyroiditis syndrome and the possibly related postpartum silent thyroiditis has raised important issues both theoretical and practical. These were outlined at the beginning of this chapter.

Is Silent Thyroiditis a New Form of Hashimoto's Thyroiditis?

Initially it was suggested that silent thyroiditis might be a new form of Hashimoto's thyroiditis because of biopsy findings of lymphocytic infiltration.[16,28] However, neither the oxyphilic change of the follicular epithelium nor the fibrosis, typical of Hashimoto's thyroiditis, have been demonstrated.[16,19,20,25,28] The nonspecificity of focal lymphocytic aggregates is easily appreciated, since this finding is common in almost any thyroid disease. There remains broad support for the suggestion that silent thyroiditis and postpartum silent thyroiditis are forms of chronic lymphocytic thyroiditis, perhaps a different kind of autoimmune response from that associated with Hashimoto's thyroiditis, or perhaps arising on the basis of some other as yet unknown pathogenetic basis.[17-20]

What Is the Evidence for Autoimmune Disease?

The suggestion that autoimmunity might play a role in silent thyroiditis and especially postpartum silent thyroiditis is based upon the finding of lymphocytic aggregates, the detection of antithyroid antibodies, and the known enhancement of immune activity in postpartum women, arising after the period of relative suppression of immune responsiveness which is associated with pregnancy itself.[22,23,25] However, the concept that these might be autoimmune diseases is not entirely satisfying. Autoimmune disease, especially of the thyroid in the form of Hashimoto's thyroiditis, tends to be chronic and progressive, not of short duration and spontaneously resolving. Particularly disturbing is the frequency with which patients recover from rather profound hypothyroidism. This is a sequence of events which is entirely inconsistent with the well-known course of the classical autoimmune disease of the thyroid, Hashimoto's thyroiditis.[18] As Hashimoto's thyroiditis advances thyroid function progressively deteriorates. The detection of antibodies per se cannot be taken as proof that the antibodies are the cause of the disease in the absence of other features of autoimmune disease. As already noted the demonstration of lymphocytic infiltrates in the tissue has no precise pathophysiologic implication. Therefore the case for an autoimmune disease is far from substantial.

Are the Silent Forms of Thyroiditis Properly Called "Chronic"?

Patients with Hashimoto's thyroiditis, a chronic disease, have lymphocytic infiltration. Is this grounds for the assumption that those who do not have Hashimoto's thyroiditis, but have lymphocytic aggregates, also have a chronic disease[29,30]? This resembles the argument that: "Gold glitters, therefore all that glitters is gold." The logical non sequitur aside, labeling "chronic" a disease which nearly always regresses more or less completely within a few months is at least a peculiar exercise in linguistics. Only in *Alice's Adventures in Wonderland* do words mean anything that one wants them to mean.

Our data do provide evidence for a persistent functional defect, less than frank hypothyroidism, in a substantially higher proportion of patients than heretofore reported. Interestingly enough, these abnormalities also occurred after typical painful subacute thyroiditis more often than is generally appreciated, although less often than in those with silent thyroiditis or postpartum silent thyroiditis. Even so, can these findings be taken as support for the designation of "chronic"? In that there seems to be some persistent residual, perhaps. However, since this residual seems to represent the end result of incomplete recovery, rather than simply a stage in a progressive deterioration, "chronic" would be unacceptable to us. Indeed the term "subacute" seems admirably suited to the description of such an entity. Unfortunately, this term has long been associated with the presumably viral thyroiditis.

Are the Silent Forms of Thyroiditis Best Called "Lymphocytic Thyroiditis"?

The term "lymphocytic thyroiditis" has been advocated in recognition of the consistent microscopic findings of lymphocytic aggregates. It has been emphasized that the microscopic anatomy is the most dependable feature upon which to base presumptions of etiology or pathogenesis.[18,19,31] But is this really the case? Lymphocytic infiltrations are seen in Hashimoto's thyroiditis, Graves' disease, with thyroid carcinomas, in later stages of subacute thyroiditis,[32-35] and in almost any thyroid gland. Clearly lymphocytic infiltration carries with it no definite pathogenetic implication. The designation "lymphocytic thyroiditis," rather than shedding light upon the pathogenesis of the disease, may have become an impediment to further thought. Those who use this designation may think that they have thereby said something important, or even definitive, as to etiology, pathogenesis, or future course. Nothing could be further from the truth. This kind of thinking becomes particularly objectionable when it is appreciated that the lymphocytic aggregates regress as the disease remits.[20,36]

The preoccupation with the lymphocytic infiltration of both forms of silent thyroiditis has led to neglect of another microscopic finding which may be more important. Biopsies have consistently demonstrated follicular disruption and destruction with extensive epithelial desquamation. These changes serve to explain both the spontaneously resolving hyperthyroidism (discharge of stored thyroid hormone) and the temporary period of hypothyroidism which follows (impaired thyroid hormone synthesizing capacity until recovery of normal follicular anatomy and function). That these dramatic and extensive follicular microscopic abnormalities clear up has been shown both by serial biopsies[20,36] and also by the fact that thyroid secretory function recovers more or less completely.

Is it mere coincidence that this is precisely the same sequence of biochemical and microscopic events which has been observed in patients with subacute thyroiditis? Does the absence of giant cell granulomas in silent thyroiditis and postpartum silent thyroiditis patients mean that these diseases could not have a similar etiology to subacute thyroiditis? In fact does the presence of giant cell granulomas in subacute thyroiditis patients tell us anything about its etiology? History teaches us the opposite. After all it was the pathologists who mistakenly assumed that these granulomas meant tuberculosis. It was only after clinical and immunologic studies indicated that a viral etiology was more likely[37,38] that this error was corrected.

Is There Any Reason to Suspect a Viral Etiology for the Silent Forms of Thyroiditis?

To these authors the serial clinical and microscopic findings suggest that these thyroid glands have been subjected to some acute toxic insult which produces extensive destruction of the follicular structures. There is more or less complete sparing of the regenerative capacity of the tissue so that elimination of the toxic agent is followed by recovery. One can conceive of a number of possible toxic agents or mechanisms which might fit the picture. One could not exclude chemical toxins, bacterial toxins, or for that matter a temporary outpouring of killer lymphocytes. However, it seems somehow easier and less fanciful to suggest that if subacute thyroiditis is a viral disease,[37,38] something which resembles it so closely both clinically and microscopically might also be a viral disease. The differences in cellular infiltrate, frequency and magnitude of antibodies, and end result may only reflect the fact that a different, perhaps new and more virulent, virus is responsible. Nikolai tested for antibodies to viruses previously associated with subacute thyroiditis.[39] His studies were negative. Those studies do not exclude the possibility of a new virus.

If the detection of a sizable number of postpartum silent thyroiditis patients in our clinic in the past few years may be taken as support for a new entity, or at least one which is much more common, and if one has the temerity to suggest (as we have done) that this may be a disease of viral etiology, then it becomes necessary to look further in two directions. First, the common link in patients with postpartum silent thyroiditis is exposure to the flora peculiar to hospitals. The discovery that the hyperthyroid phase of postpartum silent thyroiditis has its onset about 1 month after delivery is consistent with the incubation period for viral disease and the time lapse from onset of a presumed infection to the development of hyperthyroidism. It is important, therefore, to study prospectively large series of pregnant women, preferably from different locations, to ascertain the frequency of this disease and whether that frequency varies from institution to institution. Also it seems logical to check the husbands of affected women (and perhaps their children as well). If this is an infectious disease there might be more clinically inapparent victims than is currently appreciated. There is one report of a wife-husband involved with subacute thyroiditis-silent thyroiditis.[14] Whether this was coincidental or indeed if both had the same disease differing only in severity cannot be determined.

Importance of the RAIU in Silent Thyroiditis

There is one point upon which all agree. Silent thyroiditis patients should not receive conventional treatment for hyperthyroidism, for this will resolve spontaneously. However, the findings of the hyperthyroidism of silent thyroiditis are indistinguishable from those of conventional hyperthyroidism. A RAIU on all hyperthyroid patients is thus essential before treatment. A low RAIU in a patient with hyperthyroidism does not establish a diagnosis of silent thyroiditis. This occurs in subacute thyroiditis, jod-Basedow's disease, factitious hyperthyroidism, toxic stroma ovarii, on rare occasions with extensive infiltration of the thyroid gland by metastatic carcinoma,[40] and finally patients with autonomously functioning thyroid nodules which undergo acute hemorrhagic infarction.[41]

Hypothyroidism After Silent Thyroiditis May Be Temporary

It is desirable to observe these patients for a few months, expecting that hypothyroidism will regress. Patients who are quite symptomatic should be treated. About 6 months later one may reassess the continued necessity for treatment. If the goiter has regressed and antithyroid antibodies are absent or positive in low titers, withdrawal from thyroid hormone may be successful. Some patients will be seen first in the hypothyroid phase of these diseases. Even with subacute thyroiditis, whether the patient appreciates pain may be a function of the severity of the disease or the perceptivity of the patient.[42] If pain is minimal it might be unrecognized, and there may be neither pain nor tenderness when the patient is examined. A recent report of spontaneous remission from primary hypothyroidism[43] may be an example of a patient who initially had subacute thyroiditis or silent thyroiditis. This suggests that recovery should be considered possible for all patients with spontaneously developing goitrous hypothyroidism.

How Best Can Recurrent Episodes of Spontaneously Resolving Hyperthyroidism Be Prevented?

Duick has suggested prophylactic thyroid ablation, surgically or with ^{131}I therapy.[44] Would it be just as effective to introduce suppressive doses of levothyroxine during the hypothyroid phase, and maintain the treatment permanently? Would this prevent the reaccumulation of thyroid hormone stores and thus their future discharge in the event of a recurrence? Or is there enough low-grade autonomous thyroid function to assure a gradual restoration of thyroid hormone stores? We are treating one such patient with thyroid hormone to attempt to answer these questions.

COMMENTARY*

Nobuyuki Amino, M.D.

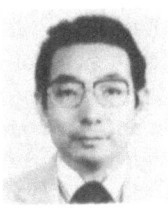

Hamburger and Meier have suggested that silent thyroiditis and postpartum silent thyroiditis differ from subacute thyroiditis only in that they represent different responses to infectious agents (probably viral), which might be more virulent than those causing subacute thyroiditis.

Experience with Destruction-Induced Thyrotoxicosis

Table 2-5 summarizes clinical data on our patients with destruction-induced thyrotoxicosis. All patients with painful thyroiditis had subacute thyroiditis. I have seen only a few patients with other types of painful thyroiditis and want to clarify the difference between silent thyroiditis and subacute thyroiditis (now believed induced by viral infection). Thyrotoxic subacute thyroiditis was diagnosed on the basis of clinical findings and high values of T_4, T_3, and resin T_3 uptake, low values of radioactive iodine uptake (RAIU), high erythrocyte sedimentation rates, and

*I am grateful to the members of the Endocrine Clinic, Osaka University Hospital, for help in examining the patients.

Table 2-5. Clinical data on patients with destruction-induced thyrotoxicosis.

	Subacute thyroiditis	Silent thyroiditis	
		Spontaneous	Postpartum
No. examined	24	11	29
Female patients	22 (92)	10 (91)	29 (100)
Age less than 30 years	1 (4)	7 (64)[b]	24 (83)[b]
Antibodies[c]			
Positive TGHA	0 (0)	5 (45)[a]	11 (38)[a]
Positive MCHA	0 (0)	9 (82)[b]	24 (83)[b]
Goiter			
Palpable at thyrotoxic state	24 (100)	10 (91)	26 (90)
Persistence	0 (0)	10 (91)[b]	26 (90)[b]

Values in parentheses indicate the percentage.
[a]Significantly different from subacute thyroiditis ($P < 0.01$; chi-square test).
[b]Significantly different from subacute thyroiditis ($P < 0.001$; chi-square test).
[c]TGHA antithyroglobulin hemagglutination antibody; MCHA antithyroid microsomal hemagglutination antibody.

negative antithyroid antibodies. As described by Hamburger and Meier, silent thyroiditis was more frequent in younger female patients. No difference in the frequencies of positive antibodies was observed between spontaneous silent thyroiditis and postpartum silent thyroiditis, and the frequencies are similar to those in autoimmune thyroid diseases.[45] Small goiters persisted in all patients with silent thyroiditis who had palpable goiter during the initial thyrotoxic state, although the size of goiter decreased significantly during the observation period. Patients with postpartum thyrotoxicosis had neither neck pain nor fever.

Evidence for Autoimmune Thyroiditis

I believe that all cases of postpartum silent thyroiditis and almost all cases of spontaneous silent thyroiditis are forms of autoimmune thyroiditis. Postpartum silent thyroiditis may be induced during the course of autoimmune thyroiditis by physiologic-immunologic changes associated with gestation. All patients who had had transient hypothyroidism in a previous postpartum period developed recurrence of postpartum transient thyrotoxicosis followed by hypothyroidism.[46] Thus, the occurrence of postpartum thyrotoxicosis could be predicted in patients who had had the postpartum syndrome once before. Silent thyroiditis was also observed after artificial or spontaneous abortion. More than 80 percent of patients with postpartum thyroiditis had positive antithyroid microsomal antibodies, suggesting an autoimmune thyroiditis. Hamburger and Meier claim that detection of antibodies per se is not proof of autoimmunity in the absence of other features of autoimmune disease, that autoimmune disease tends to be chronic and progressive, not of short duration, and that spontaneous resolution of profound hypothyroidism is entirely inconsistent with the course of Hashimoto's thyroiditis. Our recent study suggests that serum antithyroid antibodies in patients without overt thyroid disease may indicate the existence of lymphocytic infiltration in the thyroid gland, presumably reflecting subclinical autoimmune thyroiditis.[47] This type of thyroiditis is far more frequent than the classic Hashimoto's thyroiditis.[48]

All of our patients with subclinical autoimmune thyroiditis, with antithyroid microsomal antibodies more than 1:5120 before pregnancy, developed postpartum thyrotoxicosis (unpublished data). Absence of antibodies at the time of postpartum thyrotoxicosis cannot rule out autoimmune thyroiditis, since 5 to 15 % of the patients with autoimmune thyroid diseases gave a negative reaction even with the sensitive microsomal hemagglutination method.[45] Furthermore the reaction for antibody becomes negative at the time of thyrotoxicosis in some patients. A typical case is shown in Table 2-6. The titers of antithyroid microsomal antibodies decreased during pregnancy, as in other cases of autoimmune thyroid diseases,[49] and no antibody was detectable at the time of postpartum thyrotoxicosis. However, later it became detectable again and persisted. The negative reaction for antibody may be related to neutralization by antigen(s) leaking from the inflamed thyroid gland. Therefore, possible preexistent subclinical autoimmunity should be considered in patients who develop antithyroid antibodies after destruction-induced thyrotoxicosis.

Table 2-6. Changes in antithyroid antibodies in a patient with postpartum silent thyroiditis.

Time of test	T_4 (μg/dl)	T_3 (ng/dl)	Free T_4 index	TSH (μU/ml)	TGHA[a]	MCHA[a]
Six months before pregnancy	6.1	130	5.7	5.6	Negative	1280
Pregnancy						
8 weeks	14.8	252	11.3	1.8	Negative	160
20 weeks	11.0	237	5.9	3.8	Negative	40
Postpartum						
1 month	6.7	141	4.2	1.2	Negative	20
4 months	18.3	258	20.7	<1.0	Negative	Negative
5 months	8.8	135	8.5	<1.0	Negative	40
7 months	4.2	141	3.5	6.1	Negative	40
13 months	8.2	169	7.1	3.0	Negative	1280

[a]TGHA, antithyroglobulin hemagglutination antibody; MCHA, antithyroid microsomal hemagglutination antibody.

Hamburger and Meier used the hemagglutination method for detection of microsomal antibodies, but they considered titers of 1:1600 or more positive. This cutoff value is too high, and excludes many cases of mild autoimmune thyroid disease[47-49] such as a case shown in Table 2-6.

Postpartum Thyroiditis

Persistence of goiter and antithyroid antibodies suggests that postpartum thyroiditis is a "chronic" disease compatible with one of autoimmune nature, although the changes of thyroid hormones are transient. Thyroid function is normal and static in most cases of autoimmune thyroiditis, including subclinical forms.[47,48] Patients with subclinical forms often show transient aggravation induced by various factors, but rarely develop irreversible hypothyroidism.[48] Very recently we screened patients with postpartum transient thyrotoxicosis and/or transient hypothyroidism at 3 to 5 months after delivery.[50] Eleven of 250 (4.4%) postpartum subjects had transient thyrotoxicosis and two of these patients developed transient hypothyroidism. Transient hypothyroidism was also found in three other patients. Thus, in all, postpartum transient hypothyroidism was found in five of 250 subjects (2.0%) at 3 to 6 months postpartum. All but one of these patients had persistent positive antithyroid microsomal antibodies.

Seasonal Distribution of Thyroiditis

The seasonal distribution of subacute thyroiditis and postpartum silent thyroiditis is shown in Table 2-7. Postpartum thyroiditis was distributed throughout the year, whereas subacute thyroiditis was more common in the latter half of the year in

Table 2-7. Seasonal distribution of patients with subacute thyroiditis and postpartum silent thyroiditis.

	January–March	April–June	July–September	October–December
Subacute thyroiditis	0	0	2	4
Postpartum thyroiditis	4	1	3	1

Numbers indicate numbers of patients seen at the Endocrine Clinic of Osaka University Hospital in 1979.

1979. These results support the possibility of seasonal occurrence of subacute thyroiditis, but not of postpartum thyroiditis, although a final conclusion on this problem must await additional data.

Findings of Follow-up Studies Suggesting Autoimmune Disease

Follow-up studies on patients with autoimmune thyroiditis revealed amelioration during pregnancy and aggravation after delivery.[46,49] The size of goiter decreased in association with decreases of peripheral K-lymphocytes and antithyroid antibodies during pregnancy.[46] Postpartum thyroid destruction was associated with increases of antithyroid antibodies and of peripheral B- and K-lymphocytes. These data suggest that antibody-dependent cell-mediated cytotoxicity plays an important role in postpartum autoimmune thyroid destruction. Postpartum aggravation has been observed not only in autoimmune thyroiditis but also in Graves' dis-

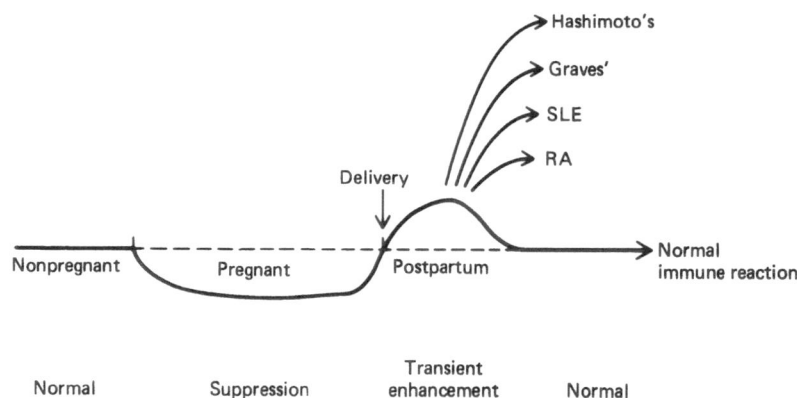

Figure 2-1. Immune rebound hypothesis regarding the postpartum onset of autoimmune diseases. Possible immunosuppression in pregnancy may disappear at delivery. "Transient enhancement" of the immune reactions may occur after delivery by a mechanism similar to the "rebound phenomenon" observed after withdrawal of immunosuppressive glucocorticoid therapy.

ease.[23,51] Amelioration during late pregnancy and relapse or aggravation 2 to 6 months postpartum have also been reported for other autoimmune diseases, e.g., rheumatoid arthritis,[52] systemic lupus erythematosus,[53] myasthenia gravis,[54] and idiopathic thrombocytopenic purpura.[55] I think that immune rebound mechanisms may induce aggravation or clinical onset of these autoimmune diseases, as illustrated in Figure 2-1. Postpartum silent thyroiditis may not be induced by viral infection.

Relationship of Spontaneous to Postpartum Silent Thyroiditis

The incidence of positive antibodies and the age distribution in cases of spontaneous silent thyroiditis were similar to those for postpartum silent thyroiditis (Table 2-5). In cases of spontaneous silent thyroiditis, persistence of goiter and antibodies were also observed. Moreover, follow-up observations revealed the occurrence of postpartum silent thyroiditis in patients who had had spontaneous silent thyroiditis before. These results suggest that a similar factor may induce both spontaneous and postpartum silent thyroiditis. Furthermore, similar increases of peripheral total- and K-lymphocytes and antithyroid antibodies were observed at the time of aggravation in spontaneous silent thyroiditis (unpublished data). In a preliminary study, no significant changes were found in viral antibodies to cytomegalovirus, adenovirus, influenza, mumps, RS, herpes, rubella, measles, ECHO, or Coxsackie viruses or in antibodies to mycoplasma during the clinical course of spontaneous silent thyroiditis. From these data, it seems likely that spontaneous silent thyroiditis is also induced by changes of immune reaction on the basis of autoimmune thyroiditis, although the trigger is unknown. If an infectious agent is the trigger for a flare of autoimmunity, it may be a new virus and one that is *less* virulent than those causing subacute thyroiditis. Clinical findings are usually milder in silent thyroiditis than in subacute thyroiditis. In autoimmune thyroiditis, the thyroid gland may be more easily damaged than normal even by a weakly virulent virus.

Responses to Queries of Hamburger and Meier

Item 1: The pattern of change in circulating levels of thyroid hormones may be similar in all types of destruction-induced thyrotoxicosis. More marked and acute thyroid destruction may induce more pronounced thyrotoxicosis, followed with prominent hypothyroidism. Similar changes of thyroid hormones, however, need not indicate similarity in etiology.

Item 2: I believe that lymphocytic infiltration and persistent antithyroid antibodies mean that spontaneous and postpartum silent thyroiditis are forms of autoimmune thyroiditis.

Item 3: Similarities of sequential microscopic changes do not suggest similar etiologies for these three types of thyroiditis.

Table 2-8. A patient with transient postpartum hypothyroidism treated with triiodothyronine.

Time of test	T_4 (μg/dl)	T_3 (ng/dl)	Free T_4 index	TSH (μU/ml)	Goiter size (cm)	Body weight (kg)	Treatment
Pregnancy							
8 weeks	5.8	163	4.4	21.0	6.8	50	None
28 weeks	12.3	216	9.4	1.4	5.8	56	None
Postpartum							
1 month	6.0	131	7.6	<1.0	7.0	51	None
2 months	<1.0	38	<0.8	239	8.8	53	None
3 months	<1.0	35	<0.7	355	7.7	54	T_3, 50 μg/day started
4 months	<1.0	222	<0.8	9.1	6.3	52	T_3, 75 μg/day
5 months	1.3	440	1.1	2.7	6.3	51	T_3, 75 μg/day
8 months	1.4	280	1.4	4.4	5.8	49	T_3, 25 μg/day
9 months	1.4	139	1.2	35.0	6.6	49	T_3 discontinued
10 months	3.9	103	3.9	12.4	6.1	49	None
12 months	5.6	121	5.5	3.8	6.2	49	None

Item 4: A RAIU is not available in all clinics and hospitals. In Japan patients must be kept on low iodine diet for 2 weeks before the RAIU. Thus, it is not practical for every patient with hyperthyroidism to have a RAIU to exclude spontaneously resolving hyperthyroidism. The T_3/T_4 ratio was helpful for differentiation of destruction-induced thyrotoxicosis from hyperthyroidism of Graves' disease,[56] although this was not confirmed by Nikolai et al.[19]

Item 5: Spontaneous recovery from postpartum hypothyroidism occurred in all patients under 30 years old who showed high RAIU and marked thyroid enlargement during the hypothyroid phase. Patients over 30 years old with slight goiter should be followed carefully for irreversible hypothyroidism, especially when the RAIU is not increased at the time of hypothyroidism. When the patients have severe symptoms of hypometabolism, treatment with T_3 may be useful, since spontaneous recovery will be detected by increase of serum T_4. Data on one such case are summarized in Table 2-8. At 5 months postpartum her serum T_4 increased from undetectable to 1.3 μg/dl during the administration of T_3, 75 μg per day. Spontaneous recovery was confirmed 7 months later.

Item 6: Thyroid ablation with ^{131}I need not be used and may in fact be contraindicated. Symptoms and signs are usually mild in the hyperthyroidism of silent thyroiditis, and lifelong treatment with thyroid hormone is inappropriate for these patients.

COMMENTARY

Colum A. Gorman, M.B., B.Ch., Ph.D.

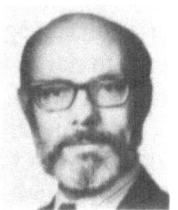

Classification of Thyroiditis

Hamburger and Meier have provided us with a thoughtful analysis of the features of several variants of thyroiditis. Since their title distinguishes between silent thyroiditis and postpartum silent thyroiditis, there is the implication that these are two different conditions. I contest that assumption. The title also distinguishes between chronic thyroiditis and viral thyroiditis. This would seem to imply that chronic thyroiditis is not caused by a virus and that there is some form of thyroiditis which we are sure is caused by a virus. Neither of these statements is known to be true.

The fact is that authors writing about thyroiditis have dropped us in a semantic quagmire. Appellations applied to various types of thyroiditis may be based on severity and duration of clinical expression (acute, subacute, chronic); on histology (lymphocytic, granulomatous, pyogenic, invasive fibrotic); or the terminology may rely on traditional eponyms which cut across the other classifications (Riedel's, de Quervain's, Hashimoto's). To this surfeit of classifications have recently been added the variant subgroups of painful, silent, or painless thyroiditis, and a chronologic association—postpartum thyroiditis. What is needed is an etiologic classification of thyroiditis. Since the information to provide such a classification does not exist, I propose a classification which includes some of the recently described forms of thyroiditis in the context of the traditional entities (Table 2-9).

Let us begin with an area in which there will be more or less general agreement. Patients with thyroiditis can usually be fitted comfortably into the acute,

Table 2-9. Thyroiditis classified in relation to traditional entities.

Thyroiditis	
Acute ——————————	Pyogenic
Subacute ⟨	Lymphocytic / Granulomatous
Chronic ⟨	Lymphocytic / Invasive fibrotic

subacute, and chronic categories (Table 2-10). Acute thyroiditis is usually bacterial and pyogenic, associated with fever and often with abscess formation. It tends to run its course in days or weeks. A variety of organisms have been cultured from the gland.

Subacute thyroiditis tends to run its course in weeks or months. No infecting organism has been consistently cultured from the gland. It is characterized initially by transient hyperthyroidism due to leakage of preformed thyroid hormone from damaged follicles, and later by transient hypothyroidism when the stores of preformed hormone have been exhausted and synthesis of new hormone in the healing follicles is not yet sufficient to restore normal serum thyroxine levels. Traditionally, this clinical course has been associated with a granulomatous reaction, particularly with giant cells. Recently, we have recognized a similar clinical course with a lymphocytic infiltrate.

Chronic thyroiditis runs its course in months or years and is accompanied by varying degrees of lymphocytic infiltration and fibrosis. Antibodies directed against thyroid microsomes and thyroglobulin are characteristically found in the

Table 2-10. Thyroiditis classification scheme.[a]

	Acute	Subacute	Chronic
Course	Days	Weeks or months	Months or years
Etiology	Infectious	Unknown, possibly viral	Unknown, autoimmune phenomena are prominent
Pathology	Polymorphonuclear infiltrates; abscess formation common	Lymphocytic infiltration or granulomatous infiltration; disrupted follicles prominent in both	Lymphocytic infiltration and fibrosis in varying proportions
Clinical features	Acutely ill patient; swollen, tender thyroid	Moderately ill patient; thyroid may or may not be painful or tender; usually painless with lymphocytic form; hyperthyroidism variably present	Typically painless, firm thyroid; usually tendency to hypofunction, but stimulatory antibodies with hyperfunction may be present; fibrosis can be severe and invasive
Termination	Complete resolution with appropriate antibiotics	Usually return to euthyroidism; occasionally persistent hypothyroidism	Eventual progression toward hypothyroidism

[a]Any form of thyroiditis may occur in painful or painless forms. Acute thyroiditis is usually painful, chronic is usually painless, and subacute is typically painless when lymphobytic and painful when granulomatous. Exceptions are frequent. Subacute lymphocytic thyroiditis is often diagnosed in the postpartum period.

serum. As lymphocytic infiltration and fibrosis progress, the patient tends to become gradually hypothyroid. Sometimes stimulating antibodies are present and hyperthyroidism is seen. In the chronic Riedel's thyroiditis, fibrosis is extensive and invasive; serum antibody levels are highly variable.

With this classification, part of the question posed in Hamburger's title becomes moot. There is no reason to attempt distinction between the conditions "silent thyroiditis" and "postpartum silent thyroiditis." According to the classification we might rephrase the question: "Do painless subacute lymphocytic thyroiditis and painless subacute granulomatous thyroiditis when diagnosed in the postpartum period differ fundamentally from the same conditions diagnosed outside the postpartum period?" I think the answer to that question would be no. It is well known that many instances of painless thyroiditis, either lymphocytic or granulomatous, are diagnosed serendipitously during routine examination for other purposes. It is likely that any condition (e.g., pregnancy and postpartum checkups) which brings the population at risk to physicians will result in more cases being diagnosed. The conclusion that thyroiditis and pregnancy are causally associated may be incorrect. The association may be purely one of chance. No firm epidemiologic evidence has yet been presented which warrants consideration of postpartum silent thyroiditis as a separate entity from thyroiditis occurring at other times. This is particularly true when one considers how loosely the term postpartum has at times been applied. About half of Hamburger's patients were first diagnosed within 3 to 12 months after the time of delivery. This represents a generous extension of the postpartum period as usually defined.

Are Patients with Painless Subacute Lymphocytic Thyroiditis Different in any Important Way from Patients with Subacute Granulomatous Thyroiditis?

Since we do not know what stimuli induce the thyroid to respond with a lymphocytic reaction and what stimuli elicit a granulomatous reaction, the answer to this question remains unsettled. Because patients with subacute lymphocytic thyroiditis have such a marked propensity to recurrence (all four of the patients we originally described have now each had three recurrences), because the thyroid histology is so strikingly different from that seen in granulomatous thyroiditis, and because pain, tenderness, and elevation of the erythrocyte sedimentation rate are so consistently absent from the patients with subacute lymphocytic thyroiditis, I tend to believe that these patients have a syndrome different from granulomatous thyroiditis.

Differences between Subacute and Chronic Lymphocytic Thyroiditis

The distinctions between subacute lymphocytic thyroiditis and chronic lymphocytic thyroiditis are more clear-cut. When hyperthyroidism is seen in chronic lymphocytic thyroiditis, the synthesis and secretion of thyroid hormone are coupled; i.e., radioiodine uptake (RAIU) by the thyroid gland and secretion of thyroid hormone are both increased. In contrast, the hyperthyroidism in subacute lymphocytic thyroiditis is associated with high thyroxine levels but a low RAIU, implying that the hyperthyroidism is due to release of preformed hormone from damaged thyroid follicles. Chronic lymphocytic thyroiditis is typically associated with evidence of autoimmunity which is characteristically absent in patients with subacute lymphocytic thyroiditis. Hypothyroidism is usually transient when it occurs in conjunction with subacute lymphocytic thyroiditis and permanent when it occurs in association with chronic lymphocytic thyroiditis. Whether some patients with subacute lymphocytic thyroiditis develop chronic lymphocytic thyroiditis is unclear.

Points of Agreement with Hamburger and Meier

Up to this point, I have been spiritedly disagreeing with Hamburger and his colleague, but we certainly do see eye-to-eye on three points. I agree that a RAIU is an essential component of the pretreatment evaluation of patients with hyperthyroidism. Without a RAIU, Graves' disease cannot always be reliably distinguished from the transient hyperthyroid states associated with subacute lymphocytic and subacute granulomatous thyroiditis. One wonders how many of the remissions, supposedly induced by antithyroid drugs in patients with "Graves' disease," were in patients with transient hyperthyroidism associated with lymphocytic or granulomatous thyroiditis. The recovery of these patients was predestined whether antithyroid drugs were used or not. Secondly, when one encounters newly diagnosed hypothyroidism, it may be reasonable to treat with thyroid hormone for 6 months and then to withdraw therapy for several months to see whether spontaneous recovery of thyroid function has occurred. Gharib et al.[57] have reported that the hypothyroidism seen in association with Addison's disease will spontaneously recover when the Addison's disease is treated with corticosteroids. Perhaps in addition to subacute lymphocytic and subacute granulomatous thyroiditis, there are other causes of transient hypothyroidism. In the patients I have seen thus far, serum thyroxine and TSH levels are diagnostic, but hypothyroidism has usually been brief and associated with few symptoms, because serum thyroxine levels return to normal before the full-blown clinical manifestations of myxedema develop. If hypothyroidism is fully expressed clinically, in my experience, the prognosis for full recovery of thyroid function must be considered poor.

I agree with Hamburger and Meier also on the potential value of thyroid hormone suppressive therapy. In patients who show a marked propensity to recurrent subacute lymphocytic thyroiditis, the symptoms produced depend upon the release of preformed hormone from damaged thyroid follicles. It follows that if the follicles can be prevented from accumulating thyroid hormone (by suppressive therapy with thyroxine between attacks), although the same recurrent insult to the thyroid may take place, it will be asymptomatic. Among the patients with subacute lymphocytic thyroiditis that I have treated with suppressive therapy, there have been no recurrent symptomatic episodes.

At present the greatest need is for good prospective studies of environmental, infectious, and chemical influences on thyroid histology and function. Until these have been done, our understanding, our terminology, and our classifications of thyroiditis will remain imperfect and probably controversial.

COMMENTARY

Mitsuo Inada, M.D.

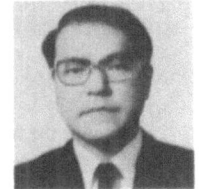

Subacute thyroiditis is characterized by transient thyrotoxicosis, painful tender goiter, fever, raised erythrocyte sedimentation rate, and low radioactive iodine uptake (RAIU). The disease almost always resolves spontaneously, passing through thyrotoxic and hypothyroid phases.[58] Recently, cases of painless thyroiditis with transient thyrotoxicosis and low RAIU were reported.[11,12,16,18-20,22,25,30,59] These cases were differentiated from subacute thyroiditis by the absence of pain, fever, an elevated sedimentation rate, and by needle biopsy findings. A substantial proportion of painless thyroiditis patients were seen in the postpartum period.[22,25,59] These patients often had postpartum recurrences.[59] However, the pathogenesis of silent thyroiditis or postpartum silent thyroiditis is still controversial.

Pathogenesis of Silent Thyroiditis

Morrison and Caplan[14] reported typical subacute thyroiditis and silent thyroiditis with thyrotoxicosis and low RAIU in a wife and husband. They suggested that transient thyrotoxicosis with low RAIU is due to silent subacute thyroiditis (presumably a viral infection), and that variable host response to a viral inflammatory reaction might be responsible for the absence of thyroidal pain and tenderness. Hamburger and Meier also suggest that silent thyroiditis and postpartum silent thyroiditis differ from subacute thyroiditis only in that they represent slightly different responses to infectious agents (probably viral) which may be more virulent than those causing subacute thyroiditis. On the other hand, Gluck et al.[16] and others[12,18,20] demonstrated that thyroid biopsy specimens from patients with silent thyroiditis were most compatible with chronic lymphocytic thyroiditis.

Biopsy Findings, Silent Thyroiditis

Recently, we reported two patients with silent thyroiditis, in whom the thyroid biopsies were performed in the thyrotoxic and recovery phases.[20] The clinical and laboratory findings were as follows:

Case 1.

A 36-year-old woman presented with typical clinical and biochemical findings of hyperthyroidism of 2 months' duration. The RAIU was less than 3% on repeated determinations, in
spite of low iodine intake. She denied having neck pain or symptoms of upper respiratory
tract infection. Surreptitious use of thyroid hormones or iodine was excluded. She had not
been pregnant for 13 years. A diffuse nontender goiter, twice normal size, was noted. The
erythrocyte sedimentation rate was 7 mm/h. The antithyroglobulin antibody was positive
(1:1000), but antimicrosomal antibody was undetectable throughout the disease. Needle
biopsy of the thyroid was performed while the patient was thyrotoxic and showed marked
lymphocytic infiltration, poorly preserved thyroid follicles, and epithelial cell damage. Ashkanazy cells were not present. Granulomatous changes of subacute thyroiditis were not found.
Neither were there changes suggestive of Graves' disease. The hyperthyroidism resolved
spontaneously within 1 month.

About 2 months after the initial examination, the RAIU was still very low, thyroid hormone levels were at the lower limit of normal, and the serum TSH level was 5 μU/ml. Moreover, she had increased fatigue and dry skin, suggesting hypothyroidism. About 2 weeks later,
values for T_4 and T_3 improved and the plasma TSH level became undetectable. Thereafter,
she remained euthyroid without treatment. The RAIU and the thyroid biopsy were repeated
3 months after the initial presentation. The RAIU was 36.9% and imaging showed uniform
distribution of radioactive iodine within the thyroid. The histologic examination revealed
well-preserved thyroid follicles, slight focal lymphocytic infiltrations, and minimal fibrosis.
The goiter was almost unchanged throughout the course of the disease.

Case 2.

A 61-year-old woman reported with clinical and biochemical findings of hyperthyroidism, but
the RAIU was less than 1%. She denied ingestion of iodine or thyroid hormone. There was
a diffuse nontender goiter, almost three times normal size. The antimicrosomal antibody was
positive (1:1280), while the antithyroglobulin antibody was undetectable. A thyroid biopsy
specimen obtained during the thyrotoxic phase revealed marked lymphocytic infiltration,
poorly preserved thyroid follicles, and epithelial cell damage. Ashkanazy cells were not present. There was no evidence of subacute thyroiditis.

About 1 month later, her symptoms had cleared spontaneously and T_4 and T_3 levels were
normal. Thereafter, she remained euthyroid. The goiter did not change during the entire
course of the disease. About 3 months after the initial examination, the antibody findings
were unchanged. The thyroid ^{99m}Tc uptake was nearly normal (0.4%) and imaging showed
uniform distribution of ^{99m}Tc within the thyroid. Histologic examination revealed slight focal
lymphocytic infiltrations and well-preserved thyroid follicles. Although mild fibrosis was
observed, there were no changes of granulomatous thyroiditis.

These patients had painless transient thyrotoxicosis with low RAIU which was
followed by hypothyroidism and finally recovery. They had thyroid autoantibodies
in serum and persistent goiters of considerable size throughout the disease. Moreover, the histologic findings during the acute phase revealed interfollicular infiltrations of lymphocytes with follicular cell damage. These findings might suggest
Hashimoto's thyroiditis.[16] However, germinal centers and Ashkanazy cells were
not present, and fibrosis was mild or minimal.

Histologic Abnormalities Spontaneously Regressed

It was remarkable that in both patients the histologic abnormalities improved
spontaneously within several months, along with spontaneous regression of clinical

and biochemical abnormalities. To our knowledge, no other reports have appeared of short-term reversible changes in the histologic abnormalities of Hashimoto's thyroiditis. As Hamburger and Meier observed, Hashimoto's thyroiditis, an autoimmune disease, tends to be progressive, not of short duration and not spontaneously resolving. Thus, the reversible abnormalities seen in the biopsy specimens in silent thyroiditis might suggest that silent thyroiditis is not a new form of Hashimoto's thyroiditis.

Pathogenetic Implications of Biopsy Findings

A recent study[19] described the histologic findings on biopsy specimens obtained from 12 patients with transient thyrotoxicosis secondary to silent thyroiditis during the thyrotoxic phase. These findings were compared to those in Hashimoto's thyroiditis. Although lymphocytic infiltrations were seen in both diseases, Ashkanazy cell change, germinal centers, and fibrosis were present more frequently in Hashimoto's thyroiditis.

On the other hand, it is very difficult to conclude that silent thyroiditis is a variant of subacute thyroiditis. Our patients had higher titers of autoantibodies than those usually seen in subacute thyroiditis, and moreover, they had persistent goiters of considerable size, in contrast to most patients with subacute thyroiditis. Four other patients with silent thyroiditis seen in our clinic had persistent goiters throughout the course of the disease. We also reported two patients with postpartum silent thyroiditis, who may have had postpartum recurrences.[59] Therefore, it is unlikely that silent thyroiditis, at least in these cases, is a variant of subacute thyroiditis. We suspect that silent thyroiditis represents a heterogeneous group of disorders, some of which may truly be a variant of subacute thyroiditis, and some of which may be lymphocytic thyroiditis of unknown origin. Although the etiology of persistent goiter and transient thyrotoxicosis in these patients is unclear, unknown factors other than infectious agents might be responsible.

Diagnostic Value of 30-min ^{99m}Tc Uptakes

In our laboratory, 30-min thyroid uptake of ^{99m}Tc is measured by using the scinticamera equipped with a 4096 channel data system. This procedure is very simple, and radiation from ^{99m}Tc to thyroid is negligible compared to that from ^{131}I. Patients with silent thyroiditis had markedly diminished thyroid uptake of ^{99m}Tc. Therefore, we measure ^{99m}Tc thyroid uptake in all patients with thyrotoxicosis. This is necessary because we cannot otherwise differentiate the hyperthyroidism of silent thyroiditis from that of Graves' disease.

Transient to Persistent Hypothyroidism

Finally, it is relatively easy to differentiate transient hypothyroidism from persistent hypothyroidism. In order to exclude the diagnosis of transient hypothyroidism, a careful history is necessary. If the patient had thyrotoxic symptoms several months earlier, he should be observed for some months prior to treatment with thyroid hormone.

COMMENTARY

Thomas F. Nikolai, M.D.

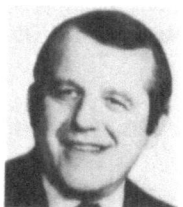

Classification of Thyroiditis

Silent thyroiditis, which I call lymphocytic thyroiditis with spontaneously resolving hyperthyroidism (a more descriptive term), has increased in frequency recently. Hamburger and Meier have tried to distinguish several syndromes associated with thyroiditis, one of which is silent thyroiditis. They made this differentiation primarily upon the clinical and laboratory findings, disregarding microscopic features. Five types of thyroiditis may be recognized:

(1) Acute thyroiditis (suppurative) (bacterial)

(2) Sclerosing thyroiditis (Riedel's struma)

(3) Chronic lymphocytic thyroiditis (Hashimoto's thyroiditis) (autoimmune)

(4) Subacute thyroiditis (de Quervain's) (granulomatous) (giant cell) (viral) (with and without spontaneously resolving hyperthyroidism)

(5) Lymphocytic thyroiditis with spontaneously resolving hyperthyroidism (silent thyroiditis)—with frequent postpartum association

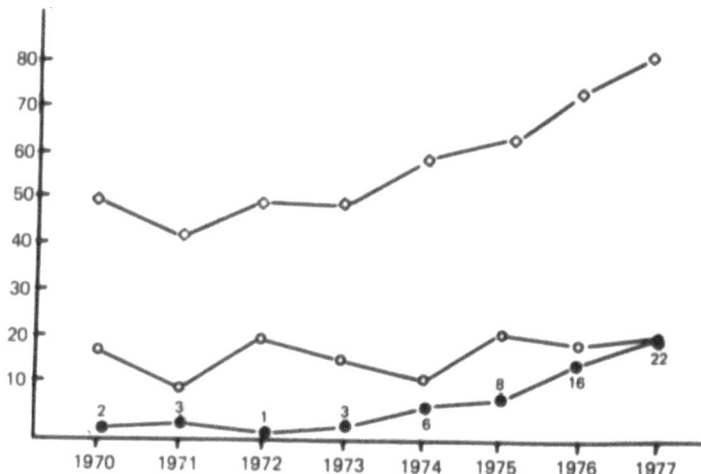

Figure 2-2. The rising frequency of spontaneously resolving hyperthyroidism. ◇—◇: hyperthyroidism; ○—○: subacute thyroiditis; ●—●: spontaneously resolving hyperthyroidism.

I will deal primarily with the differentiation of types 4 and 5 and attempt to answer the six questions posed by Hamburger and Meier.

Subacute thyroiditis generally presents in one of three different ways: (1) asymptomatic goiter without hyperthyroidism—frequently a single cold thyroid nodule recognized only after excision to rule out malignancy; (2) as a painful tender thyroid with spontaneously resolving hyperthyroidism; or (3) as a painful tender thyroid without spontaneously resolving hyperthyroidism.

Lymphocytic thyroiditis with spontaneously resolving hyperthyroidism was first described in 1974 and since has been recognized by a number of workers.[11-20] I observed my first case in 1968 followed by a few cases per year through 1974. Then the frequency increased, most cases having been seen since 1975 (Fig. 2-2). This is also the experience of Hamburger and Meier. I am sure we had not overlooked the disease earlier, because of unfamiliarity, since radioactive iodine uptakes (RAIU) were done on almost all our hyperthyroid patients after 1960.[19]

Clinical Differentiation of Painful and Painless Forms of Thyroiditis with Spontaneously Resolving Hyperthyroidism

Subacute thyroiditis (painful) with spontaneously resolving hyperthyroidism and lymphocytic thyroiditis with spontaneously resolving hyperthyroidism have nearly identical acute clinical courses, evolving from transient hyperthyroidism, through a temporary hypothyroidism, to recovery. The principal finding differentiating these diseases in the acute hyperthyroid phase is the neck pain and thyroid tenderness of subacute thyroiditis, which is rare in lymphocytic thyroiditis. I have not seen subacute thyroiditis with spontaneously resolving hyperthyroidism without neck pain and thyroid tenderness. In lymphocytic thyroiditis with spontaneously resolving hyperthyroidism, only five of over 100 patients had thyroid tenderness and only two had neck pain—all equivocal or mild. These five patients had biopsy-proved lymphocytic thyroiditis. Thirty patients with hyperthyroidism presenting with neck pain and thyroid tenderness had granulomatous or giant cell thyroiditis demonstrated by biopsy. Granted, subacute thyroiditis without hyperthyroidism may present with only mild pain and tenderness or as an asymptomatic goiter or nodule, as shown by surgical series.[6] Therefore, the clinician can almost always differentiate between subacute thyroiditis with spontaneously resolving hyperthyroidism and lymphocytic thyroiditis with spontaneously resolving hyperthyroidism by the presence or absence of neck pain and thyroid tenderness. Other features, such as age and sex of patient and history of preceding viral prodrome or respiratory infection, are not helpful.

Laboratory Findings

Laboratory testing is useful but not definitive in separating these entities. The sedimentation rate in lymphocytic thyroiditis with spontaneously resolving hyperthyroidism is rarely over 50 mm/h, whereas in subacute thyroiditis with spontaneously resolving hyperthyroidism it is usually over 50 mm/h.[19] Antithyroid antibody tests are negative, or positive in low titer, more often in subacute thyroiditis with spontaneously resolving hyperthyroidism than in lymphocytic thyroiditis with spontaneously resolving hyperthyroidism. However, the overlap is so great that commonly used antibody tests are not helpful in the differential diagnosis.

Value of Biopsy Findings

Hamburger and Meier discount the diagnostic value of biopsy. Here I must strongly disagree, as I believe the pathologic changes are of prime importance. They state that only focal lymphocytic infiltration is found and that features of chronic lymphocytic thyroiditis (i.e., Hashimoto's thyroiditis), such as oxyphilic change, fibrosis, and germinal centers, are absent in lymphocytic thyroiditis with spontaneously resolving hyperthyroidism. They further observe that lymphocytic infiltrates are common in most thyroid diseases. However, I have found distinctive features of a lymphocytic thyroiditis in these patients, different from the granulomatous reaction of subacute thyroiditis with spontaneously resolving hyperthyroidism. Thyroid biopsies in over 40 patients in the early through late stages of lymphocytic thyroiditis with spontaneously resolving hyperthyroidism show evidence of lymphocytic thyroiditis, not just focal lymphocytic infiltrates.[16,18,19,36,60] There are moderate focal or diffuse lymphocytic infiltration, areas of follicle collapse with papillary infolding and intrafollicular cellular debris, occasional oxyphilic changes (present in only 15–20%), and minimal or no fibrosis. However, two recent patients had the above findings plus marked fibrosis, germinal centers, and generalized oxyphilic change, characteristic findings of advanced Hashimoto's thyroiditis. Our pathologists had no trouble differentiating subacute thyroiditis with spontaneously resolving hyperthyroidism from lymphocytic thyroiditis with spontaneously resolving hyperthyroidism, except in one specimen which showed features of both diseases.

Differentiation from Graves' Disease

My main diagnostic difficulty is differentiating lymphocytic thyroiditis with spontaneously resolving hyperthyroidism from the hyperthyroidism of Graves' disease. In many instances where I initially suspected Graves' disease, I was surprised to find a RAIU of 2% or less. Biopsy demonstrated lymphocytic thyroiditis with no evidence of Graves' disease.[19] I strongly concur with Dorfman[61] that once a clinical diagnosis of hyperthyroidism is confirmed by elevated serum levels of l-thyroxine and triiodothyronine, the next step should be the RAIU (unless the patient is pregnant). Lymphocytic thyroiditis with spontaneously resolving hyperthyroidism accounts for 10–20% of all cases of hyperthyroidism in our experience.[19] Treating hyperthyroid patients as having Graves' disease without the RAIU may be inappropriate.[19] In a few pregnant hyperthyroid women I have used needle biopsy to differentiate Graves' disease from lymphocytic thyroiditis with spontaneously resolving hyperthyroidism.

Primary Hypothyroidism May Be Transient

I have seen several cases closely resembling case 3 of Hamburger and Meier. These patients, initially euthyroid, subsequently developed transient hypothyroidism. I have also noted several cases of transient hypothyroidism similar to those of Amino et al.[21] Therefore, the long-held notion that primary hypothyroidism is always permanent must be reevaluated.

Recurrent Episodes

It has been my experience that approximately 10–15% of patients with lymphocytic thyroiditis with spontaneously resolving hyperthyroidism have recurrent episodes within 6 months to 4 years. Relapses are rare in subacute thyroiditis, except in the first few months after initial presentation.[60]

Several patients with biopsy-proved lymphocytic thyroiditis with spontaneously resolving hyperthyroidism, placed on suppression therapy because of gradually enlarging goiters months or years after recovery from transient hyperthyroidism, had recurrent episodes of transient hyperthyroidism and increase in thyroid gland size. This also occurred in two patients with chronic lymphocytic thyroiditis (i.e., Hashimoto's thyroiditis) on thyroid suppression. Thus, suppression therapy with thyroid hormone may not prevent recurrent episodes of spontaneously resolving hyperthyroidism. We resorted to total thyroidectomy in two patients who had multiple episodes of transient hyperthyroidism with suppressed RAIU, as did Gorman et al.[18]

Relation to Hashimoto's Thyroiditis

Finally, are lymphocytic thyroiditis with spontaneously resolving hyperthyroidism and chronic lymphocytic thyroiditis (i.e., Hashimoto's thyroiditis) different diseases or different expressions of the same disease? I have reported features of lymphocytic thyroiditis with spontaneously resolving hyperthyroidism which resemble chronic lymphocytic thyroiditis (Hashimoto's thyroiditis), while other features were quite different (Table 2-11). Long-term follow-up study shows that patients with subacute thyroiditis with or without spontaneously resolving hyperthyroidism rarely develop permaent thyroid disease.[60] Subacute thyroiditis patients with spontaneously resolving hyperthyroidism, but not those without it, may have augmented response of TSH to TRH stimulation up to 15 years later, indicating loss of thyroid reserve due to the severity of the initial thyroiditis. These patients rarely develop hypothyroidism or goiter, because the thyroiditis is usually

Table 2-11. Relationship between silent thyroiditis and chronic lymphocytic thyroiditis.

	Silent thyroiditis	Chronic lymphocytic thyroiditis
Family history	Low	High
Female to male ratio	Low (2–3:1)	High (10:1)
Postpartum association	Common (10%)	Occasional
Histology		
Oxyphilic change	Infrequent	Usual
Fibrosis	Mild	Mild, moderate, or severe
Lymphoid germinal centers	Rare	Frequent
Progressive thyroid disease	50%	Usual course

a single episode of short duration and not a progressive disease. Approximately 50% of our lymphocytic thyroiditis with spontaneously resolving hyperthyroidism group after 1 to 10 years had permanent thyroid abnormality, including one or more of the following: hypothyroidism, goiter, elevated baseline TSH, augmented TRH response, positive antithyroid antibodies, and histologic evidence of lymphocytic thyroiditis.[60] Therefore, using biopsy to differentiate patients with thyroiditis, it appears that subacute thyroiditis with or without spontaneously resolving hyperthyroidism is a benign nonprogressive thyroid disease, while lymphocytic thyroiditis with spontaneously resolving hyperthyroidism is persistent and progressive, often leading to permanent thyroid disease quite similar to Hashimoto's thyroiditis.

What is the Cause?

The big unanswered question is what is the precipitating factor for transient hyperthyroidism in these thyroiditis patients. Although virsues appear to play a role in subacute thyroiditis with or without spontaneously resolving hyperthyroidism,[37,38] I found no evidence of acute and/or convalescent viral antibody response to a wider range of viruses[19] than those studied in subacute thyroiditis by Volpé et al.[37] No other viral studies or thyroid viral cultures have been done in lymphocytic thyroiditis with spontaneously resolving hyperthyroidism to my knowledge. Therefore, the cause of the transient hyperthyroidism in lymphocytic thyroiditis with spontaneously resolving hyperthyroidism remains unknown. Possibilities include an unknown virus, an autoimmune phenomenon, other infectious agents, high dietary iodide levels, or a combination of these factors.

Hamburger and Meier distinguish the postpartum form of silent thyroiditis from other forms of painless thyroiditis with hyperthyroidism by a higher incidence of antithyroid antibodies, goiter, and hypothyroidism. Needle biopsies in postpartum silent thyroiditis (10% of my patients with silent thyroiditis) show no appreciable differences in microscopic findings from other patients with lymphocytic thyroiditis with spontaneously resolving hyperthyroidism. I agree that the postpartum disease is due to the known enhancement of immune activity at that time.[22,23]

My Responses to Questions Posed by Hamburger and Meier

(1) Subacute thyroiditis with and without hyperthyroidism is a different disease from lymphocytic thyroiditis with spontaneously resolving hyperthyroidism (including postpartum). They can be differentiated by clinical findings, biopsy, and long-term follow-up.

(2) Thyroid biopsy is the most important diagnostic tool in differentiating these forms of thyroiditis. Without biopsy data Hamburger and Meier may have reached erroneous conclusions about these diseases.

(3) Whether lymphocytic thyroiditis with spontaneously resolving hyperthyroidism is an early stage of Hashimoto's thyroiditis or a different disease is unknown. However, our long-term follow-up studies suggest that the former may be the case, or that the disease occurs in genetically susceptible people.

(4) Every hyperthyroid patient, except pregnant females, should have a RAIU to differentiate transient hyperthyroidism of throiditis from Graves' disease. In pregnant women, needle biopsy will make this differentiation.

(5) Some patients with goitrous and nongoitrous primary hypothyroidism have transient disease. If the hypothyroidism is not too severe observation for 3 to 6 months before starting treatment may be indicated. However, temporary therapy of the hypothyroidism for 3 to 6 months and then withdrawal and observation for 2 to 3 months is another method. Further clinical study is needed in this area.

(6) Approximately 10–15% of patients with lymphocytic thyroiditis with spontaneously resolving hyperthyroidism have recurrent episodes. Several patients have even had recurrent episodes while on thyroid suppression therapy. Therefore, I believe that subtotal thyroidectomy or thyroid ablation with ^{131}I may be indicated in the occasional patient with significant disability from recurrent episodes.

COMMENTARY

Robert Volpé, M.D.

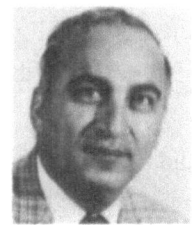

Painless Thyroiditis is Neither Chronic Nor New

This reviewer is in partial agreement with Hamburger and Meier that painless ("silent") thyroiditis is usually not a form of chronic autoimmune thyroiditis. Indeed, as suggested by these authors, it is probably not a new or different form of thyroiditis; painless thyroiditis has been observed for many decades.[1,62] Older reports indicate that histologic sections from thyroidectomies performed on painless goiters sometimes showed a typical pseudogranulomatous picture of subacute (de Quervain's) thyroiditis.[15,62] Moreover, I have carried out biopsies at intervals in patients with painful thyroiditis and have shown that in a later phase of their disorder a lymphocytic infiltration transiently appears (unpublished data).

It is nevertheless true that the number of patients with such painless thyroiditis seems to have markedly increased over the last several years; moreover, certain features of this variant are clearly different from the painful form of thyroiditis.

Histology of Painless Thyroiditis

The most cogent difference in the histologic picture, found in most biopsies obtained during the course of this painless disorder, is that lymphocytic infiltration predominates (as compared to the pseudogranulomatous appearance of the painful condition).[19,39] This has led some authors to conclude that this malady represents an unusual form of chronic lymphocytic thyroiditis. However, as Nikolai and his colleagues[19,39] point out, only about one-third of the specimens showed evidence of Hürthle cells, which when present were generally infrequent as well. Fibrosis was usually absent or minimal. In chronic lymphocytic thyroiditis, Hürthle cells and fibrosis are common features.

Antibodies in Painless Thyroiditis

Hamburger and Meier state that thyroid autoantibodies are frequently detectable in "silent" thyroiditis. However, this has not been the general experience when ordinary serological techniques are employed, although such antibodies have been detected by radioassay.[17] In fact, there is a discrepancy between the results of serological procedures for the antibodies to thyroglobulin and the findings by radioassay, and this has been clearly shown to be due to interference by excessive amounts of thyroglobulin liberated during the course of the thyroiditis.[63,64] Such increases in thyroglobulin will give artifactual levels of antithyroglobulin by radioassay. Thus there is no certainty that significant thyroid autoantibodies appear often in this entity.

It is of concern to me that some of the patients cited by Hamburger and Meier did have high levels of antimicrosomal antibody which persisted. In my experience such antibodies are very rare in the "silent" form of subacute thyroiditis, and do not persist. Their Case 3 had transient hypothyroidism which recovered. In my view this case does not belong in the category of painless thyroiditis or, if it does, it makes the disorder much more heterogeneous in its presentation and etiology. Almost certainly this case has Hashimoto's thyroiditis, which can be marked by remissions and exacerbations.[65]

Course of Painless Thyroiditis

It is certainly now known that in subacute lymphocytic (painless) thyroiditis, there is complete histological resolution upon recovery.[36] It thus would appear that this condition does not represent chronic autoimmune thyroiditis, since recovery is quick, and there is doubt that there are significant thyroid autoantibodies present throughout the course of this illness. Thus, while the etiology of this condition is not yet clear, it still may be a variant of subacute (de Quervain's) thyroiditis, or may be yet another form of thyroidal inflammatory response to viral or other etiological agents.

Postpartum Thyroiditis

However, the form of this condition seen commonly in the postpartum period conceivably could be autoimmune in nature, despite the fact that clinically and pathologically it resembles the form of painless thyroiditis referred to in the paragraph above. In 1976, Amino and his colleagues[21] found that pregnancy and delivery strikingly influenced the clinical course of autoimmune thyroid diseases. They reported patients with transient postpartum hypothyroidism and autoimmune thyroiditis, and subsequently described transient postpartum hyperthyroidism in Graves' disease and in autoimmune thyroiditis. (See the preceding Commentary by Dr. Amino for further discussion of this point.)

Case 2 of Hamburger and Meier would fit into this category, and in my opinion clearly does represent chronic autoimmune thyroiditis, with very high titers of antimicrosomal antibody.

Conclusion

It thus may well be that painless ("silent") thyroiditis (subacute lymphocytic thyroiditis) may be clinically and pathologically homogeneous, but etiologically heterogeneous. It is entirely possible that cases not associated with pregnancy have no autoimmune basis, whereas it seems probable that patients who suffer recurrent painless thyroiditis following pregnancy belong in a different category, and may well be due to the transient rebound of autoimmune processes following cessation of pregnancy, as suggested by Amino et al.

Until more is known about the true nature of this interesting condition, it would be imprudent to impute a specific etiology to all those with a similar presentation. While one can accept that those cases not associated with pregnancy who have no significant thyroid autoantibodies present and who go on to full recovery cannot be considered in the category of chronic autoimmune thyroiditis, it would be equally unwise to contend that they are definitely due to the same viral etiology (or even different viruses) as in the case of subacute painful (de Quervain's) thyroiditis. We need a good deal more information before we can be certain that this entity does represent a variant of the painful condition.

COMMENTARY*

Paul G. Walfish, M.D.

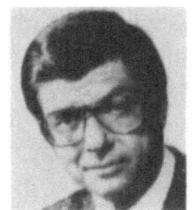

Etiology of Silent Thyroiditis and Postpartum Thyroiditis

Subacute thyroiditis, silent thyroiditis, and postpartum thyroiditis nearly always evolve through similar changes in thyroid function. There is an initial spontaneously resolving thyrotoxicosis followed by temporary hypothyroidism before recovery to euthyroidism. Although this similarity in course might imply a common pathophysiologic inflammatory process, it is possible that there are different etiologic mechanisms for these syndromes.

Possible Virus Etiology

Although a viral etiology has been proposed for typical painful subacute thyroiditis, proof is lacking.[66] However, frequent association of a preceding upper respiratory infection and a prodrome of muscular aches, malaise, fever and increased sedimentation rate, often related to a local outbreak of a specific viral infection, is strong evidence for viral etiology. After weeks or months, recovery is the rule. These clinical features are often absent in painless thyroiditis and postpartum thyroiditis.[19]

A search for specific evidence of viral infections has indicated a wide variety of possible agents. A similar spectrum of viruses may occur in control groups with or without previous clinical evidence of viral disease.[66] However, many typical subacute thyroiditis patients have no evidence of virus infection. Furthermore, various viruses isolated in some of these subjects are not known to cause typical subacute thyroiditis.[66] Changes in Coxsackie viral antibody titers were most common after typical subacute thyroiditis.[66] Although any of a variety of viruses might be an etiologic agent, these viral antibodies might merely reflect an anamnestic response to an inflammatory thyroid lesion.[66] Also, subacute thyroid-

*The secretarial assistance of Mrs. D. Goodman and Miss E. Sinclair and the support of this work from the Research Funds of the Department of Medicine, Mount Sinai Hospital and the Mount Sinai Institute, Toronto, Ontario, Canada are gratefully acknowledged.

itis might represent a thyroid inflammatory response common to different etiologic agents, of which viruses are only one. In contrast to typical subacute thyroiditis, viral antibodies have not been found in silent thyroiditis.[19]

Evidence for Possible Nonviral Infectious Causes

Q fever and malaria have been implicated.[66] Recently reports from several countries[67–69] have shown agglutinating antibodies to *Yersinia enterocolitica* in a number of thyroid diseases including subacute thyroiditis. A cross reactivity between *Y. enterocolitica* antigen and a thyroid antigen against which antibody was formed has been postulated to explain this association.[69,70] No specific infectious agent has been established for most patients with either typical subacute thyroiditis or silent thyroiditis. A new form of unrecognized viral thyroiditis, although possible, is speculative. A new type of anamnestic response to viral or other infectious agents could also account for these syndromes.

Evidence from Comparative Pathology Between Subacute Silent and Postpartum Silent Thyroiditis Syndrome

In contrast to the pseudogranulomas of typical subacute thyroiditis, Gluck et al. emphasized that biopsy in painless thyroiditis showed a lymphocytic thyroiditis, possibly autoimmune,[16] findings confirmed by others for silent thyroiditis or postpartum thyroiditis.[16,18,20,36,39,59,71,72] However unless biopsy is performed in the thyrotoxic phase, results may be nonspecific, since findings suggesting lymphocytic thyroiditis may be obtained later in typical subacute thyroiditis.[66] Lymphocytic thyroiditis is nonspecific and may occur in many thyroid diseases. A recent report has emphasized the presence of coexisting focal atrophy and involution of thyroid follicles which correlated with observed thyroid functional status in silent thyroiditis.[36] To show typical pseudogranulomas of de Quervain's thyroiditis, a core from a large bore needle biopsy, rather than a fine needle biopsy, may be needed.

The typical fibrosis and atrophy of Hashimoto's chronic thyroiditis have not been found in silent thyroiditis. Also, inadequate mention has been made of plasma cell and Hürthle cell involvement, which may occur in patients with either typical subacute thyroiditis or silent (lymphocytic) thyroiditis. The degree of focal lymphocytic infiltration frequently correlates with the magnitude of antithyroid antibody titers in silent and postpartum thyroiditis, suggesting autoimmune disease. Although a correlation of structure and etiology can be hazardous, differences in histocytology between typical subacute and silent thyroiditis have stimulated renewed interest in the etiology of these syndromes. It is possible that a variety of agents can produce similar microscopic findings of thyroidal injury.

Electron microscopy has not shown viral inclusion bodies in typical subacute thyroiditis.[73] However, during a mumps epidemic, mumps virus was grown in cultures of thyroid tissue obtained at biopsy from patients with subacute thyroiditis, without clinical evidence of mumps.[74] No similar findings have been reported for tissue culture studies in silent thyroiditis.

Evidence for Possible Autoimmune Mechanisms in the Inflammatory Thyroiditis Syndromes

Since 1967, there have been many reports concerning autoimmunity in the pathogenesis of typical painful subacute thyroiditis. However, antithyroid antibodies are not always found. When found (20–30% of patients) the rise in titer is usually transitory, correlates poorly with the onset of the thyrotoxic phase, and usually disappears in a few months.[66] Permanent hypothyroidism is rare after painful subacute thyroiditis.[66] A few patients have an evanescent rise in thyroid-stimulating immunoglobulins. This is a response to release of thyroglobulin, which occurs in subacute thyroiditis, and interferes nonspecifically "in vitro" with the radioreceptor assay.[66] Alternatively, a transiently positive test for thyroid-stimulating immunoglobulin could indicate sensitization of T-lymphocytes against thyroid antigen in an appropriate immune response to the liberation of antigen during the inflammation.[66] Since the presence or absence of thyroid-stimulating immunoglobulin does not correlate with the hyperthyroid phase of the condition, it cannot be an important pathogenic factor.[75]

Positive antithyroid antibody titers occur in 20–30% of painless thyroiditis patients and persist during the course of the illness. About 20–25% of patients followed for 12 to 18 months after the thyrotoxic phase of silent thyroiditis had persistent antibodies, goiter, and a continuing hyperreactive TSH response to TRH, suggesting a chronic process.[39,71,72] Two of our first five patients with silent postpartum thyroiditis[22,24] had persistent antithyroid antibodies; one had persistent hypothyroidism 2 years later. Hence, some patients with postpartum silent thyroiditis may have laboratory evidence suggesting chronic autoimmune thyroiditis either early or late in the disease and ultimately require permanent thyroid hormone therapy. A high incidence of persistent antithyroglobulin antibodies, measured by radioimmunoassay, suggests autoimmunity in silent thyroiditis.[17]

Evidence for Autoimmune Mechanisms in Postpartum Silent Thyroiditis

Amino and co-workers reported transient postpartum hypothyroidism.[21,76] Most of their patients had antithyroid antibodies. That some of Amino's patients may have had silent thyroiditis, with a missed thyrotoxic phase, was suggested by our five postpartum patients with transient hyperthyroidism followed by transient hypothyroidism[22,24] and other similar cases.[25,77–81] Moreover, Nikolai[19,39,71] as well as Hamburger, previously[72] and in the present report, cited an unusually high frequency of postpartum silent thyroiditis patients. About half of our women with silent thyroiditis had episodes within 6 months of pregnancy. Fine needle biopsy in the thyrotoxic phase showed lymphocytic thyroiditis[22] and large needle biopsy showed focal involution of epithelium without pseudogranulomas.[16,18,20,36,59,71]

The occurrence of silent thyroiditis in the postpartum period indirectly suggests an autoimmune process. Several presumably autoimmune disorders, i.e., rheumatoid arthritis and systemic lupus erythematosus, have antenatal remissions and postpartum relapse.[53,82,83] Moreover, antithyroid antibody titers fall during pregnancy and rebound postpartum.[84] A reduction of goitrous hypothyroidism during pregnancy has been reported.[85] Changes in cell-mediated immunity relating to T-

and B-lymphocytes and alterations in autoimmunity during pregnancy are reversed several months postpartum, with activation of a previously suppressed autoimmune process.[86] Patients with autoimmune thyroiditis and transient postpartum thyroiditis have decreased total lymphocytes, K-cells, and antithyroid antibodies during pregnancy, which increase after delivery.[46] These findings indirectly support a possible autoimmune etiology for silent postpartum thyroiditis, involving an antibody-dependent cell-mediated cytotoxic process.

Evidence from Recurrences of Silent Postpartum or Nonpostpartum Thyroiditis

Recurrences of painful subacute thyroiditis are uncommon.[66] However, silent (unrelated to pregnancy) thyroiditis may produce recurrent episodes of transient thyrotoxicosis.[18,19,39] Recurrent episodes of postpartum thyroiditis have been suspected[59,79] and now confirmed.[87] Findings for three patients are outlined in Table 2-12. Two patients had initial episodes unrelated to pregnancy, while second episodes occurred several years later, after the first subsequent pregnancies. The third patient, case 3 of our original report,[22] had two postpartum episodes. All these patients had spontaneous resolution to euthyroidism after their first episode and none had clinical evidence of antenatal thyroid dysfunction. Relapses following pregnancy favor autoimmune disease,[87] rather than coincidental recurrent infection.

Evidence from Reports of Other Autoimmune Disease in Silent Thyroiditis Patients

Case reports have described a previous episode of postpartum or nonpostpartum Graves' disease before a silent postpartum or nonpostpartum thyroiditis episode.[25,80] Also reported is postpartum onset of painless thyroiditis, followed by

Table 2-12. A summary of clinical and laboratory features of 3 patients with postpartum recurrences of the transient thyrotoxic and painless thyroiditis (TTPT) syndrome[87]

Clinical and Laboratory Features	No. of patients
1. Recurrent (2 episodes) of the TTPT syndrome	3 of 3
2. First and second TTPT episodes occurred postpartum	1 of 3
3. Only second TTPT episode occurred postpartum	2 of 3
4. Serum thyroid antibodies	
antithyroglobulin antibody negative ($< 1:100$)	3 of 3
antimicrosomal antibody positive ($1:400-1600$)	2 of 3
5. Needle biopsy: lymphocytic thyroiditis	2 of 3 tested
6. Thyroid stimulating IgG by thyroid displacing antibody and thyroid stimulating antibody	Negative for 2 tested
7. HLA typing: DRw3 and/or DRw5 haplotype	3 of 3

transient Graves' disease, which evolved spontaneously to permanent hypothyroidism, and biopsy findings of Hashimoto's thyroiditis.[81]

Years ago Roberton[88] and later Cooke[89] described postpartum myxedema. One of Cooke's cases also had systemic lupus erythematosus, demonstrating a spectrum of autoimmune disease in the same patient. This is additional indirect evidence of an autoimmune mechanism, especially for postpartum silent thyroiditis patients who have postpartum relapses.

Evidence for Possible Genetic Susceptibility for Patients with Inflammatory Thyroiditis

Genetic HLA susceptibility in patients with autoimmune thyroid disease, i.e., Hashimoto's thyroiditis and Graves' disease, has been reviewed.[66,90] An association of subacute thyroiditis and HLA-Bw35 has been claimed for Caucasians.[91,92] In Japanese with Graves' disease there is an increased incidence of HLA-Bw35[93]; however, in Caucasians HLA-B8 is more common.[90] More recently an increased frequency of DRw5 for goitrous thyroiditis and DRw3 for atrophic thyroiditis has been noted in Caucasians.[94,95] One report showed a wide variety of HLA types including some patients with postpartum silent thyroiditis.[96] HLA studies in three of our patients with recurrent postpartum thyroiditis are shown in Table 2-13. Patients 1 and 2 (initial episode unrelated to pregnancy but a second episode after their first subsequent pregnancy) had either a DRw3 or DRw5 haplotype. Patient 3 (two postpartum episodes) had both a DRw5 and DRw3 haplotype. Perhaps patients with DRw3 or 1-5 haplotypes have a genetic predisposition for recurrent postpartum thyroiditis. Our first patient with postpartum painless thyroiditis was recognized after her infant was recalled for low cord serum T_4 that subsequently reverted to normal. The mother had spontaneously resolving thyrotoxicosis and progressed rapidly to symptomatic hypothyroidism. Transient neonatal hypothyroidism may result from transplacental passage of maternal TSH-binding inhibitor immunoglobulin,[97] and supports the concept that autoimmune mechanisms are involved in some patients with the postpartum thyroiditis syndrome. However, this did not explain the hypothyroidism in our infant who had a low cord TSH concentration.

Table 2-13. Results of HLA locus haplotypes* for 3 patients with postpartum recurrences of silent thyroiditis.

TTPT patient	HLA locus typing results		
	A	B	DRw
No. 1 (S.S.)	2, w26	w39, 35	1, 3
No. 2 (S.C.)	1, 11	35, 16	5, 7
No. 3 (C.F.)	2, w31	w49, 40	3, 5

*Courtesy Dr. N. R. Farid, Health Sciences Center, Memorial University, St. John's, Newfoundland, Canada.

Interplay of Nonautoimmune Triggering Factors with Genetic Susceptibility and Autoimmune Mechanisms

Interplay between environmental triggering factors, autoimmunity, and genetic susceptibility may make it difficult to isolate a precise etiology for silent thyroiditis. Alterations in autoimmune defense mechanisms may be directed by a genetic susceptibility to triggering toxic, infectious, or even chemical agents, e.g., iodides, either related or unrelated to pregnancy. These could induce changes in autoimmune mechanisms favoring either a transient or a persistent (chronic) autoimmune thyroiditis-like process.

Clinical Assessment and Management

Diagnostic Testing

To differentiate the thyrotoxicosis of thyroiditis from conventional thyrotoxicosis, a radioactive iodine uptake (RAIU)[22,24] is essential. Contrary to one report,[56] the T_3/T_4 ratio has been unreliable.[39,98] In view of reports of postpartum thyroiditis years after an episode of Graves' disease,[25,80] and vice versa, RAIU is needed for each thyrotoxic episode.

Management of Postpartum Thyroid Disease

Postpartum Thyrotoxicosis. The differential diagnosis of postpartum thyrotoxicosis with diffuse goiter is summarized in Table 2-14. Table 2-15 gives differential diagnostic points and Table 2-16 presents an approach to the management of the syndrome. Other causes of thyrotoxicosis with low RAIU were discussed by Hamburger and Meier. Treatment with propranolol and barbiturates may be given as required. Serial follow-up examinations will confirm spontaneous resolution and also show whether hypothyroidism (temporary or permanent) develops.

Postpartum Hypothyroidism. Patients with postpartum hypothroidism, particularly if a similar episode occurred with a previous pregnancy, require further study (Table 2-17). All antithyroid foods or drugs should be excluded. When the gland is smaller than 40 g, nontender, and Graves' ophthalmopathy is absent,

---

Table 2-14. Possible causes of postpartum thyrotoxicosis with a diffuse goiter.

1. Graves' disease: first attack vs. recurrence
2. Painless thyroiditis: first attack vs. recurrence
   Subgroups: (A) Transient—subacute thyroiditis?
   (B) Persistent—chronic thyroiditis?
   Differential diagnosis: (A) Graves' disease and iodine contamination
   (B) Thyrotoxicosis factitia
3. Painful (typical) thyroiditis

Table 2-15. Differential diagnostic points in the assessment of the postpartum thyrotoxicosis syndromes.

1. Previous history:	thyroid and autoimmune disease
2. Drug history:	rule out iodides; thyroid hormone
3. Clinical signs:	thyroid gland size and tenderness; Graves' exophthalmopathy
4. Best lab tests:	$^{131-}$I or $^{123-}$I thyroid uptake
5. Other lab tests:	T_3/T_4?; urine I?; needle biopsy?; serial T_4, T_3, TSH, thyroid antibody, TRH stimulation

Table 2-16. Approach to the management of postpartum thyrotoxicosis.

I. With high thyroid ^{131}I uptake
  Standard treatment for primary persistent hyperthyroidism
II. With low ^{131}I thyroid uptake
  Conservative therapy for transient hyperthyroidism:
    propranolol, barbiturates, serial lab tests
III. Watch for subsequent hypothyroidism
  If asymptomatic: No thyroid hormone treatment; frequent follow-up
  If symptomatic: T_3 and/or T_4 treatment for 6–8 months; serum T_4 and TSH
    response on T_3; stop after 6–8 months and reassess

Table 2-17. Possible causes of postpartum hypothyroid syndromes.

1. Chronic autoimmune thyroiditis:	(a) initial or recurrent
	(b) transient or persistent
2. Painless subacute thyroiditis:	(a) initial or recurrent
	(b) transient or persistent
3. Hypothyroid Graves' disease:	evolved to persistent
4. Drug-induced hypothyroidism:	iodides, lithium, etc.
5. Painful subacute thyroiditis:	(a) initial or recurrent
	(b) transient or persistent

Table 2-18. Differential diagnosis of postpartum hypothyroidism.

1. Previous history:	thyroid and autoimmune disease
2. Drug history:	rule out iodide, propylthiouracil, lithium, etc.
3. Clinical signs:	thyroid gland size and tenderness, Graves' exophthalmopathy, etc.
4. Best lab tests:	serial T_4, TSH, thyroid antibody, and TRH tests for determining transient vs. persistent
5. Other lab tests:	serum T_4 and TSH on T_3 treatment?

Table 2-19. Approach to management of postpartum hypothyroidism.

I. If large goiter and definite autoimmune thyroiditis
    Standard treatment for primary persistent hypothyroidism
II. If possible transient hypothyroidism
    If asymptomatic: No thyroid hormone treatment; frequent follow-up
    If symptomatic: T_3 or T_4 treatment for 6–8 months; serum T_4 and TSH tests on
        T_3 treatment; stop treatment after 6–8 months and reassess

---

thyroiditis may have evolved from thyrotoxic to hypothyroid phase. Table 2-18 gives the differential diagnosis. Table 2-19 summarizes management of postpartum hypothyroidism. If hypothyroidism is not too severe and the goiter not large, thyroid hormone may be withheld pending follow-up examinations over a 6- to 8-month period during which it will be evident whether there is spontaneous improvement.

Comments on Therapeutic Issues in the Management of the Silent Thyroiditis Syndromes

Patients with a previous history of postpartum hypothyroidism merit thyroid hormone therapy withdrawal and reassessment to determine if hypothyroidism is persistent. Although it was proposed that thyroid hormone therapy might minimize the inflammatory process of typical subacute thyroiditis and prevent relapses[99] this remains to be proved and may not apply to silent thyroiditis. It is not known whether recurrences of silent thyroiditis while on thyroid hormone therapy will enhance the likelihood of thyrotoxicosis being induced or unmask an otherwise subclinical episode. If intermittent thyroid hormone replacement therapy during episodes of transient hypothyroidism is indicated, a later withdrawal and reassessment would be indicated whenever there is no persistent enlargement of the thyroid gland (greater than 30 g) and/or no strongly positive antithyroid antibody titers.

The suggestion that radioactive iodine therapy be used during the recovery phase for patients who have had several relapses of this syndrome appears to be too radical a routine therapy and is probably unjustified on the basis of current knowledge, particularly for young patients in the childbearing years.

Prednisone has been a useful therapeutic and diagnostic aid in the treatment of the typical acute painful thyrotoxic phase of subacute thyroiditis,[66] producing relief of pain and swelling within 24 to 48 h. In the absence of pain, the thyrotoxic phase of the painless (silent) thyroiditis syndrome can be effectively treated with propranolol and barbiturates. Although prednisone therapy may be of diagnostic value by rapidly reducing the size of the goiter,[100] the low RAIU value and the clinical course provides equivalent information without the accompanying risks of prednisone therapy.

Silent thyroiditis and postpartum silent thyroiditis patients are at a greater risk for long-term persistent small goiters, positive antithyroid antibodies, abnormal TRH tests indicating persistent subclinical hypothyroidism, and recurrent spontaneously resolving thyrotoxicosis after a variety of clinical stress situations including the postpartum period. Regular follow-up observations at 6- to 12-month intervals for changes in goiter, thyroid antibody titers, or biochemical evidence of hypothyroidism is recommended. Female patients who have an episode of silent thyroiditis unrelated to pregnancy should be observed for later postpartum recurrences. These recurrences can be quite subtle and may be missed or misinterpreted by both patients and physicians as representing nonthyroidal postpartum disorders unless appropriate studies are performed.

We agree that surveys of postpartum thyroid function are indicated to determine the incidence of various postpartum thyroid disorders.

SUMMARY—CHAPTER 2

Modern Classification of Thyroiditis

The comments of our panel of experts have served to highlight and (more than I had hoped) to clarify the issues raised by the intriguing entities of silent thyroiditis and postpartum thyroiditis. Gorman perceptively calls attention to the "semantic quagmire" in which many of us have been bogged down. I should like to propose (Table 2-20) a modification of his simplified classification of thyroiditis which

Table 2-20. Modern classification of thyroiditis.

Clinical course	Pathologic process	Microscopic anatomy	Etiology
Acute	Infection	PMN; abscess	Bacterium; fungus
Subacute	Infection?	Giant cell granuloma; follicle destruction	Virus?
	Immunologic	Lymphocytes; follicle destruction	?
Chronic	Immunologic Hashimoto's	Lymphocytes; germinal centers; fibrosis; Hürthle cell change	?
	Silent postpartum	Lymphocytes; follicle destruction	?
	Invasive fibrotic (Riedel's)	Fibrosis; lymphocytes	?

retains his idea that clinical, pathologic (pathophysiologic), and etiologic features of these diseases must be considered independently.

The clinical side of this classification is one with which most authorities could live. It indicates that granulomatous thyroiditis is subacute in the sense that there is almost always complete recovery. The silent forms of thyroiditis, on that basis, are also subacute in many instances, but some patients (especially those postpartum) have chronic disease evidenced by persistent goiter, hypothyroidism, or both. From the etiologic standpoint there should also be little ground for dispute. The association of viral infection with typical painful granulomatous thyroiditis if not proved (as Gorman indicates) is at least strongly suggested. The etiologies for the other forms of subacute and chronic thyroiditis are unknown. Also, the microscopic findings should not present problems.

Autoimmunity as a Pathogenetic Mechanism

There may be argument with the center column, "Pathologic Process." That autoimmunity plays a role in the pathogenesis of Hashimoto's thyroiditis seems well established. In my opinion the preponderance of evidence, in particular the detailed studies of Amino, makes a strong case for autoimmunity in both forms of silent thyroiditis as well (Volpé's reservations with respect to the nonpostpartum form notwithstanding). However, one should not confuse pathogenesis (e.g., autoimmunity) with etiology (e.g., virus, bacterium, chemical, inherited enzyme deficiency, etc.).

Gorman says that the postpartum patients might have been identified not because of any pathogenetic relationship to the pregnancy, but rather because pregnant patients are examined. When Gorman has the opportunity to review the detailed immunologic data of Amino he might be inclined to reconsider. (Incidentally, he misreads our data when he says, "About half of Dr. Hamburger's patients were first detected within 3 to 12 months after the time of delivery." To be included in the postpartum group, our patients had to have evidence of disease within 6 months of delivery. After the initial evaluation these patients were examined serially. Table 2-4 includes data from multiple testings in the same patients.)

The Relevance of Biopsy Findings

The absence of generalized oxyphilic cell change in the silent thyroiditis syndromes, as well as the absence of a prominent fibrotic change, provide a histologic basis for the inference that the silent thyroiditis syndromes are in some way different from Hashimoto's thyroiditis. These differences may not be apparent unless biopsy specimens are obtained. The clinical features can be identical, i.e., diffuse firm goiter, hypothyroidism, and positive antithyroid antibodies. Thus, Volpé considers our Case 3 as an example of Hashimoto's thyroiditis, whereas Nikolai observes that using needle biopsy he has identified the microscopic features of silent lymphocytic thyroiditis in several similar cases. Whether these microscopic differences denote different stages in the same pathologic process or fundamentally different processes (at least etiologically if not pathogenetically) is unclear. However, the extreme frequency of typical Hashimoto's thyroiditis in which the spontaneously resolving hyperthyroidism is absent, and hypothyroidism is chronic and progressive rather than remitting, contrasts with the much less frequent silent thyroiditis. This alone would make it unlikely that silent thyroiditis is only a (heretofore unappreciated) phase in the genesis of Hashimoto's thyroiditis.

It seems clear that Nikolai is correct in suggesting that without biopsy data confusion is possible between the chronic forms of silent thyroiditis and Hashimoto's thyroiditis, as well as between viral subacute thyroiditis (which may be painless) and the painless subacute thyroiditis with lymphobytic infiltration. Hence all of the reports of patients with painless subacute thyroiditis who were not biopsied are suspect, and so are those of Hashimoto's thyroiditis when the diagnoses were based upon the presence of goiter, hypothyroidism, and antithyroid antibodies. However, biopsy data do not define either pathogenesis or etiology (as Inada observes).

Probably there are only a limited number of ways in which the thyroid gland can respond to the various insults to which it may be exposed. Therefore it is reasonable to conclude (as Volpé suggests) that thyroid disorders with similar clinical courses, and even similar microscopic findings, may have different etiologies. Also (assuming that immunologic diseases do not arise de novo), the acceptance of an immunologic basis for the development of a disease does not address the issue of etiology.

If it is agreed that one cannot classify these thyroiditis patients precisely without biopsy data, does this mean that biopsies are necessary for all of these patients? I can readily agree with Nikolai that biopsy is useful in pregnant patients (for whom the radioactive iodine uptake is not done) to differentiate Graves' disease from the hyperthyroidism of thyroiditis. This differentiation is important, for the former group requires antithyroid therapy, whereas the hyperthyroidism of the latter group will subside spontaneously. Otherwise I am not convinced that needle biopsy data provide important information with regard to either etiology or management of these thyroiditis patients. As Gorman's simplified approach implies, the clinical course and thyroid functional status are the determinants of treatment. Nevertheless, we are appreciative of the efforts of those who have performed biopsies for they have helped us immeasurably to expand our understanding of these diseases.

Treatment of Recurrent Episodes of Spontaneously Resolving Hyperthyroidism

The experts disagree on the treatment of patients with recurrent episodes of spontaneously resolving hyperthyroidism resulting from silent thyroiditis. Gorman has had success with long-term thyroid hormone administration beginning, presumably, when the patient enters the hypothyroid phase of the episode. By suppressing TSH this treatment should suppress reaccumulation of stored thyroid hormone so that in the event of another inflammatory event there would be too little hormone available for discharge to produce hyperthyroidism. Unfortunately Nikolai has found that this does not work for some patients, and for them he has advised thyroidectomy. Of course, radioactive iodine could be given during the recovery phase of the disease when the radioactive iodine uptake level is usually quite high. Amino, on the other hand, does not consider it necessary to employ any of these measures, because in his experience the hyperthyroidism has been mild and transient. Walfish agrees. They are right for most patients, but we have seen several for whom recurrent episodes of hyperthyroidism have been unpleasant enough to indicate that prophylactic treatment was in order. I would try thyroid hormone first, and if that failed, I would use radioactive iodine.

Joel I. Hamburger, M.D.

REFERENCES

1. Crile G Jr, Rumsey EW: Subacute thyroiditis. JAMA 458, 1950
2. Bergen SS Jr: Acute nonsuppurative thyroiditis. Arch Intern Med 102:747, 1958
3. Hamburger JI: Subacute thyroiditis: Evolution depicted by serial ^{131}I scintigram. J Nucl Med 6:560, 1965
4. Lewitus Z, Rechnic J, Lubin E: Sequential scanning of the thyroid as an aid in the diagnosis of subacute thyroiditis. Isr J Med Sci 3:847, 1967
5. McConahey WM: Treatment of granulomatous (subacute) thyroiditis. Mod Treatment 1:168, 1964
6. Cassidy CE: The diagnosis and treatment of subacute thyroiditis. In Astwood EB, Cassidy CE (eds): Clinical Endocrinology II. New York, Grune & Stratton, 1968, pp 220–231
7. Volpé R: Treatment of thyroiditis. Mod Treatment 6:474, 1969
8. Skillern PG, Nelson HE, Crile G Jr: Some new observations on subacute thyroiditis. J Clin Endocrinol Metab 16:1422, 1956
9. Hamburger JI: Occult subacute thyroiditis: diagnostic challenge. Mich Med 70:1125, 1971
10. Hamburger JI: Subacute thyroiditis: diagnostic difficulties and simple treatment. J Nucl Med 15:81, 1974
11. Papapetrou PD, Jackson IMD: Thyrotoxicosis due to "silent" thyroiditis. Lancet 1:361, 1975
12. Woolf PD, Daly R: Thyrotoxicosis with painless thyroiditis. AM J Med 60:73, 1976
13. Blonde L, Witkin M, Harris R: Painless subacute thyroiditis simulating Graves' disease. West J Med 125:75, 1976
14. Morrison J, Caplan RH: Typical and atypical ("silent") subacute thyroiditis in a wife and husband. Arch Intern Med 138:45, 1978
15. Harland WA, Frantz VK: Clinico-pathologic study of 261 surgical cases of so-called "thyroiditis." J Clin Endocrinol Metab 16:1433, 1956
16. Gluck FB, Nusynowitz ML, Plymate S: Chronic lymphocytic thyroiditis, thyrotoxicosis, and low radioactive iodine uptake. N Engl J Med 293:624, 1975

17. Dorfman SG, Cooperman MT, Nelson RL, Depuy H, Peake RL, Young RL: Painless thyroiditis and transient hyperthyroidism without goiter. Ann Intern Med 86:24, 1977

18. Gorman CA, Duick DS, Woolner LB, Wahner HW: Transient hyperthyroidism in patients with lymphocytic thyroiditis. Mayo Clin Proc 53:359, 1978

19. Nikolai TF, Brosseau J, Kettrick MA, Roberts R, Beltaos E: Lymphocytic thyroiditis with spontaneously resolving hyperthyroidism (silent thyroiditis). Arch Intern Med 140:478, 1980

20. Inada M, Nishikawa M, Oishi M, Kurata S, Imura H: Transient thyrotoxicosis associated with painless thyroiditis and low radioactive iodine uptake. Arch Intern Med 139:597, 1979

21. Amino N, Miyai K, Onishi T, Hashimoto T, Ari K, Ishibashi K, Kumahara Y: Transient hypothyroidism after delivery in autoimmune thyroiditis. J Clin Endocrinol Metab 42:296, 1976

22. Ginsberg J, Walfish PG: Postpartum transient thyrotoxicosis with painless thyroiditis. Lancet 1:1125, 1977

23. Amino N, Miyai K, Yamamoto T, Kuro R, Tanaka F, Tanizawa O, Kumahara Y: Transient recurrence of hyperthyroidism after delivery in Graves' disease. J Clin Endocrinol Metab 44:130, 1977

24. Walfish PG, Ginsberg J: Postpartum thyroid disease (Letter to the Editor). Ann Intern Med 88:128, 1978

25. Eckel RH, Green WL: Postpartum thyrotoxicosis in a patient with Graves' disease. Association with low radioactive iodine uptake. JAMA 243:1454, 1980

26. Hamburger JI: Clinical Exercises in Internal Medicine, Vol. 1. Thyroid Disease. Philadelphia, Saunders, 1978, pp 6–18

27. Peake RL, Willis DB, Asimakis GK Jr, Deiss WP Jr: Radioimmunologic assay for antithyroglobulin antibodies. J Lab Clin Med 84:907, 1974

28. Gorman CA, Duick DS, Woolner LB: The various forms of thyroiditis. N Engl J Med 294:53, 1976

29. Gluck FB, Nusynowitz ML, Plymate S: The various forms of thyroiditis. N Engl J Med 294:53, 1976

30. Woolf PD: Painless thyroiditis as a cause of hyperthyroidism. Arch Intern Med 138:26, 1978

31. Gluck FB, Plymate SR, Nusynowitz ML: "Silent" subacute thyroiditis (Letter to the Editor). Arch Intern Med 138:1024, 1978

32. Fraser R: Subacute thyroiditis. Lancet 1:382, 1952

33. Stein AA, Hernandez I, McClintock JC: Subacute granulomatous thyroiditis: a clinicopathologic review. Ann Surg 153:149, 1961

34. Vanderlinde RJ, Milne J: Subacute thyroiditis. JAMA 173:97, 1960

35. Steinberg FU: Subacute granulomatous thyroiditis: a review. Ann Intern Med 52:1014, 1960

36. Inada M, Nishikawa M, Naito K, Ishi H, Tanaka K, Imura H: Correlation of the histological abnormalities of the thyroid with the stage of transient thyrotoxicosis associated with painless thyroiditis. Paper number 168. Program of the Seventh International Thyroid Congress, Sidney, Australia, 1980

37. Volpé R, Row VV, Ezrin C: Circulating viral and thyroid antibodies in subacute thyroiditis. J Clin Endocrinol Metab 27:1275, 1967

38. Swann NH: Acute thyroiditis: Five cases associated with adenovirus infection. Metabolism 13:908, 1964

39. Nikolai TF: Lymphocytic thyroiditis with spontaneously resolving hyperthyroidism (silent thyroiditis). Thyroid Today 2:1, 1979

40. Hamburger JI: Pitfalls in the laboratory diagnosis of atypical hyperthyroidism. Arch Intern Med 139:96, 1979

41. Hamburger JI, Taylor CI: Transient thyrotoxicosis associated with acute hemorrhagic infarction of autonomously functioning thyroid nodules. Ann Intern Med 91:406, 1979

42. Larsen PR: Serum triiodothyronine, thyroxine, and thyrotropin during hyperthyroid, hypothyroid, and recovery phases of subacute nonsuppurative thyroiditis. Metabolism 23:467, 1974

43. Yamamoto T, Sakamoto H: Spontaneous remission from primary hypothyroidism. Ann Intern Med 88:808, 1978

44. Duick DS: Management of thyrotoxicosis with a low radioactive iodine uptake. Arch Intern Med 140:469, 1980

45. Amino N, Hagan SR, Yamada N, Refetoff S: Measurement of circulating thyroid microsomal antibodies by the tanned red cell hemagglutination technique: its usefulness in the diagnosis of autoimmune thyroid disease. Clin Endocrinol 5:115, 1976

46. Amino N, Mori H, Yabu Y, Kuro R, Yamada T, Hisa Y, Tanizawa O, Miyai K: Mechanisms of occurrence of transient postpartum hypothyroidism in autoimmune thyroiditis. Paper number 167. Program of the Seventh International Thyroid Congress, Sidney, Australia, 1980

47. Yoshida H, Amino N, Yagawa K, Uemura K, Satoh M, Miyai K, Kumahara Y: Association of serum antithyroid antibodies with lymphocytic infiltration of the thyroid gland: studies of 70 autopsied cases. J Clin Endocrinol Metab 46:859, 1978

48. Amino N, Miyai K: Autoimmune thyroiditis and Hashimoto's disease. Lancet 2:585, 1978

49. Amino N, Kuro R, Tanizawa O, Tanaka F, Hayashi C, Kotani K, Kawashima M, Miyai K, Kumahara Y: Changes of serum antithyroid antibodies during and after pregnancy in autoimmune thyroid diseases. Clin Exp Immunol 31:30, 1978

50. Amino N, Mori H, Iwatani Y, et al.: (Unpublished)

51. Yabu Y, Amino N, Mori H, Miyai K, Tanizawa O, Takai S, Kumahara Y, Matsuzuka F, Kuma K: Postpartum recurrence of hyperthyroidism and changes of thyroid stimulating immunoglobulins in Graves' disease. J Clin Endocrinol Metab 51:1454, 1980

52. Hench PS: The potential reversibility of rheumatoid arthritis. Proc Staff Mayo Clin 24:167, 1949

53. Friedman EA, Rutherfold JW: Pregnancy and lupus erythematosus. Obstet Gynecol 8:601, 1956

54. Fraser D, Turner JWA: Myasthenia gravis and pregnancy. Lancet 2:417, 1953

55. Lorz HM, Frumin AM: Spontaneous remission in chronic idiopathic thrombocytopenic purpura during pregnancy. Obstet Gynecol 17:362, 1961

56. Amino N, Yabu Y, Miyai K, Fujie T, Azukizawa M, Onishi T, Kumahara Y: Differentiation of thyrotoxicosis induced by thyroid destruction from Graves' disease. Lancet 2:344, 1978

57. Gharib H, Hodgson SF, Gastineau CF, Scholz DA, Smith LA: Reversible hypothyroidism in Addison's disease. Lancet 2:734, 1972

58. Volpé R, Johnston MW, Huber N: Thyroid function in subacute thyroiditis. J Clin Endocrinol Metab 18:65, 1958

59. Inada M, Nishikawa M, Oishi M, Kurata S, Imura H: Postpartum transient thyrotoxicosis: report of two cases. Endocrinol Jpn 26:611, 1979
60. Nikolai TF, Coombs GJ, McKenzie AK: Lymphocytic thyroiditis with spontaneously resolving hyperthyroidism (silent thyroiditis) and subacute thyroiditis—long-term follow-up. Arch Intern Med (in press) 1981
61. Dorfman SG: Hyperthyroidism—usual and unusual (Editorial). Arch Intern Med 137:995, 1977
62. Volpé R, Johnston MW: Subacute thyroiditis: a disease commonly mistaken for pharyngitis. Can Med Assoc J 77:297, 1957
63. Pinchera A, Fenzi GF, Bartalena L, Chiovata L, Marcocci C, Pacini F: Thyroid antigens involved in autoimmune thyroid disorders. In Klein E, Horster FA (eds): Autoimmunity and Thyroid Diseases. Stuttgart, FK Schattauer Verlag, 1979, pp 49–67
64. VanHerle AJ, Vassart G, Dumont JE: Control of thyroglobulin synthesis and secretion. N Engl J Med 301:239, 307, 1979
65. Rallison ML, Dobyns BM, Keating FR, Rall JE, Tyler FH: Occurrence and natural history of chronic lymphocytic thyroiditis in childhood. J Pediatr 86:675, 1975
66. Volpé R: Subacute (de Quervain's) thyroiditis. Clin Endocrinol Metab 8:81, 1979
67. Bech K, Larsen HJ, Hansen JM, Nerup J: *Yersinia enterocolitica* infection and thyroid disorders. Lancet 2:951, 1974
68. Shenkman L, Bottone EJ: Antibodies to *Yersinia entercolitica* in thyroid disease. Ann Intern Med 85:735, 1976
69. Weiss M, Rubinstein E, Bottone EJ, Shenkman L, Bank H: Isr J Med Sci 15:553, 1979
70. Bech K, Clemmensen D, Larsen HJ, Nerup J: Cell-mediated immunity to *Yersinia enterocolitica* serotype 3 in patients with thyroid disease. Allergy 33:82, 1978
71. Nikolai TF, Parr S, Otteson C, Kopp D: Long-term follow-up of patients with subacute thyroiditis with and without spontaneous resolving hyperthyroidism and lymphocytic thyroiditis with spontaneous resolving hyperthyroidism (silent thyroiditis). Program of the Endocrine Society, 61st Annual Meeting, Anaheim, California, June 1979, pp 240 (abstract No. 671)
72. Hamburger JI: The clinical spectrum of thyroiditis. Thyroid Today 3(4):1, 1980
73. Basteine PA, Ermans AM: Thyroiditis and thyroid function. Clinical, morphological and physiological studies. International Series of Monographs in Pure and Applied Biology: Modern Trends and Physiological Sciences, Vol. 36. Oxford, Pergamon Press, 1972
74. Eylan E, Zmucky R, Sheba C: Mumps, virus and subacute thyroiditis. Evidence of a causal association. Lancet 1:1062, 1957
75. Strakosch CR, Joyner D, Wall JR: Thyroid stimulating antibodies in patients with subacute thyroiditis. J Clin Endocrinol Metab 46:345, 1978
76. Amino N, Miyai K, Kuro R, Tanizawa O, Azukizawa M, Takai S, Tanaka F, Nishi K, Kawashima M, Kumahara Y: Transient postpartum hypothyroidism: 14 cases with autoimmune thyroiditis. Ann Intern Med 87:155, 1977
77. Hoffbrand BI, Webb SC: Postpartum thyroiditis. Postgrad Med J 54:793, 1978
78. Kurhara H, Takamatsu M, Ogawa S, Watanabe T: Transient thyrotoxicosis different from subacute thyroiditis. Program of the Eighth International Thyroid Congress, Sydney, Australia (Abstract No. 128), February 3–8, 1980
79. Dailey GE: Recurrent postpartum transient hyperthyroidism. Ann Intern Med 90:719, 1979

80. Check JH, Avellino J: Painless thyroiditis and transient thyrotoxicosis after Graves' disease. JAMA 244:1361, 1980
81. Sartani A, Feigl D, Zaidel L, Ravid M: Painless thyroiditis followed by autoimmune disorders of the thyroid. A case report with biopsy. J Endocrinol Invest 3:169, 1980
82. Oka M: Effect of pregnancy on the onset and course of rheumatoid arthritis. Ann Rheum Dis 12:227, 1953
83. Garsenstein M, Pollak VE, Kark RM: Systemic lupus erythematosus and pregnancy. N Engl J Med 267:165, 1962
84. Parker RH, Beierwaltes WH: Thyroid antibodies during pregnancy and in the newborn. J Clin Endocrinol Metab 21:792, 1961
85. Nelson JC, Palmer FJ: A remission of goitrous hypothyroidism during pregnancy. J Clin Endocrinol Metab 40:383, 1975
86. Editorial: Immunological changes in women. Lancet 1:909, 1974
87. Walfish PG, Green N: Postpartum recurrence of the transient thyrotoxicosis and painless thyroiditis syndrome. Program and Abstracts of the 62nd Annual Meeting of the Endocrine Society, Washington, D.C., June 18–20, 1980, pp 203 (abstract No. 513)
88. Roberton HEW: Lassitude, coldness and hair changes following pregnancy and their response to treatment with thyroid extract. Br Med J (Suppl) 2:93, 1948
89. Cooke RT: Myxedema in young women. J Coll Gen Practit 6:626, 1963
90. Volpé R: The role of autoimmunity in hypoendocrine and hyperendocrine function: with special emphasis on autoimmune thyroid disease. Ann Intern Med 87:86, 1977
91. Bech K, Lumholtz B, Nerup J, Thomsen M, et al.: HLA antigens in Graves' disease and subacute thyroiditis. Proceedings of the European Thyroid Association, Helsinki, June 29–July 1, 1976
92. Nyulassy S, Hnilica P, Buc M, Guman M, Hirschova V, Stefanovic J: Subacute (de Quervain's) thyroiditis: association with HLA-Bw35 antigen and abnormalities of the complement system, immunoglobulins and other serum proteins. J Clin Endocrinol Metab 45:270, 1977
93. Grumet FC, Konishi J, Payne RO, Kriss JP: Association in Japanese of Graves' disease with HLA specificity w5. In Robbins J, Braverman LE (eds): Thyroid Research.International Congress Series 378. Amsterdam, Excerpta Medica, 1976, pp 376–379
94. Moens H, Farid NR: Hashimoto's thyroiditis is associated with HLA-DRw3. N Engl J Med 299:131, 1978
95. Farid NR, Moens H, Sampson L, Barnard JM: The association of HLA-DRw5 with goitrous autoimmune thyroiditis. Clin Res 28:672A, 1980
96. Jenkins H, Farid NR: Subacute thyroiditis-like syndromes relation to HLA. Tissue Antigens 13:167, 1979
97. Matsura N, Yamada Y, Nohara Y, Konishi J, Kasagi K, Endo K, Kojima H, Wataya K: Familial neonatal transient hypothyroidism due to a maternal TSH-binding inhibitor immunoglobulins. N Engl J Med 30:738, 1980
98. Walfish PG: T$_3$/T$_4$ ratio in thyroid disease. Lancet 2:1056, 1978
99. Higgins HP, Bagley TA, Diosy A: Suppression of endogenous TSH. A treatment of subacute thyroiditis. J Clin Endocrinol Metab 23:235, 1963
100. Nikolai TF, Schwieso JA: Lymphocytic thyroiditis with spontaneously resolving hyperthyroidism (silent thyroiditis). Frequency 1978 and 1979 and response to corticosteroid therapy. Program of the 62nd Annual Meeting of the Endocrine Society, Washington, D.C., June 18–20, 1980 (abstract No. 458)

Chapter 3

Should All Autonomously Functioning Thyroid Nodules Be Ablated to Prevent the Subsequent Development of Thyrotoxicosis?

Joel I. Hamburger, M. D.

INTRODUCTION

Solitary Autonomously functioning thyroid nodules (AFTN) are discrete thyroid lesions which are independent of pituitary stimulation for function and growth. The availability of radioactive iodine permitted the demonstration, in vitro, of an inverse relationship between the functional activity of AFTN and the extranodular thyroid tissue.[1] These observations have been confirmed by in vivo studies using manual[2] and mechanical detecting devices.[3,4]

Laboratory criteria for the diagnosis of AFTN are well established.[4,5] These include persistent nodular function (autonomous function) in spite of the administration of suppressive doses of thyroid hormone and the preferential responsiveness of suppressed extranodular thyroid tissue to parenteral TSH. Wider application of these criteria has permitted the diagnosis of smaller AFTN and the appreciation that nontoxic AFTN are much more common than the toxic form.[5-7]

Nevertheless, the solitary AFTN is an uncommon thyroid lesion in the United States. Only 0.9% of patients referred to the Northland Thyroid Laboratory (NTL) had AFTN.[8] Higher incidences have been reported from Brazil[9,10] (2.4% and 6%) and Holland[11] (9%). In Switzerland[12] one-third of all patients with hyperthyroidism have toxic AFTN, whereas at NTL only one toxic AFTN is seen for every 50 patients with toxic diffuse goiter.

Because AFTN are uncommon, and some physicians have preferred to ablate all AFTN prophylactically, there are limited data on the natural history of these lesions. This chapter will address the following issues relative to the nontoxic AFTN, issues which bear decisively on decisions relative to patient management.

(1) How often and how rapidly do nontoxic AFTN become toxic?

(2) Which patients with nontoxic AFTN should have prophylactic ablative treatment?

(3) When prophylactic treatment is indicated, should it be[131] I therapy or operation?

EXPERIENCE OF NORTHLAND THYROID LABORATORY

Between 1961 and 1980, 42,076 patients have been referred to NTL for diagnosis and management of thyroid problems. Diagnostic methods for the confirmation of a diagnosis of an AFTN have been described in detail in earlier publications.[4,5] Criteria for a diagnosis of AFTN were met by 361 patients (0.9%). Ten percent of patients with solitary nodules had AFTN.

Thyroid nodule size was estimated by palpation in conjunction with thyroid imaging. AFTN sizes cited throughout refer to average diameter in centimeters.

Patients were classified as "hyperthyroid" if there were clinical features of hyperthyroidism and elevations of serum concentrations of T_4, T_3, or both. Patients were classified as "borderline hyperthyroid" if clinical features of hyperthyroidism were lacking, but the serum concentrations of T_4, or more often T_3, were at the upper level of the normal range or slightly elevated, and the response of the serum TSH concentration to 100 μg of TRH intravenously was negligible. These patients also had AFTN 2.5 cm or larger in diameter. Patients were classified as "euthyroid" if they were clinically and biochemically euthyroid. Some of these patients also responded negligibly to TRH, but serum concentrations for neither T_3 nor T_4 were near the upper level of the normal range.

Serum total T_4 values were corrected for abnormal concentrations of binding globulins by the calculation of a free thyroxine index (FTI).[13] The normal range for NTL is 1.4–4.0. Serum T_3 concentrations were measured by RIA using the T_3(RIA) PEG kit method from Abbott Laboratories (Chicago, IL). The normal range for NTL is 80–220 ng/dl. Serum TSH concentrations were measured by RIA using the TSH(RIA) kit method from Pantex Company (Santa Monica, CA). The normal range for NTL is less than 8 μU/ml.

Ablative therapy (surgical or ^{131}I) was advised for all patients with toxic AFTN and, in the early years, for many nontoxic AFTN as well, particularly when observed in older patients or when thyroid function tests were at the upper level of the normal range. Thus between 1961 and 1970, 24 (35.3%) of 68 nontoxic AFTN were subjected to prophylactic ablation. However, from 1971 to 1980 prophylactic ablation was more selectively employed, and only 15 (6.8%) of 216 nontoxic AFTN were so treated.

Selected case reports which exemplify the important issues relative to management of nontoxic AFTN will be presented, followed by data on the 361 patients.

CASE 1: LONG-TERM FOLLOW-UP OF A LARGE NONTOXIC AFTN
April 1964. A 24-year-old woman came for a sixth opinion about a thyroid nodule discovered 1.5 years earlier while she was pregnant. During the pregnancy the nodule doubled in size.

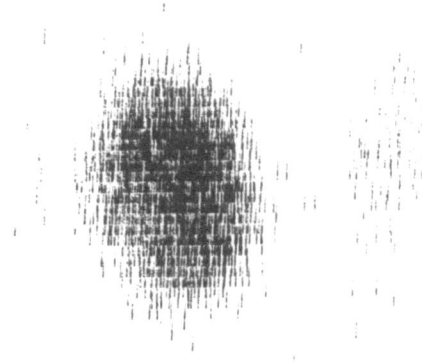

Figure 3-1. Thyroid image showing a 3-cm "hot" nodule in the right lobe of the thyroid. Function in the left lobe is incompletely suppressed.

No treatment had been given. Five other physicians had advised surgical removal. However, the patient was determined to find a physician who agreed with her that operation was unnecessary. There was no history of thyroid dysfunction and the physical findings were unremarkable with the exception of a 3-cm firm nodule in the right lobe of the thyroid. A 24-h radioactive iodine uptake was 22%. The thyroid image revealed a hot nodule with considerable suppression of function in the left lobe (Fig. 3-1). Suppression imaging confirmed a diagnosis of a nontoxic AFTN. Observation was advised.

The patient returned annually for the next 16 years. She remained clinically euthyroid. In July 1980 the FTI value was 2.1 and the serum T_3(RIA) concentration was 140 ng/dl. There was no response of the serum TSH(RIA) to 100 μg of TRH intravenously. The thyroid image (Fig. 3-2) suggested that nodular degeneration had taken place inferiorly and medially. However, complete suppression of the left lobe had been present for the previous 8 years. At no time during the 16 years had she had any symptoms from the nodule, nor had she altered her adamant opposition to surgical treatment.

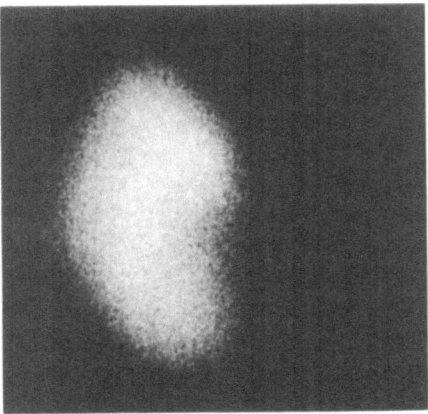

Figure 3-2. Thyroid image showing a 3-cm "hot" nodule with an area of lesser activity inferomedially. Function in the left lobe is now well suppressed.

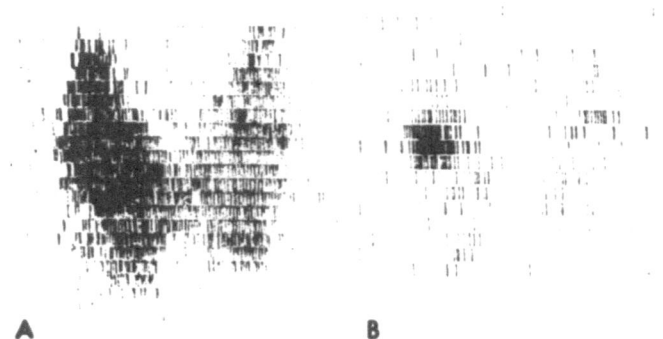

A   **B**

Figure 3-3. A Thyroid image reveals diffuse uniform function in a goiter 2.5 times normal size. **B** A suppression image reveals a small autonomous nodule in the right lobe.

CASE 2   LONG-TERM FOLLOW-UP OF A SMALL NONTOXIC AFTN

A 26-year-old woman was referred with a diffuse goiter 2.5 times normal size (Fig. 3-3A). She was euthyroid. Treatment with levothyroxine 0.2 mg daily was advised to shrink the goiter.

In 18 months the goiter regressed excepting only a 1-cm nodule in the right upper pole. Imaging revealed persistent uptake of the tracer in the location of the nodule, while function elsewhere in the thyroid was well suppressed (Fig. 3-3B). Thyroid hormone was discontinued and the patient was asked to return for annual evaluations. Over the next 11 years the nodule gradually enlarged to 3 cm. The patient remained euthyroid with the FTI value 2.5 and the serum T_3(RIA) level 200 ng/dl (NR 80–220). However, the response of the serum TSH(RIA) level to 100 μg of TRH intravenously was blunted, i.e., baseline value 3.2 μU/ml, post-TRH value 3.7 μU/ml. Observation was continued. Imaging (Fig. 3-4) revealed the enlarged hot nodule on the right, some persistent activity in a small nodule in the inferior pole of the right lobe, and also in a small nodule in the left upper pole.

CASE 3:   PROGRESSION FROM A NONTOXIC TO A TOXIC AFTN

A 67-year-old woman was referred for the evaluation of a 5-cm mass in the right lobe of the thyroid which had been present for 20 years, but had gradually been enlarging. She was

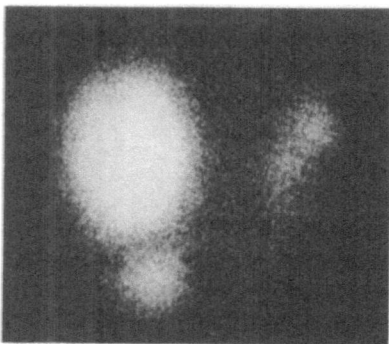

Figure 3-4. Thyroid image reveals a 3-cm "hot" nodule in the right lobe of the thyroid, and smaller functional nodules in the lower pole of the right lobe and the upper pole of the left lobe.

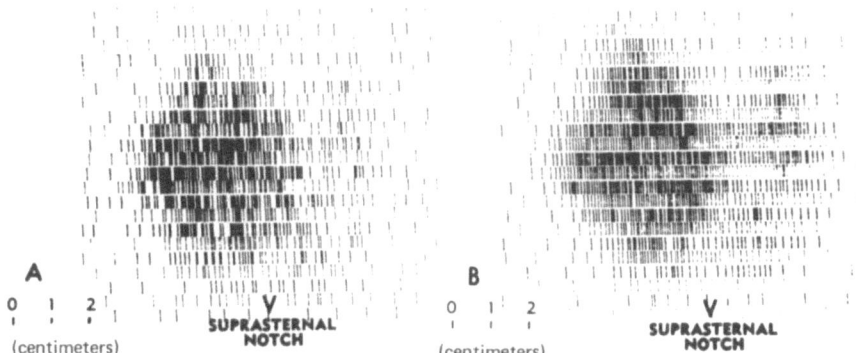

Figure 3-5. A Thyroid image reveals a 5-cm "hot" nodule in the right lobe of the thyroid. B Repeat imaging after TSH stimulation reveals activation of previously partially supressed thyroid tissue in the left lobe.

clinically euthyroid. The FTI value was 2.5 and the serum $T_3(RIA)$ concentration was 100 ng/dl. Imaging (Fig. 3-5A) revealed a large hot nodule in the right lobe, with minimal activity in the left lobe. Imaging after TSH administration (Fig. 3-5B) showed that the suppressed left lobe could function. Observation was advised. During the following 6 years the nodule remained stable in size, but the secretory activity increased. At 5.5 years the $T_3(RIA)$ level was 223 ng/dl. Six months later the $T_3(RIA)$ was 386 ng/dl, and the FTI was 6. She was treated with ^{131}I.

CASE 4: PAPILLARY CARCINOMA DEVELOPING IN THE EXTRANODULAR THYROID TISSUE AFTER TREATMENT OF A NONTOXIC AFTN WITH RADIOACTIVE IODINE

A 58-year-old euthyroid woman with paroxysmal tachycardia had a 3.5-cm nodule in the lower pole of the left thyroid lobe. Imaging revealed a hot nodule with incomplete suppression of extranodular tissue (Fig. 3-6A). Suppression imaging (Fig. 3-6B) confirmed autonomous function. A dose of 30 mCi of ^{131}I was given for ablation of the AFTN, primarily for prophylactic purposes, but also hoping this might improve her paroxysmal tachycardia. Suppression of extranodular tissue was maintained by exogenous thyroid hormone (continued for 1 week after the ^{131}I therapy) to confine uptake of ^{131}I to the AFTN, thus preserving extranodular tissue as a source of future thyroid hormone. Three months later she was euthyroid. The thyroid image revealed bilateral functional activity, although the function in the nodule was irregularly reduced (Fig. 3-6C). She was reevaluated annually and remained euthyroid. Paroxysmal tachycardia had ceased.

Three years and nine months after the ^{131}I therapy a 3×1.5 cm mass was detected lateral to the right lobe of the thyroid (Fig. 3-6D). The left lower pole, the site of the AFTN, was hypofunctional. Operation was advised. The right neck mass was a papillary carcinoma in continuity with the right upper pole of the thyroid. There were other foci of papillary carcinoma in the right lower pole, isthmus, and left lobe. The remnant of the AFTN was free of carcinoma. In an earlier publication[14] we suggested that although the supplemental thyroid hormone administered to suppress extranodular tissue function might have minimized beta radiation to that tissue from the ^{131}I therapy, there was still a substantial exposure of the extranodular tissue to the gamma component of the radiation emitted by ^{131}I concentrated in the AFTN. As the function of the intensely irradiated AFTN deteriorated, TSH secretion by the pituitary recovered and stimulated the less heavily irradiated extranodular thyroid tissue to produce thyroid hormone. It was postulated that this TSH stimulation of previously irra-

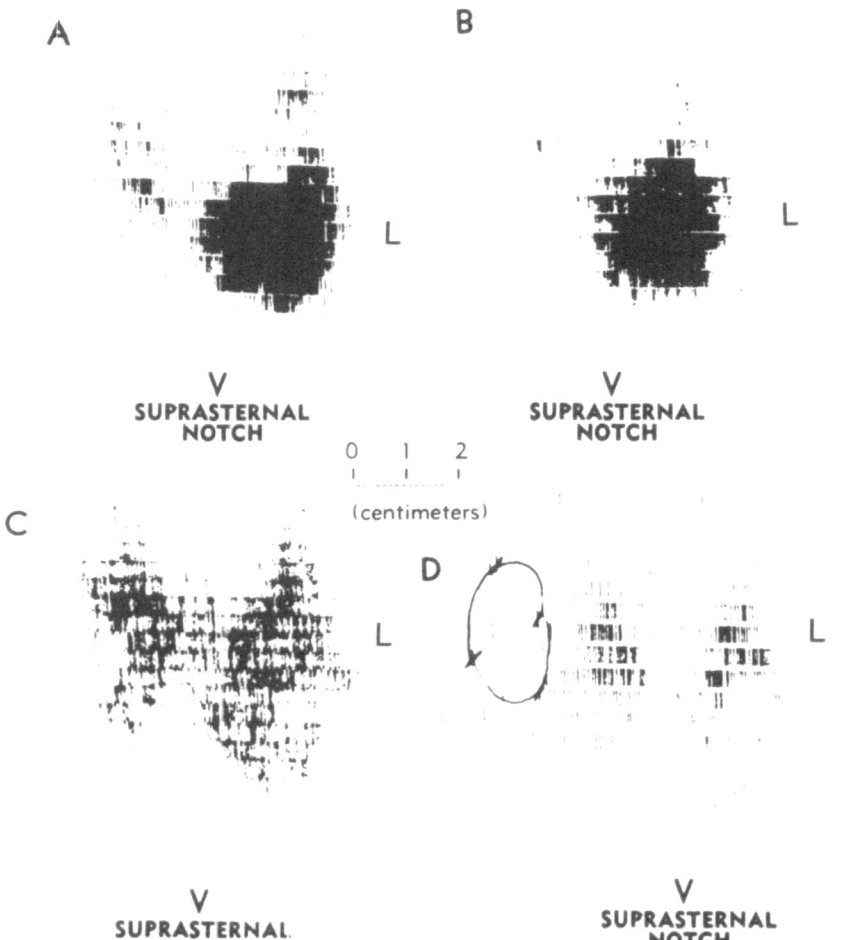

Figure 3-6. A Thyroid image revealing a 3.5-cm "hot" nodule in the left lobe. **B** A suppression image confirms autonomous function. **C** After ^{131}I therapy function in the extranodular thyroid tissue recovered, while the nodule has irregularly reduced function. **D** Three years and 9 months after the ^{131}I therapy a "cold" mass is detected in the right side of the neck.

diated, but not destroyed, thyroid tissue simulated the conditions one creates when he wishes to deliberately induce thyroid cancer in the experimental animal.[15]

CASE 5:   RECOVERY FROM TRANSIENT TOXICITY AFTER AN ACUTE HEMORRHAGIC EPISODE IN AN AFTN; RECURRENT TOXICITY ONE YEAR LATER

A 28-year-old woman abruptly developed a 4-cm painful mass in the right lobe of the thyroid. She also noted increasing nervousness and mild palpitation. She was first evaluated 2 weeks after the onset of the swelling. The mass was round, firm, smooth, and resilient. The heart

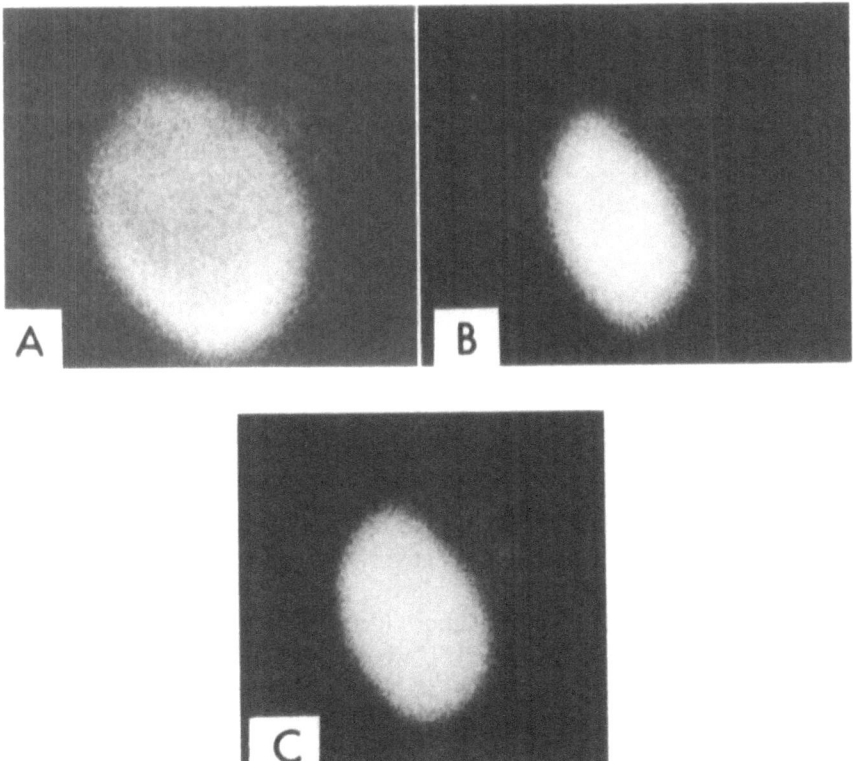

Figure 3-7. A Thyroid image revealing a 4-cm mass concentrating all of the tracer, but having relatively reduced activity centrally and superiorly. **B** The "hot" nodule is smaller with more uniform function. **C** The "hot" nodule is slightly larger.

rate was 108/min and there was a mild hand tremor. The FTI was 3.3 and the serum T_3 (RIA) concentration was 275 ng/dl. A baseline serum TSH(RIA) concentration was 1.2 μU/ ml, and a repeat value 20 min after the intravenous administration of 100 μg of TRH was 1.7 μU/ml. Thyroid imaging (Fig. 3-7A) revealed a large hot nodule with reduced activity centrally. Four ml of blood was aspirated followed by a 50% reduction in nodule size.

Three months later she was euthyroid. Imaging (Fig. 3-7B) revealed intense activity in a 2.5-cm nodule. Six months later, although the nodule had not enlarged, and the patient felt well, the serum FTI and T_3(RIA) values were 3.8 and 283 ng./dl, respectively. Over the next 6 months the hot nodule enlarged (Fig. 3-7C) and frank toxicity developed. She was treated surgically.

Table 3-1 gives the age and sex distribution for the 361 AFTN patients, classified as nontoxic, borderline toxic, and toxic at the time of the latest examination. There were 69 (19.1%) toxic AFTN, 18 (5%) borderline toxic, and 274 (75.9%) nontoxic AFTN. The toxic and borderline toxic groups include AFTN which were so classified when first evaluated, or progressed to states of toxicity or borderline toxicity under observation. The age cited for the toxic and borderline toxic

Table 3-1. Age and sex distribution of toxic, borderline toxic, and nontoxic AFTN.

Age (years)	No. of patients	Females			Males			% Toxic and borderline toxic
		Nontoxic AFTN	Border-line	Toxic AFTN	Nontoxic AFTN	Border-line	Toxic AFTN	
11–19	31	22	3	5	1	0	0	25.8
20–29	70	56	5	6	2	0	1	17.1
30–39	76	61	3	10	2	0	0	17.1
40–49	69	55	2	7	4	0	1	14.5
50–59	68	48	1	12	4	2	1	23.5
60–69	35	13	1	13	3	0	5	54.3
70 +	12	3	1	6	0	0	2	75
Total	361	258	16	59	16	2	10	24.1

patients is the age at which these states of function were first evident. Of the 274 nontoxic AFTN, 130 (47.4%) were in patients 40 years old or older. Of 87 toxic and borderline toxic AFTN, 54 (62%) were in patients 40 years old or older. Of the 47 AFTN in patients 60 years old or older, 28 (59.6%) achieved functional levels of toxicity or borderline toxicity. If we exclude four patients seen only one time, and two who were prophylactically ablated, there were 68.3% toxic or borderline toxic AFTN in patients 60 years old or older. Only 59 (18.8%) patients younger than 60 years had toxic or borderline toxic AFTN. This is a highly significant difference (chi-square analysis, $P < 0.001$).

The female to male ratio for nontoxic AFTN was 16.1:1; but this ratio for toxic and borderline toxic was 6.3:1, more nearly resembling the sex ratio for Graves' disease. The proportion of AFTN in males which were toxic or borderline toxic was 42.9%; for females it was only 22.5%, again a highly significant difference (chi-square analysis, $P < 0.001$).

These data indicate that AFTN which become toxic are most common in elderly males. However, it is of considerable interest to observe that those with the next highest proportion of toxic or borderline toxic AFTN were the patients less than 20 years old. Eight (25.8%) were toxic or borderline toxic. Four of these younger patients had had prophylactic surgical ablation, one because of an associated cold nodule, one because of a history of thymic radiation, and two because of large size of the nodules. Nine others were seen only once. If these 13 patients are excluded, 44.4% of the remaining AFTN in patients less than 20 years old had achieved toxic or borderline toxic state.

Table 3-2 presents data on the functional status of AFTN after observation for various periods of time, by age range. Of 147 AFTN followed for up to 6 years, 31 (21%) became toxic or borderline toxic. In contrast, none of the 21 patients followed 7 to 15 years became toxic and only three became borderline toxic. This difference may be the result of a policy of prophylactic surgical or ^{131}I ablation for large AFTN before 1971.

Table 3-2. Functional status of initially untreated nontoxic AFTN after varying periods of observation, by age.

Age (years)	Duration of follow-up (years)								
	0.5–2			2–6			7–15		
	Still nontoxic	Border-line	Toxic	Still nontoxic	Border-line	Toxic	Still nontoxic	Border-line	Toxic
11–19	4	1	3	4	1	1	1	0	0
20–29	7	1	2	18	2	1	6	2	0
30–39	9	0	2	17	2	4	3	0	0
40–49	8	0	0	19	1	0	3	1	0
50–59	4	1	1	18	2	2	3	0	0
60 +	1	1	1	6	1	1	2	0	0
Total	33	4	9	83	9	9	18	3	0

In an earlier report[8] it was shown that toxic AFTN were all 2.5 cm or larger, and almost always were at least 3 cm. It was these larger lesions which progressed from the nontoxic to the toxic or borderline toxic state. No AFTN less than 2 cm progressed to the toxic state in up to 15 years of observation. One reached borderline toxicity after 12 years, having enlarged from 1.5 to 2.5 cm (Case 2). Also the first sign of impending toxicity was an elevation of the serum T_3 concentration in 10 of the 18 AFTN which progressed from nontoxic to toxic; three of these subsequently developed hypersecretion of both T_3 and T_4. These data suggest that nontoxic AFTN are most likely to become toxic within 6 years if they are 2.5 cm or larger, are in patients less than 20 or more than 60 years old, and if the output of T_3 is already at the upper limit of normal.

Prophylactic therapy was pursued for 39 patients: 32 had surgical excision and seven received [131]I. Sixty-two of the 69 patients with toxic AFTN had treatment under our supervision, 43 with ^{131}I and 19 surgically. Surgically treated patients ranged in age from 11 to 62 years (average 22.6) and ^{131}I-treated patients ranged in age from 37 to 86 years (average 60.4).

Younger patients were treated surgically because successful ^{131}I treatment of AFTN may require doses as high as 30 to 50 mCi.[5,16] There was a reluctance to administer high doses of ^{131}I to young people for benign disease. The development of a multifocal carcinoma in one patient after ^{131}I therapy (Case 4) has further reduced enthusiasm for ^{131}I in younger AFTN patients. Finally, surgical treatment is simpler than for Graves' disease since nodulectomy is all that is required. One of the surgically treated patients had a 0.5-cm occult sclerosing papillary carcinoma in the center of a 3.5-cm AFTN. No other malignancies were found in this group. In addition to the patient described in Case 4 who developed cancer after ^{131}I therapy, there were four patients who gave histories of prior radiation therapy to the head and neck area who had thyroidectomies. Two patients had only benign AFTN. A third had a 1-cm lymph node metastasis from papillary carcinoma in the neck on the side contralateral to the AFTN. At operation a small focus of papillary carcinoma was found in the ipsilateral lobe. The AFTN was benign. The fourth irradiated patient had a 3-cm AFTN in the right lobe and a 1-cm cold nodule in the isthmus. The cold nodule was a follicular carcinoma; the AFTN was benign. Sixteen additional AFTN patients had received prior radiation therapy. Three patients had toxic lesions which were treated with ^{131}I. The remaining 13 are being observed.

Five patients had prophylactic operations because imaging revealed zones of reduced function, raising concern for cancer on the part of the patients or other physicians. These were all areas of degeneration. Finally, three patients were operated upon because of associated cold nodules. All were benign, as were the AFTN.

Of the 50 ^{131}I-treated patients, seven are known to be dead from other causes. One patient had surgical removal of a hard nodular remnant which was benign. The one patient who subsequently developed multifocal cancer in the extranodular tissue has already been described. No malignancies have been observed in the 41 remaining patients in the follow-up up to 14 years.

DISCUSSION

Frequency of AFTN

Although AFTN are uncommon, they have generated considerable interest, especially since radioactive iodine, imaging devices, and commercial preparations of TSH have become readily available. These new tools were necessary for the performance of the dynamic in vivo studies which have both confirmed speculations of earlier researchers as to the underlying pathophysiologic relationships and permitted the reliable diagnosis of AFTN in clinical practice. The more recent development of practical clinical methods for the assay of T_3 in the serum and the availability of TRH have made possible more complete observations on the functional changes which take place in the untreated AFTN, thus providing semi-quantitative guidelines of value in the prediction of the future course which a given AFTN may take.

The application of modern diagnostic methods has led to the appreciation that most AFTN are less than 2 cm.[5-7] These small lesions never secrete enough hormone to produce hyperthyroidism. Few of them change much within at least a 10-year period.[8] Curiously these small AFTN occurred about 20 times as often in women as in men. Men usually have the larger AFTN which are more often toxic. One might speculate that small AFTN in men rapidly enlarge. But this seems not to be the case, for the few small AFTN in men which have been followed have behaved just like those in women. Younger patients must be informed of the possiblilty that some small AFTN eventually increase in size and become toxic. Since many undergo degeneration, eliminating the potential for future hyperthyroidism, we advise observation for smaller AFTN.

Relation of AFTN Size to Function

When an AFTN reaches the size of 2.5 cm or larger, and has not undergone degeneration, the functionaly activity will usually be great enough to suppress extranodular function. A thyroid image will reveal a hot nodule with little activity elsewhere. A negligible response to TRH testing will be obtained and the serum T_3 level will be at least high normal. Because one AFTN is larger than another it need not be producing more thyroid hormone. Also, the larger the AFTN the greater the chance of central degeneration. Inspection of the thyroid image will reveal areas of reduced activity within the nodule: these cold areas do not signify malignancy. None of the patients subjected to thyroidectomy with these findings had cancer. All were degenerated AFTN. Also suggestive of degeneration is a large hot nodule with persistent function in the extranodular tissue. One can infer that such a nodule has a low probability of future toxicity.

Relation of Age to AFTN Function

Untreated larger nontoxic AFTN frequently become toxic within a few years. This progression seemed to be particularly common when sizable AFTN were discovered in teenagers or elderly patients. In the younger patients perhaps growth was too rapid to allow time for degeneration, or it may be that degeneration is less common in young people. Pediatric reports indicate correctly that AFTN are not common in children. Our youngest patient was 11 years old. However, 9% of our patients were less than 20 years old when first seen. Five patients developed toxicity and three are borderline. Of those followed 6 months or longer and not prophylactically ablated 44.4% reached toxic or borderline toxic levels of function. In patients over 50 years old borderline toxic AFTN may increase hormone secretion and precipitate atrial fibrillation and congestive heart failure. Therefore, for the teenager and the elderly patient larger, potentially toxic AFTN should be treated prophylactically.

What should be done for patients between 20 and 50 years old with these larger AFTN? The younger the patient the less the danger from a subsequent episode of hyperthyroidism and the greater the opportunity for degeneration. Therefore it seems that observation or prophylactic ablation are options of about equal merit.

Transient Toxicity After Hemmorhagic Infarction

Sudden enlargement with the onset of the features of hyperthyroidism should not be assumed to be the result of progression of the lesion. This may occur as a transient phenomenon associated with acute hemorrhagic infarction of the AFTN.[17] This process may eliminate the potential for future sustained toxicity, but as Case 5 demonstrates this does not always happen.

Methods for Prophylactic Ablation of AFTN

If one plans prophylactic ablation of a nontoxic AFTN, should this be done surgically or with ^{131}I? Our preference has been operation for patients less than 40 to 50 years old and ^{131}I for those who are older. Although some patients may respond to ^{131}I doses which deliver less than 5 mCi to the nodule, others require 15 mCi or more.[16,18] Having undertreated an elderly patient with a toxic AFTN with a 20 mCi dose of ^{131}I, and having observed her development of atrial fibrillation and congestive heart failure, I have been sensitive about this point. However, if one subscribes to the high dose theory he is faced with certain technical and theoretical problems. In the United States patients given doses higher than 30 mCi require hospitalization. This is one of the major inconveniences of operation which ^{131}I therapy ordinarily avoids. Also the appropriateness of such high doses of ^{131}I in younger patients for benign disease may be argued. As greater experience with cancer doses of ^{131}I in young people has accumulated this concern has been somewhat reduced.

The unavoidable gamma radiation delivered to the extranodular thyroid tissue, tissue which then comes under endogenous TSH stimulation, reproduces the conditions most favorable to the induction of thyroid cancer in experimental animals. Whether the cancer in our patient was coincidental or radiation induced is arguable. Most radiation-related thyroid cancers have appeared more than 10 years after the radiation exposure. The development of cancer in our patient only 3 years and 9 months after her therapy makes it somewhat less likely that the tumor was radiation induced. However, the multifocal nature of the cancer, involving only sites of low level radiation, in a patient whose thyroid tissue was exposed to a surge of TSH as the pituitary suppression produced by the excess secretion of the AFTN was relieved is a combination of features which cannot easily be dismissed. There is only one other similar report in the literature which I have been able to find.[19] This observation provides some comfort for the ^{131}I therapist.

If one is concerned about this problem there are two things which might be done to reduce the potential risk. First, one could stimulate the extranodular tissue with parenteral TSH just prior to the therapy and attempt to ablate all of the thyroid tissue. Second, if one is successful in ablating the AFTN one could administer suppressive doses of thyroid hormone to prevent the release of TSH from the pituitary. If the first of these steps is taken, the second will be needed in any event. However, the latter can be done without the former.

COMMENTARY

Manfred Blum, M.D.

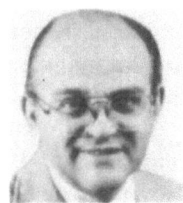

Autonomously functioning thyroid nodules (AFTN) are uncommon growths of the thyroid gland which are almost always benign and are not dependent on normal neuroendocrine, thyrotropin-mediated (TSH) regulatory mechanisms. AFTN may occur at any age, affecting females more often than males, and contrary to previous belief are more often associated with euthyroidism than with hyperthyroidism. Before discussing treatment, we must understand the natural history of this disorder, the subject of ongoing investigation.

An Incomplete Portrait

Because an AFTN may be asymptomatic for many years, and the disorder is relatively rare, and patients change physicians during a period of years, the natural course of the AFTN has not been documented in an adequate population.[1,3,5–8,20] A time course can be simulated by compiling sequential data on a particular patient from several clinics, by inferences drawn from medical histories, and by statistical sampling of characteristics from patients in various age groups. This indirect data can supplement more reliable information that is derived from the long-term observation of a small population of patients. Our current incomplete portrait of the patient with an AFTN suggests that an asymptomatic nodule may be detected in youth or early in adult life before it is important clinically. A microscopic or preclinical macroscopic hyperfunctioning nodule which could be autonomous or supersensitive to TSH may be the precursor of the small AFTN. A small AFTN produces little thyroid hormone and is not detectable with routine imaging procedures, unless function of the extranodular thyroid is suppressed by sufficient exogenous thyroid hormone. Larger nodules produce sufficient thyroid hormone to supply the individual's metabolic requirement, extinguishing the TSH stimulus to be extranodular tissue, and are seen on scans as solitary functioning nodules. A third group of nodules produces an excessive amount of thyroid hormones and causes hyperthyroidism. There appears to be a functional continuum rather than three distinct groups of nodules.

Size and Function: Concomitant Growth and Degeneration

The increase in size of an AFTN appears to be a dynamic process consisting of tissue growth and involutional changes. The degenerated portions of a nodule are hemorrhagic and cystic and are detectable on an isotope scan as areas of reduced activity within the nodule[5,20] and on echography as irregular fluid-filled zones.[5,20,21] In the past there was concern that a "cold" area in a "hot nodule" might be an area of malignancy. This concern has been allayed because cancers have not been detected in these degenerated areas when AFTN were resected.

Generally, hormone production is roughly proportional to nodular tissue mass.[5,6,8,16,20,22,23] Nodules less than 2.5 cm in diameter are almost never toxic. However, patients with larger nodules may be euthyroid or hyperthyroid. Larger nodules tend to degenerate.[5,20] As a result, thyroid hormone levels depend upon which of two concommitant processes predominates: growth or degeneration. By the time a nodule has achieved a 2.5-cm diameter of solid tissue, it produces adequate T_4 and T_3 to suppress TSH. Hyperthyroidism occurs when the solid component exceeds 3 cm.[8,20] In contrast, sudden swelling of a nodule to considerable size is usually accompanied by pain, a cold area on the thyroid scan, the echographic appearance of fluid, and no increase in the production of thyroid hormones. Repeated small hemorrhages may be asymptomatic resulting in a complex nodule that is heterogeneous on isotopic and ultrasonic imaging. Very large complex nodules tend to be hyperthyroid but may be euthyroid.[20] Function by an AFTN may deteriorate considerably after degeneration. I reported spontaneous infarction of an AFTN causing its complete clinical disappearance followed by resumption of function by the previously dormant portions of the thyroid.[24]

The Effect of Iodide and Other Environmental Factors

The level of function of an AFTN is not only dependent on size but also on the amount of iodine available.[25-27] Increased hormone output may occur after exposure to inorganic or organic iodides, e.g., radiographic contrast media and iodinated medications. Other environmental factors influence the situation. There is an appreciable difference in AFTN incidence in various parts of the world. The incidence in Brazil, Holland, and Switzerland is several times higher than in the United States.[9-12] Repletion of iodide in certain parts of the world results in hyperthyroidism (Jodbasedow) which suggests autonomous nodular disease rather than Graves' disease. The reason for these discrepancies is unknown but may in part be related to the environmental abundance of iodine and goitrogens.

Although current data suggest an increased incidence of benign and malignant nonfunctioning nodules in patients exposed to therapeutic x ray in their youth, there does not seem to be such a relationship to AFTN. Nevertheless, such a history may have therapeutic implications, as will be discussed later.

Hormone Productivity

Autonomous nodules produce T_4 and T_3. Most patients with toxic AFTN exhibit elevation of both hormones, but isolated elevation of T_3 or T_4 may occur. Early reports suggested that preferential hypersecretion of T_3 was a sporadic occurrence and the exception rather than the rule.[5,28] I reported a 20% incidence of T_3 toxicosis, mainly in middle-aged patients with AFTN.[20] T_3 toxicosis has also been observed in children with AFTN.[29] Hamberger subsequently reported a 46% incidence of T_3 toxicosis in a large series.[7] T_3 toxicosis may be transient, followed by a euthyroid state,[5] or progress to elevation of both T_3 and T_4.[8,20] These observations have led to the inference that elevated T_3 levels may precede hyperproduction of T_4 as a phase in the development of classic hyperthyroidism. Isolated elevation of T_4 has been observed in at least one elderly patient with a toxic AFTN.[30] The literature suggests that elevation of T_4 with a normal T_3 occurs mainly in sick or elderly people, and may reflect deficient T_3 production or conversion.[31]

Age and Gender

Hamburger reported that AFTN were "distributed about equally in patients older and younger than 40 years of age."[28] However, in his series of 349 patients, three-quarters of the toxic patients were in an older age group and more than half of those 60 years of age and older were hyperthyroid. Several authors have suggested a relationship between nodule size and patient age.[5,7,8] I reported a linear correlation between these two factors,[20] and virtually all patients older than age 60 were hyperthyroid.

AFTN in children have been considered uncommon, and hyperthyroidism rare.[32] It was suspected that careful screening might detect more youngsters who were hyperthyroid.[33] Hamburger reported that four of 25 patients between the ages of 11 and 19 years (13.8%) were hyperthyroid, an incidence that was similar to that for all age groups under 60 years.[8] One wonders whether factors other than nodule size may be operative in the production of thyroid hormone in younger patients. Information on iodine exposure in toxic as contrasted with euthyroid patients would be important.

There is a strong preponderance of females among patients with AFTN. Burman et al.[7] reported only four males in 54 patients (7.4%), compared to five of 35 (11%) reported by myself[20] and 27 of 349 (8%) by Hamburger.[8] However, hyperthyroidism appears to be more common in men than women. Some 33% of men are hyperthyroid contrasted with 16.5% of women according to Hamburger. In my series of 111 patients there are 14 males; 13 were hyperthyroid when first seen or became hyperthyroid later.[30]

Progression to Hyperthyroidism

Early papers reported very few AFTN patients who progressed from euthyroidism to hyperthyroidism. In 1975 I reported this sequence in four patients and hyperthyroidism following iodine exposure in a fifth, among 13 with euthyoid AFTN.[20] Wiener and DeVries showed progression in six of 58 Dutch patients within 1 to

11.8 years.[11] Fourteen of Hamburger's 159 patients from the north central United States became hyperthyroid, nine within 2 years and the other five within 6 years.[8] Currently eight of 49 of my patients observed for 1 to 10 years have progressed to hyperthyroidism.[30] Progression was most likely when an AFTN was 3 cm in diameter or larger, and particularly common in the elderly. Hamburger's series suggests that teenagers are at risk for progression to hyperthyroidism.[8] The interval between onset of observation and hyperthyroidism is variable. Hamburger suggests that hyperthyroidism generally occurs within 6 years.[8] My experience is somewhat different.[30] Perhaps the point of departure is the definition of "the period of observation." Most of our AFTN patients reported as asymptomatic nodule discovered years earlier and not treated prophylactically. Furthermore, chest roentgenograms taken many years previously may reveal indentation of the trachea by a nodule long before the diagnosis of AFTN was entertained. This type of historical data indicate that the onset of hyperthyroidism may be delayed by many more years than published reports suggest. A number of factors may influence the time when an asymptomatic patient is first examined, and they will affect these data. Nevertheless, it is apparent that most euthyroid patients with an AFTN do not become hyperthyroid for many years, particularly patients younger than age 50.

Other Factors

One additional consideration in the natural history of AFTN relates to nonmetabolic consequences. Pressure symptoms due to an AFTN obstructing the thoracic inlet may be observed. Although many patients complain of local fullness, I have seen true obstruction in only one patient with a large degenerated AFTN which required prompt surgical intervention.[34] A more frequent consideration is the effect of actual or potential hyperthyroidism on someone with another disease process. The elderly, the frail, and those with cardiovascular disease can ill afford the additional burden of hyperthyroidism. Severe weight loss, myopathy, aggravation of neurologic or psychiatric disease, congestive heart failure, or myocardial infarction may be the consequences. These considerations are especially applicable to the elderly who are more likely to have underlying disease and in whom evidence of hyperthyroidism may be subtle, "masked," or "apathetic."

When to Treat AFTN

There are two complications of an AFTN which require treatment. Pressure symptoms usually necessitate surgery, and hyperthyroidism requires ablation surgically or with ^{131}I.

Controversy relates to treatment of nontoxic AFTN. Some physicians advise prophylactic ablation of all AFTN. An understanding of the natural history of the disease will perhaps permit more selective treatment.

The Risk of Malignancy

The consensus has been that carcinoma is extremely uncommon in functioning thyroid nodules. However, there is semantic confusion about the heterogeneous classification, "functioning nodule." Various terms have been used including hyperfunctioning, hot, warm, autonomous, hypertrophic, and reactive. The problem is compounded because a scan may show more or less activity in the region of a palpable nodule which could be caused by normal tissue underlying a small, poorly functioning nodule to produce a "cool" nodule or a slight increase in thickness of tissue resulting in mildly enhanced activity of a "warm" nodule. The terms "warm" or "cool" offer no pathophysiologic insight. Perhaps it would be wise to abandon these euphemistic thermal terms for thyroid nodules; but they seem so firmly entrenched in our lexicon that they probably will continue to be used. I classify functioning nodules (they may be hyperfunctioning or isofunctioning) as autonomous or TSH-dependent. Function by the former is not suppressible by thyroid hormone, and extranodular tissue is stimulable by TSH. In the latter, nodular function is suppressible and extranodular tissue is not responsive to additional TSH, basal levels of that neurohumor already being abundant. The incidence of cancer among functioning nodules as defined above is very small. Fisher has calculated an incidence of 0.7% in a total of 4280 reported cases of single or multiple "hyperfunctioning" thyroid nodules.[35] However, carcinomas are observed occasionally.[5,33,36–39]

Occult thyroid cancer, remote from a benign AFTN and discovered accidentally, has been reported.[37] In this volume, Hamburger reported two cancers in extranodular tissue in a population of 361 patients with AFTN, 39 of whom were treated surgically. Both had a history of prior irradiation. One of the cancers was occult. There was a third patient whose cancer was discovered after an AFTN had been treated with [131]I. In my series of 111 AFTN patients, 21 were treated surgically and none had cancer in the AFTN or elsewhere.[30]

The question of occult thyroid malignancy in association with AFTN has been raised by several observers. Since occult malignancies are generally considered not to adversely affect health or longevity, this is not an important factor in the management of AFTN.[40]

The Effect of the Natural History of the AFTN on the Need for Therapy

Local Pressure
Obstruction of the thoracic inlet due to an AFTN is very rare. When it occurs, surgery is required.

Progression to Hyperthyroidism and Age of the Patient
Progression to hyperthyroidism is gradual and takes many years. Most patients remain euthyroid. However, hyperthyroidism is clearly more common in patients

with nodules whose average diameter exceeds 3 cm and in those over age 50. Indeed, most elderly patients with AFTN are hyperthyroid. Therefore, prophylactic management may be appropriate for these.

The progression of thyroid function to hyperthyroidism during youth may be more common than previously thought. In addition, AFTN may grow more rapidly in the young. Furthermore, prophylactic treatment may be appropriate for AFTN in younger patients because of their long survival, the uncertain long-term prognosis of the nodule, and the relative safety of treatment in this group. Therefore, the consensus favors prophylactic treatment for children and adolescents with AFTN. I prefer surgery to radioiodine for this purpose.

Gender

AFTN are less common in men than women. However, more of the men are hyperthyroid. It is unclear whether the AFTN develops later in life in men than women or whether asymptomatic euthyroid nodules are less often discovered in men than women. I believe that a nontoxic AFTN in a man may be managed the same as in a woman.

History of Exposure to Therapeutic X Rays in Youth

There is no known association between exposure to therapeutic x rays and subsequent AFTN development. However, about two-thirds of patients irradiated during youth have thyroid nodules and one-third of these are malignant. Surgery is generally advised for a solitary nonfunctioning nodule in previously irradiated patients, and some investigators recommend suppressive therapy for all patients with this history. The presence of an AFTN in an irradiated gland complicates follow-up in this very important group of patients, and therefore I favor excision of AFTN in patients previously irradiated.

The Influence of Associated Disease

The elderly and those with cardiovascular disease can ill afford the untoward physiologic effects of hyperthyroidism. Therefore, I recommend prophylactic ablation of non toxic AFTN in these people.

The Influence of Iodides

The production of thyroid hormone by an AFTN may be potentiated by inorganic or organic iodides. Therefore, AFTN patients should avoid iodides. However, this may be impossible if radiologic procedures utilizing iodinated contrast media are needed. Prior temporary blockade of iodine organification with thionamides is reasonable.

How to Treat the Patient with an AFTN

Generally the nontoxic AFTN does not require symptomatic relief. With a toxic AFTN propranolol may be used to ameliorate toxic symptoms and the thionamides will reduce thyroid hormone levels to normal prior to surgery. Inorganic iodide should not be used unless organification has been blocked for reasons already discussed.

The thionamides play no role in the definitive management of nontoxic or toxic AFTN. Although these drugs reduce T_4 and T_3 temporarily, one cannot expect elimination of the AFTN. I have seen three patients given long-term thionamide treatment who years later had large toxic AFTN. One of these had severe obstruction of the thoracic inlet and another had cardiac complications.

Treatment of an AFTN requires destruction of tissue by surgery or ^{131}I. Simple lobectomy is adequate for an AFTN, and some surgeons are content with "nodulectomy." Damage to the laryngeal nerves is uncommon unless the mass is very large. Since the procedure is unilateral, hypoparathyroidism is not anticipated. I advise surgery in patients less than 50 years old, in those with very large nodules, and always for obstruction. However, a young patient with heart disease may be treated with ^{131}I, and an old person concerned about the cosmetics of the mass may elect surgery.

Selective ablation of an AFTN with radiation is accomplished with ^{131}I. External irradiation cannot deliver the required dose without serious untoward effects on the skin and trachea. Since AFTN are relatively radiation resistant, compared to diffuse toxic goiter, an ^{131}I dose of 10 to 15 mCi absorbed by the nodule is required to destroy it. Smaller doses may reduce hormone output and cause some AFTN shrinkage. Since the uptake of iodine by an AFTN is usually high normal or only slightly elevated, the dose of ^{131}I administered to the patient may be very large to ensure adequate AFTN treatment. Isolation in the hospital for several days is required if more than the 30 mCi must be given. I am reluctant to administer more than 30 mCi at one time, but agree that a fractional dose regimen may reduce the uptake of iodine appreciably and complicate subsequent therapy. Using a fractional approach, several treatments over several months to a year may be required and the patient must be informed of this. Fortunately, there is no urgency to treat because an AFTN progresses slowly. Indeed, ^{131}I does not result in rapid reduction of T_4 or T_3, and when amelioration of thyrotoxicosis is needed other methods must be given. A fractional dose regimen usually converts a toxic AFTN to a smaller nontoxic one. In my experience complete destruction of a nontoxic AFTN by ^{131}I is uncommon, although function may be reduced sufficiently to elicit TSH activation of the previously dormant extranodular thyroid. Another risk of ^{131}I is swelling of the AFTN and release of preformed hormone caused by irradiation thyroiditis, a dose-related phenomenon. There are problems mainly with unusually large, almost obstructive AFTN, or in patients with severely compromised coronary vascular or cardiac functional reserve. The former should probably be treated surgically. In the latter group, and only in this group of patients, one should lower T_4 and T_3 to normal with thionamides and then administer ^{131}I.

It is ironic that the single large ablation dose of ^{131}I would be suitable for prophylactic treatment of a modest-size AFTN in a healthy, euthyroid or mildly hyperthyroid, young person. Unfortunately, this is the very patient one would like to spare the risks of a large gamma radiation dose to extranodular thyroid, marrow, and gonads.

Radioiodine therapy is simple and many physicians prefer it to surgery for routine use. Hypothyroidism is not a consequence because the extranodular tissue is spared the destructive beta radiation. Furthermore, serious complications have not been reported when moderate doses of ^{131}I were given. I prefer it to surgery in those over age 50 and in selected younger patients. The management of AFTN should be individualized.

COMMENTARY

N. David Charkes, M.D.

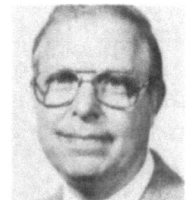

How Often Do Nontoxic AFTN Become Toxic?

Until very recently, it had been assumed that euthyroid persons with autonomously functioning thyroid nodules (AFTN) rarely became hyperthyroid and, in fact, were more likely to undergo spontaneous improvement by cystic degeneration or infarction of the nodule. The available data[8,11] suggested that the probability of developing hyperthyroidism from an AFTN over a period of up to 12 years following diagnosis was about 5%, less than half the likelihood that the nodule would spontaneously degenerate or disappear completely. It was commonly recommended, therefore, that no prophylactic treatment be undertaken in these patients, but rather that they be observed for signs of toxicty, cancer, or mechanical complaints.[11] There was a nagging suspicion, however, that hyperthyroidism was being underdiagnosed, especially in the elderly. In one series, for example, serum PBI was not elevated in 20% of 85 clinically toxic patients over the age of 60.[41] Furthermore, the majority of older patients present with cardiovascular symptoms, including angina pectoris, congestive heart failure, or tachyarrhythmias,[41] so that missing the diagnosis of hyperthyroidism could expose the patient to potentially life-threatening complications. Other thyroidologists,[8] including this author, therefore recommended prophylactic removal or radioiodine ablation to elderly, euthyroid persons with AFTN.

Hamburger now reports that 21% of 147 patients with AFTN followed up to 6 years became toxic or borderline toxic, a four-fold increase over the earlier reports. Furthermore, the first sign of impending toxicity in ten of the 18 patients who became hyperthyroid was T_3 toxicosis. In the over-60 subgroup, 4 of 11 patients (36%) became overtly toxic during the follow-up period. It thus seems clear that elderly patients with AFTN 2.5 cm or larger in diameter are at high risk of developing thyrotoxicosis, usually with serious cardiovascular complications and, more often than not, without elevation of the serum thyroxine concentration initially. The onus would now appear to be upon those who would not treat this subgroup of patients with AFTN prophylactically.

What Are the Risks of Observing Nontoxic AFTN?

First of all, the development of hyperthyroidism with serious cardiovascular manifestations is possible in the elderly. Of 27 patients with AFTN I treated with ^{131}I, half presented with tachyarrhythmias, congestive heart failure, or angina pectoris of recent onset. The mean age of this group was 64. Plummer himself noted the tendency to cardiovascular manifestations in his original description of the disease, and stressed it in later reports.[42,43] Of considerable importance is the fact that T_3 toxicosis appears to be common in these patients, so that the unwary physician who relies on the serum thyroxine alone or resin uptake will miss the diagnosis of hyperthyroidism.

A second complication of nontreatment is acute hemorrhagic infarction of the AFTN[17,24] (Hamburger's Case 5). The outcome may be thyroid storm from sudden release of stored hormone into the bloodstream, with fatal results, as in one of our patients. In a second patient, also an elderly female, serum T_4 rose abruptly to 25.6 μg%, but fortuitously she had been on propranolol for hypertension and ran a mild clinical course. Although this complication is rare, it is justly feared, and completely preventable by adequate prophylaxis.

A third complication is iodine-induced hyperthyroidism (jodbasedow), which has been reported in two persons with AFTN inadvertently given radiographic contrast agents.[11,27] Other patients may become thyrotoxic from ingestion of thyroid hormone, often prescribed by physicians who are unaware of the earlier diagnosis of AFTN.

What Are the Risks of Treatment of Nontoxic AFTN?

Surgical treatment in younger patients is technically simpler than for Graves' disease. We have reserved ^{131}I for those over the age of 50. In my series, 14 of 17 patients given 30,000 rads or more (beta) to the AFTN had complete functional ablation of the nodule, but this required a mean administrered dose of 57 mCi (the average dose deposited in this "high-dose" group was 18.4 mCi). This dose is considerably greater than that for Graves' disease, which is the reason for the age restriction. One possible complication of this high-dose treatment is transient radiation thyroiditis, but this was observed only once in our series, in a patient who received an estimated 205,000 rads—too high a dose, in retrospect, but given before the importance of the total radiation dose was fully appreciated. Another potential complication is leukemia—not yet reported under these circumstances.

A final possible complication of ^{131}I therapy is the development of thyroid cancer. Although Hamburger reports such a sequence of events in Case 4, it is very unlikely, in my opinion, that the circumstances were those of cause and effect. In the first place, thyroid cancer is a very common disease at autopsy, affecting 1–4% of the population of this country. Thus, in Hamburger's series, of 115 patients over the age of 50 (Table 3-1), we would expect up to four cases of thyroid cancer, and it is not surprising that he found them. In the case reported, and from additional data given elsewhere,[14] if we assume an effective half-life for ^{131}I of 6 days (average for AFTN in my series), I would calculate an estimated beta dose of 26,600 rads to the nodule and, therefore, about 2660 rads to the extranodular tissue. This latter radiation dose is even less than that to the thyroid in Graves' disease using so-called low dose ^{131}I treatment (50 μCi deposited per gram of gland). In the Cooperative Thyrotoxicosis Followup Study of 34,684 patients, there was no statistical difference in the incidence of thyroid cancer in those patients following subtotal thyroidectomy and in the group which had received ^{131}I treatment for Graves' disease previously.[44] On these grounds alone a cause-and-effect relationship is highly unlikely.

Furthermore, there is little if any evidence to date of a role for TSH in the development of thyroid cancer after ablative ^{131}I therapy of AFTN. In the first place, if the ^{131}I treatment is given correctly, permanent hypothyroidism is very uncommon. Transient hypothyroidism 3 to 6 months later does occur, but is of the secondary (hypopituitary) variety (low TSH), entirely analogous to the transient hypopituitarism which occurs after discontinuation of long-term thyroid hormone administration to normal subjects.[45] In our own series, all eight patients with transiently low RAI uptake in extranodular tissue following complete ablation of the nodule had a normal response to exogenous TSH administration, and equal to the pretherapy response (unpublished), indicative of hypopituitary hypothyroidism.

A complete review of the relationship of TSH to thyroid cancer is beyond the scope of this discussion, but a few points are in order. Although TSH seems to be important in the induction of thyroid cancer in rodents, workers in the field have cautioned against extrapolation of these findings to humans.[46] In areas of the world where thyroid cancer is common, e.g., Hawaii and Iceland, TSH-induced endemic goiter is rare; conversely, some areas of endemic goiter such as Finland and the Himalayas also have very low thyroid cancer rates. Thyroid cancer is also uncommon in adults with longstanding TSH-induced goiter for dyshormonogenesis or Hashimoto's disease. Finally, in 234 patients with a history of childhood neck irradiation, there was no significant difference in TSH levels in the group of patients with thyroid nodules and those without nodules.[47] The same was true, incidentally, of patients without a history of prior irradiation.[47] Although these points may not allay the fears of the ultracautious, they suggest to me that the relationship of TSH to thyroid cancer induction in adult humans is conjectural at best and cannot be used as evidence against a valuable treatment modality.

Conclusions

Recent evidence suggests that ^{131}I treatment of AFTN prophylactically in certain circumstances is good management. Patients over the age of 50 with nodules larger than 2.5 cm are ideal candidates. Younger patients could be treated surgically or observed periodically, and the serum T_4, total T_3, and RAI uptake and scan are the appropriate means of follow-up. There are few disorders where diagnosis is so specific, using readily available diagnostic measures, and the risks of nontreatment so easily avoided by prophylactic treatment, as the autonomously functioning thyroid nodule.

COMMENTARY

N. Demeester-Mirkine, M.D.

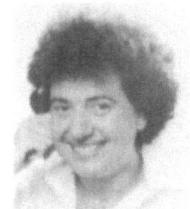

Diagnosis of AFTN

We agree with Hamburger's criteria, which provide a physiologic definition of AFTN based upon an inhibition test using thyroid hormones and a stimulation test using TSH.[48] However, since the introduction of new examining techniques there is a tendency in clinical practice to avoid such tests because they are time consuming for the patient and involve the administration of drugs which are sometimes poorly tolerated.

When hot nodules are visible with ^{99m}Tc pertechnetate, we make a scan with [131]iodine to rule out the slight possibility of a nodule in which defective organification would give a hot image with ^{99m}Tc pertechnetate and a cold one with [131]iodine.[49]

In the case of hot nodules with no active extranodular parenchyma, if PBI[131] is high and the TRH stimulation test is flat, the diagnosis seems clear to us. In patients in whom the hot nodule is surrounded by active extranodular parenchyma, an inhibition test must be performed to distinguish a hot nodule from a suppressible or nonsuppressible asymmetric goiter. As we did not perform inhibition tests in all cases of nodular goiter, we undoubtedly missed small hot nodules with little inhibition of the thyroid parenchyma, since all the 38 observed hot nodules were more than 2.5 cm in diameter.

The TSH stimulation test, allowing differential diagnosis between an isolated nodule and agenesis of one thyroid lobe, may be replaced by thyroid echography which allows easy recognition of a normal thyroid lobe. In any case, the clinical appearance of a single thyroid lobe is different from that of a hot nodule because the lobe is enlarged but retains its elongated shape and normal consistency. In cases of euthyroidism, PBI[131] and TRH give normal results. The TSH stimulation test seems indispensable in difficult cases where the gland is asymmetric and the image of the hot nodule does not appear clearly.

Usefulness of Echography in Follow-up

Compound or real time echography is useful to observe the evolution of a hot nodule. Size changes are estimated more precisely than by palpation or scanning. The centronodular echographic image is often heterogeneous and in half the cases shows echo-free zones corresponding to cystic degeneration. This technique should theoretically allow a centronodular degeneration process, giving a cystic image, to be distinguished from the very unlikely formation of a cancer which would give a more solid image. During the 3 years that we have been performing thyroid echography we have had no opportunity to observe an evolving hot nodule. But in other cases of mixed solid and liquid nodules, we have clearly established that the size increase of a clinically palpated nodule was due to an increased quantity of liquid whereas the solid content remained unchanged.

Criteria for Toxicity in an AFTN

What we found particularly problematic was defining the boundary between the nontoxic and the toxic hot nodule, because the diagnosis rests mainly on a determination of what level of T_3 is pathologic. The TRH test is often flat, even when T_3 and T_4 levels are normal. We are concerned about leaving patients in an uncomfortable state of early hyperthyroidism with T_3 levels around 200 $\mu g/dl$. It is possible that because of low-iodine diet in Europe this transitional period might last longer. Iodine supplementation may rapidly cause hyperthyroidism in euthyroid cases of hot nodules.[50]

Treatment of AFTN

From the therapeutic standpoint we agree with the approach proposed by Hamburger. Recently we have favored surgery if the patient's condition permits it. Of the 11 patients treated with [131]iodine which we have observed, there were two cases of hypothyroidism (4 to 17 mCi were delivered to the nodule; two patients received two doses). Surgery would seem to offer a cure with little risk and no sequelae.

COMMENTARY

Thomas S. Reeve, M.B.

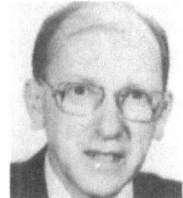

Although Plummer described functioning thyroid nodules in 1913,[42] it was not until the more widespread use of isotope scanning devices[4,51] that visualization of AFTN or "hot" thyroid nodules became possible in clinical practice. It has taken even longer to develop an understanding of the natural history of this lesion.[8] The natural history may be different in different locations, as incidence data on AFTN indicate.[9]

Royal North Shore Hospital Experience

In the Royal North Shore Hospital Thyroid Clinic a review of surgery for 1567 clinically single thyroid nodules was made between 1966 and 1979 (1393 females and 174 males). Of those, 91 had AFTN (74 females, 17 males).

Most of these 91 patients presented for a lump in the neck, a small number with nervousness, and even fewer with weight loss. Thirty-seven had clinical thyrotoxicosis confirmed by laboratory tests, while 44 patients were considered thyrotoxic on clinical grounds.

Total thyroid lobectomy was carried out in 66 instances. Bilateral subtotal thyroidectomy was performed 18 times and subtotal lobectomy seven times, because unexpected nodules were encountered in the nonfunctional segment of the thyroid. These nodules were neither detected by palpation nor "seen" on isotope scanning. This situation seems more common since TSH stimulation of the nonfunctional tissue has become less often used. Scanning of the thyroid with ultrasound[52] may detect small nodules which are both impalpable and not visualized isotopically prior to surgery. The thyroid must be fully mobilized to find nodules which can be clearly demonstrated on ultrasound scanning.

In attempting to detect unsuspected nodular tissue, it is also possible to demonstrate thyroid tissue other than an apparent AFTN on the ipsilateral and opposite sides of the gland. The use of ultrasound also gives a good idea of the extent of surgery necessary to achieve the desired objective. This should prevent removal of one lobe when no other lobe exists, e.g., hemiagenesis, without knowledge of having done so. An isotope scan after TSH stimulation would still be useful if ^{131}I ablation is planned.

Treatment of AFTN

Hamburger's material[4] suggests that patients with AFTN less than 3 cm in size should be observed, and that these patients usually will not develop thyrotoxicosis.

This has been confirmed by others in the United States.[7] As in all such studies it is important to show that patients are not disadvantaged by such a program.

Observation of Nontoxic AFTN

Having established a diagnosis of AFTN it is then incumbent upon the physician to ensure that there will be regular follow-up until there is either common agreement to follow no more, or treatment becomes necessary. Unfortunately, not all people are prepared to be followed at regular intervals for such a long period of time. That it is important to diagnose thyrotoxicosis is shown in the following case history.

CASE 1:   A "NONTOXIC" AFTN WHICH BECAME TOXIC WITHIN FOUR
          YEARS

A 20-year-old white male was diagnosed as having an AFTN. He had an elevated protein-bound iodine level but was not clearly hyperthyroid. He was told that such lesions rarely become toxic. He next presented some 4 years later with profound hyperthyroidism. The size of his lesion was 3 cm. The major reason that led to return was that in the previous year a relatively minor trauma caused a fractured humerus. The long-term high turnover of hormone affected his skeleton, in a manner not necessarily manifest, and the profound implications of this disturbance of calcium function did not occur to his physicians until he became frankly thyrotoxic. The patient did not recognize the early signs of toxicity as they had merged indistinguishably with what he had come to expect from his body day by day.

It has been suggested that degeneration of these lesions may well lead to their dissolution; however, degeneration, although common, often leaves a rim of surrounding tissue which is quite active. Hyperthyroidism in association with a partly degenerated nodule has been seen on 26 occasions. The use of ultrasound also has shown highly active lesions with central cystic degeneration which maintain the thyrotoxic state.

If one observes an AFTN, a time limit should be established beyond which the patient should not be expected to keep returning for follow-up. A size limit should be determined, and a growing nodule should probably be removed.[53] A distinct cutoff time for watching a lesion grow to a 3-cm limit should be given to the patient so that he understands the plan. Prolonged observation with no end point does not provide the patient with an anxiety-free existence. Although long-term follow-up is very satisfactory in a research situation, it has limited practical application. Patients who come from long distances and who have difficulties of communication cannot be expected to make their own judgments or to watch their own necks. The program requires overseeing by the attending physician.

Although long-term follow-up is justified to establish the natural history of a disease, before it is recommended for large numbers of patients the morbidity of follow-up should be defined. If surgery can be done with a low complication rate, or if we can develop our ^{131}I techniques to a level where the results are equivalent to surgery, it may be that these methods are simpler than long-term follow-up in terms of cost-benefit analysis. This would not only cure the patients' problem but would relieve them of the anxiety of having a lump in the neck, a lump for which the risk of malignancy, although extremely small, is not nonexistent.

Surgical Treatment of AFTN

Hamburger states that it is usually possible to remove only the nodule itself at thyroidectomy. We found that the surrounding tissue is usually so well suppressed by the nodule that total lobectomy is more practical. Total lobectomy leaves at least one side of the neck clear, simplifying subsequent evaluation of the remaining tissue, while providing for the eventuality (albeit unlikely) of an associated carcinoma with the AFTN. The isthmus should also be removed to leave the trachea clear in case of any overnight problems after surgery.

^{131}I Treatment of AFTN

The use of ^{131}I to ablate the thyroid has not had a high degree of acceptance in this unit and it is interesting to note that Hamburger expresses the same view. The method he advises is the same that we have used. In this series ten patients have been treated this way: paranodular suppression is produced with thyroxine and a large dose of ^{131}I is given (usually 15 mCi). The autonomy has been destroyed in all cases, but the nodule remained in six. In these six patients the nodule was removed to eliminate the possibility of malignancy.

We agree that the radiation dose in Hamburger's Case 4 has not been proved related to the development of thyroid cancer. The incidence of malignancy in AFTN is rare and has almost always been in the paranodular tissue. Hence our interest in visualizing that tissue after one or more doses of TSH or by performing ultrasound on patients for whom ^{131}I therapy is considered.

COMMENTARY

Jan D. Wiener, Ph.D.

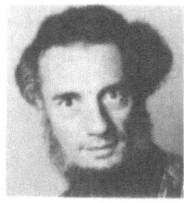

The observations and conclusions put forward in this chapter leave little room for serious dissent. My commentary will largely deal with differences of findings rather than opinion, part of which is probably due to differences in patient selection and in appreciation between observers.

We recently presented findings in a group of 58 patients, reexamined after 1 to 12 years,[11] These patients, like Dr. Hamburger's, were a selected group, i.e., those with little or no complaints at first presentation. It has been recognized from the first studies on this disorder[42] that goiter precedes symptoms by many years. Probably, therefore, the pattern described was typical of the evolution for most of our patents.

Divergent Findings: Geographic Factors?

The title of the chapter does not contain the term "solitary," but it is clear from the text that solitary or predominant nodules were present in most if not all patients. Judging from the literature, glands with multiple autonomous areas* are uncommon in the United States. In our experience two or more discrete autonomously functioning nodules or "patchy" autonomy are common. In our recent study,[11] a solitary or predominant AFTN was present in only 33 (57%) of 58 cases, and at first presentation the proportion is similar.

Before combining these two groups of patients, we should be reasonably sure that they have the same disorder. I think there is little evidence suggesting that they don't, if we remember that "toxic (multi)nodular goiter" is a confusing term, including patients with AFTN and those with Graves' disease and coincidental (nonhyperfunctioning) nodules. Actually, a spectrum of forms can be found, ranging from solitary nodules to numerous small autonomous areas ("patchy" scintigram).[54,55] Transition in a patient from a solitary AFTN to multiple "hot spots" has only rarely been documented.[11] Some extranodular autonomy has been observed in 75% of patients with a single AFTN also in the United States.[54] Signs and symptoms are the same in those with solitary AFTN or with multiple autonomous areas. The (usually very slow) evolution doesn't seem to be appreciably different either.[11] The same holds true for the response to treatment. I have found the age of those with solitary nodules to be slightly lower (55.1 vs. 60.2 years). Whether this reflects progression from solitary to multiple autonomous areas in the same patients, or the decreasing incidence of (multi)nodular goiter in this region (probably a result of increased iodine supply), is uncertain. Furthermore, borderline hyperthyroidism was present more often with multifocal autonomy (20 of 65) than with solitary AFTN (12 of 81). Finally, there was a difference in sex distribution: 18 of 81 patients with solitary AFTN were males, but only two of 65 with multifocal autonomy. The latter finding although remarkable (and unexplained) is not sufficient to reject the hypothesis that the two groups represent different forms of the same disease. This view is shared by others.[54,56] We now apply the term Plummer's disease to these two groups, a name casually introduced by Miller[57] and adopted by others.[54,58]**

---

*Since the autonomy doesn't always coincide with palpable nodules, I prefer "areas" as a more general term in the description of scintigraphic findings.

**There has been some dispute over the definition of Plummer's disease. Selby and McClellan[58] described only hyperthyroid patients, and it has been proposed[59] to restrict the designation to these patients. But as discussed above and elsewhere,[55,60] euthyroid and hyperthyroid patients (including the many borderline cases) clearly have the same disease, be it in different stages.

Even if we consider only patients with solitary AFTN, our incidence is about five times that at NTL. If we look at hyperthyroid patients, the difference is greater. Excluding borderline cases, about one in seven of our hyperthyroid patients have solitary AFTN, compared to one in 50 at NTL. This may in part reflect the greater incidence of nodular goiter in general in our region. In a series of 181 consecutive patients with solitary or predominant nodules 29 (16%) had an autonomous nodule (toxic or nontoxic), compared to 5% in the NTL.[8] Remarkably, however, only 1% of our patients were less than 21 years of age,[61] compared to 9% of the patients at NTL (Table 3-1). Both at NTL and our hospital patients less than 21 years old with Plummer's disease constitute only 0.1% of all patients referred for thyroid evaluations.

Also, many more of our patients were hyperthyroid. Admittedly, the diagnosis is sometimes subtle in borderline cases. But even if all borderline cases in our original study[55] are regarded as euthyroid, 107 of 224 patients (48%) were hyperthyroid, compared to 19% (plus 5% borderline) at NTL. If multifocal autonomy is excluded from our series, the discordance is still greater. This observation is more remarkable in view of the much lower iodine intake in our region (around 100–150 μg/day).

Finally, and most important, the association of functional autonomy with malignancy may not be the same in different parts of the world. Whereas an incidence of over 10% was reported in the United States,[5] it was only 1.2% in five large European series.[62] However, this comparison is complicated by several factors, discussed elsewhere.[62] Autonomy and malignancy can be associated in several ways. The autonomous nodule itself is very rarely malignant. Autonomy with contralateral malignancy is also rare. The patients at NTL, and at least one other center,[63] had received previous irradiation, which was not the case for our patient.[62] More often a carcinoma is found in or near an AFTN. In 36 reports there were 29 cancers in 1200 operated patients (2.4%).[62,64] Not always, however, was functional autonomy of "hot" nodules unequivocally established. Furthermore, some series contain solitary AFTN only, and the incidence of malignancy is not necessarily the same in these cases as in those with multifocal autonomy. Also, criteria for selecting patients for surgery differ in different centers. If only the AFTN is removed, a small contralateral carcinoma may go undetected. On the other hand, "occult" papillary carcinomas appear to be fairly common in clinically normal thyroid glands (4.2% in an American autopsy series).[65]

Rate of Progression: Influence of Age and Iodine Excess

An important practical point is the incidence and rate of progression of the disorder, and the possible relationship between progression and age at first presentation. Patients becoming toxic at NTL did so within 6 years, which was interpreted as due to the tendency to employ prophylactic ablation for large AFTN in the early years. In a large European series, on the other hand, it was also observed that progression (clinical, scintigraphic, and/or biochemical) most often occurred in the first few years.[66] Although patient selection will have influenced the results, the overall incidence of toxicity developing during the follow-up period was about 10% in both the European series and at NTL.

In our follow-up study,[11] progression toward hyperthyroidism or important growth of the nodule was seen in eight patients averaging 44 years of age; the mean age of the other 50 patients was 56 years. It can be calculated from Table 3-2 that of NTL patients followed for 6 years, 16% of those under age 40 became toxic, compared to only 7% of the older patients. Reinwein et al.,[66] on the other hand, found progression to be independent of age. From Table 3-1 it appears that teenagers are particularly prone to developing hyperthyroidism. Our own material points in the same direction.[11,61] Of four patients under age 21, one was mildly toxic when first seen, one was surgically treated (prophylactically), one was hyperthyroid 9 years later, and the fourth was operated on 2.5 years after first presentation because of nodule growth and difficulties with swallowing.

Iodine excess, not mentioned by Dr. Hamburger, can bring about rapid although reversible progression to toxicity and even thyroid storm.[27] Coindet, who was the first to use iodine in the treatment of (nodular) goiter, called attention to its potential dangers 160 years ago,[67] giving an amazingly complete enumeration of signs and symptoms of what we now call hyperthyroidism.[68] Usually the toxicity regresses spontaneously in parallel with the iodine excess, which however can take months when the iodine has been given as a radiopaque medium or in a drug with a long biologic half-life. Given chronically, 0.5 mg inorganic iodide or less per day may produce toxicity in these patients in regions with low iodine intake.[50,69]

Which Patients Should Be Treated?

I agreee that these nodules, particularly the larger ones, are best removed prophylactically in teenagers. It also seems wise not to wait for cardiac symptoms to develop in elderly patients with larger (not clearly degenerated) nodules. However, as described above, multifocal autonomy is common in these patients, and the amount of autonomously functioning tissue may be very difficult to estimate. The serum concentration of thyroid hormone, particularly (free) triiodothyronine, may be the best guide, treatment being advised when a high-normal value is found.

In other cases, particularly those with small amounts of autonomously functioning tissue, I wonder if reevaluation needs to be as frequent as once a year. Progression is usually very slow. Of course, the patients should be informed of the possibility of (functional and/or mechanical) progression, and asked to come back if they (or the family doctor) think such a change is occurring.

Mode of Treatment and Risk of Recurrence

Few specialist will disagree with the view that younger patients should have surgery and older patients should be treated with [131]I. I think we are slightly more reluctant to give high doses of ^{131}I to patients under 50 years of age. There is also agreement that only the AFTN need be removed. Indeed, a recurrent (toxic) nodule within a few years after nodulectomy (or hemithyroidectomy) is exceptional.[11] It was recognized by pioneers in the field over 20 years ago[70] that if there are more than one AFTN, recurrence may not be so improbable if only the well-delineated AFTN is excised. Actually, although we don't see many recurrences, we do see patients with Plummer's disease and a history of thyroidectomy for "goiter" or "hyperthyroidism." This fact has received little attention. I know of only one paper on the subject,[71] describing five patients, all euthyroid, with autonomous nodules diagnosed 3–30 (average, 15) years after thyroid surgery. Data on 20 such patients from our files, diagnosed 2–45 (average, 20) years after thyroid surgery, are given in Table 3-3. They constitute about 4% of all patients with the disease—possibly slightly less than the proportion of previously operated cases in all our newly referred thyroid patients (about 5%).

Table 3-3. Patients with previous thyroidectomy.

Patient no.	Sex	Age at present diagnosis	Years after therapy	Indication for therapy[a]	Present thyroid function[b]	Involved area[c]
1	f	68	15	?	h	s
2	f	61	32	?	e	s
3	f	69	42	h	h	s
4	f	80	14	h	h	m
5	f	30	1.9	h[d]	h	s
6	f	62	23	h	h	m
7	f	49	22	?	b	m
8	f	59	21	?	e	s
9	f	40	10	g	b[e]	m
10	f	50	32	?	h	m
11	f	75	33	?	e	m
12	f	68	45[f]	?	e	m
13	m	52	4	g	e	s
14	f	48	14	?	b	s
15	f	56	2.1	h	h	s
16	f	64	22	h	h	s
17	f	55	16	h	e	m
18	f	75	26	h	h	m
19	f	67	9	h	h	s
20	f	68	14	?	b	s

f, female; m, male.
[a]?, unknown; h, hyperthyroidism; g, goiter.
[b]h, hyperthyroid; e, euthyroid; b, borderline.
[c]s, solitary or predominant nodule; m, two or more autonomous areas.
[d]AFTN (cf. ref. 11).
[e]Hyperthyroid, 3.5 years later.
[f]"Irradiated" prior to operation.

The pathogenesis of postoperative recurrent Plummer's disease is unknown, but three possible mechanisms can be envisaged.

(1) Preoperatively there was a solitary AFTN, which was incompletely excised. The nodules are sometimes only partly encapsulated,[62] and it is probably not unusual that some autonomously functioning tissue remains in situ—possibly too little to be seen by the naked eye but detectable by scintigraphy (ref. 11, Fig. 7).

(2) Preoperatively there was some autonomously functioning thyroid tissue outside circumscribed AFTN, and the former was not removed.

(3) Preoperatively there was no autonomously functioning thyroid tissue; the present disorder arose de novo after surgery, possibly triggered by the intense stimulation of (endogenous) TSH following thyroidectomy.

The first of these mechanisms most probably caused the recurrent toxic nodule in patient no. 5 of our present series,[11] although the second possibility cannot be excluded. Two of the patients of Guinet et al.[71] had a hemithyroidectomy followed by the appearance of an AFTN in the other lobe (mechanism 2 or 3). If the third mechanism is the rule, our therapeutic policy need not be changed. But if a post-operative recurrence of this disease is not so exceptional as we have thought, we may more often favor ^{131}I treatment (or a modified surgical approach). Clearly, this is an important point to be settled. One approach will be the clinical and scintigraphic reevaluation of patients after surgical treatment for Plummer's disease.

All five of Guinet's patients and all but one of ours were female, which may be accidental. More intriguing is the fact that the average age at the time of the present diagnosis, 60 years, hardly surpasses that of all patients with Plummer's disease (58 years). In other words, if a substantial part of these patients had Plummer's disease before operation (mechanism 1 or 2), they were relatively young at that time; average about 40 years. (Some may have been selected for surgery precisely because of their age, but half of them were operated before the advent of ^{131}I therapy.) This could reflect a relatively rapid progression of disease that (as discussed above) may occur in patients under 40 years of age.

SUMMARY—CHAPTER 3

Neither Hamburger nor the discussants have documented morbidity or mortality caused by observing AFTN. We have observed one death from thromboembolism in a patient with a toxic AFTN whose nodule had been known for 20 years. These observations antedated scanning identification of such lesions, however. Since no other evidence has been presented that all AFTN should be ablated, we might rephrase the question to ask if any AFTN should be prophylactically destroyed, and if so which ones and how?

There seems to be agreement that an appreciable number of AFTN will become toxic while being observed, that this is very unlikely in nodules 2.5 cm in diameter or less, that this transformation is an undesirable occurrence in patients over 40 to 45 years of age, and that it occurs more frequently in males. A group of nodules for prophylactic ablation is thus identified.

A further group for such therapy includes patients whose radionuclide images suggest that near total suppression of extranodular tissue has occurred and whose response of TSH to TRH is flat. The nodules in juveniles which Hamburger marks for therapy have in my experience usually had these functional characteristics.

The interesting observation by Hamburger and by Emrich (personal communication) that toxicity usually occurs during the first 2 to 5 years of observation suggests the existence of two groups of AFTN. Those which manifest physical or functional growth during a short period of observation have a much higher risk of eventual toxicity. Those which manifest no change or produce only enough T_4 and T_3 to partially suppress TSH, if watched for 5 years, can in our experience be watched for 20 years.

The choice of either ^{131}I or surgical therapy is probably not of great consequence. We would reiterate the following:

(1) The chances of surgical misadventure are those of anesthetic morbidity and mortality.

(2) The doses of ^{131}I necessary for AFTN of 3 cm or over do not have the documented safety record that is available for the smaller doses used in Graves' disease, thus necessitating age discrimination for large doses of ^{131}I.

(3) Although the AFTN is microscopically a multiple disease in many instances, recurrences after lobectomy have not been of great practical importance.

(4) Radiation of uninvolved thyroid tissue is not only from gamma rays from the AFTN dose but also from beta particles, since the uptake in the suppressed lobe is often not zero.

(5) We have observed just as many incidental cancers in the glands of surgically removed AFTN as have been reported to occur subsequent to ^{131}I therapy.

J. Martin Miller, M.D.

REFERENCES

1. Cope O, Rawson RW, McArthur JW: The hyperfunctioning single adenoma of the thyroid. Surg Gynecol Obstet 84:415, 1947.
2. Dobyns BM, Skanse B, Maloof F: A method for the preoperative estimation of function in thyroid tumors. Its significance in diagnosis and treatment. J. Clin Endocrinol Metab 9:1191, 1949
3. Sheline GE, McCormack K: Solitary hyperfunctioning thyroid nodules. J. Clin Endocrinol Metab 20:1401, 1960.
4. Miller JM, Hamburger JI: The thyroid scintigram. I. The hot nodule. Radiology 84:66, 1965

5. Hamburger JI: Solitary autonomously functioning thyroid lesions. Am J. Med 58:740, 1975

6. Silverstein GE, Burke G, Cogan R: The natural history of the autonomous hyperfunctioning thyroid nodule. Ann Intern Med 67:539, 1967

7. Burman KD, Earll JM. Johnson MC, Wartofsky L: Clinical observations on the solitary autonomous thyroid nodule. Arch Intern Med 134:915, 1974

8. Hamburger JI: Evolution of toxicity in solitary nontoxic autonomously functioning thyroid nodules. J Clin Endocrinol Metab 50:1089, 1980

9. Lobo LCG, Rosenthal D, Fridman J: Evolution of autonomous thyroid nodules. In Cassano C, Andreoli M (eds): Current Topics in Thyroid Research, New York, Academic Press, 1965, p 892

10. Ferraz A. Medeiros-Neto GA, Toledo AC, Kieffer J: Autonomous thyroid nodules. I. A clinical classification and the use of a diagnostic index. J Nucl Med 13:733, 1972

11. Weiner JD, DeVries AA: On the natural history of Plummer's disease. Clin Nucl Med 4:181, 1979

12. Horst W, Rosler H, Schneider C, et al.: Three hundred six cases of toxic adenoma. J Nucl Med 8:515, 1967

13. Hamburger JI: Clinical Exercises in Internal Medicine, Vol. 1. Thyroid Disease. Philadelphia, Saunders, 1978, pp 5–10

14. Hamburger JI, Meier DA: Cancer following treatment of an autonomously functioning thyroid nodule with sodium iodide I-131. Arch Surg 103:762, 1971

15. Lindsay S, Nichols CW, Chaikoff IL: Induction of benign and malignant thyroid neoplasms in the rat. Arch Pathol 81:308, 1966

16. Skillern PG, McCullagh EP, Clamen M: Radioiodine in diagnosis and therapy of hyperthyroidism. Arch Intern Med 110:888, 1962

17. Hamburger JI: Transient thyrotoxicosis associated with acute hemorrhagic infarction of autonomously functioning thyroid nodules. Ann Intern Med 91:406, 1979

18. Miller JM: Radioiodine therapy of the autonomous functioning thyroid. Semin Nucl Med 1:432, 1971

19. Scandellari C: [131]I treatment of toxic autonomous adenoma of the thyroid. In Fiorentino M, Vangelisto R, Grigiolette E (eds): Thyroid Tumors, Lymphomas, and Granulocytic Leukemia. Padova, Piccin, 1972, p 89

20. Blum M, Shenkman L, Hollander CS: The autonomous nodule of the thyroid: correlation of patient age, nodule size, and functional status. Am J Med Sci 269:43, 1975

21. Blum M, Goldman AB, Herskovic A, et al.: Clinical applications of thyroid echography. N Engl J Med 287:1164, 1972

22. Molnar GD, Wilber RD, Lee RE, et al.: On the hyperfunctioning solitary thyroid nodule. Mayo Clin Proc 40:665, 1965

23. Miller JM: Hyperthyroidism from the thyroid follicle with autonomous function. Clin Endocrinol Metab 7:177, 1978

24. Blum M, Norcero MA Jr: Spontaneous resolution of a euthyroid autonomous nodule of the thyroid. Am J Med Sci 264:49, 1972

25. Ermans HM, Camus M: Modifications of thyroid function induced by chronic administration of iodine in the presence of "autonomous thyroid tissue." Acta Endocrinol (Kbh) 70:463, 1972

26. Blum M, Weinberg U, Shenkman L, Hollander CS: Hyperthyroidism after iodinated contrast medium. N Engl J Med 291:24, 1974

27. Blum M, Kranjac T, Park CM, Engleman RM: Thyroid storm after cardiac angiog-

raphy with iodinated contrast medium. Occurrence in a patient with a previously euthyroid autonomous nodule of the thyroid. J Am Med Assoc 235:2324, 1976

28. Hollander CS, Mitsuma T, Nihei N, Shenkman L. Burday SZ, Blum M: Clinical and laboratory observations in cases of triiodothyronine toxicosis confirmed by radioimmunoassay. Lancet 1:609, 1972

29. Popma BH, Cloutier MD, Hayles AB: Thyroid nodule producing T_3 toxicosis in a child. Mayo Clin Proc 48:273, 1973

30. Blum M: Unpublished data

31. Birkhäuser M, Busset, R, Burer, T, Burger A: Diagnosis of hyperthyroidism when serum thyroxine alone is raised. Lancet 2:53, 1977

32. Hayles AB, Kennedy RLS, Woolner LB, et al.: Nodular lesions of the thyroid gland in children. J Clin Endocrinol Metab 16:158, 1956

33. Hopwood NS, Carroll RG, Kenny FM, Foley TP Jr.: Functioning thyroid masses in childhood and adolescence. Pediatrics 89:710, 1976

34. Blum M, Biller BJ, Bergman DA: The thyroid cork, obstruction of the thoracic inlet due to retroclavicular goiter. J Am Med Assoc. 227:189, 1974

35. Fisher DA: Thyroid nodules in childhood and their management. Pediatrics 89:866, 1976

36. Johnson PC, Beierwaltes WH: Reliability of scintiscanning nodular goiters in judging presence or absence of carcinoma. J Clin Endocrinol Metab 15:865, 1955

37. Meadows PM: Scintillation scanning in the management of clinically autonomous nodules. J Am Med Assoc 177:229, 1961

38. Molnar GD, Child DS, Woolner LB: Histologic evidence of malignancy of the thyroid gland bearing a "hot" nodule. J Clin Endocrinol Metab 181:1132, 1958

39. Becker FO, Economou PG, Schwartz TB: The occurrence of carcinoma in "hot" thyroid nodules. Ann Intern Med 58:877, 1963

40. Woolner LB, Lemmon ML, Beahrs DH, Black BM, Keating FR Jr: Occult papillary carcinoma of the thyroid. Study 140 cases observed in a 30-year period. J Clin Endocrinol Metab 20:89, 1960

41. Davis PJ, Davis FB: Hyperthyroidism in patients over the age of 60 years. Medicine 53:161, 1974

42. Plummer HS: The clinical and pathological relationship of simple and exophthalmic goiter. Am J Med Sci 146:790, 1913

43. Mayo CH, Plummer HS: The Thyroid Gland. St. Louis, Mosby, 1926

44. Dobyns BM, Sheline GE, Workman JB, et al.: Malignant and benign neoplasms of the thyroid in patients treated for hyperthyroidism: a report of the Cooperative Thyrotoxicosis Therapy Followup Study. J Clin Endocrinol Metab 38:976, 1974

45. Vagenakis AG, Braverman LE, Azizi F, et al.: Recovery of pituitary thyrotrophic function after withdrawal of prolonged thyroid-suppression therapy. N Engl J Med 292:681, 1975

46. Lindsay S: The experimental production of thyroid neoplasms in the rat by irradiation. In Young S, Inmer DR (eds): Thyroid Neoplasia. New York, Academic Press, 1968, pp 279–287

47. Okerlund M, Sommers J, Beckmann A, et al: Studies on the pathogenesis of radiation-induced thyroid tumors. Paper presented at Annual Meeting of the American Thyroid Association, Cleveland, Sept 7–10, 1977

48. Demeester-Mirkine N, Ermans AM: Euthyroid hot nodules: a physiological approach. In Irvine WJ (ed): Thyrotoxicosis. Edinburgh, Livingstone, 1968, pp 68–75

49. Demeester-Mirkine N, VanSande J, Corvilain J, Dumont JE: Benign thyroid nodule

with normal iodine trap and defective organification. J Clin Endocrinol Metab 41:1169, 1975

50. Ermans AM, Camus M: Modifications of thyroid function induced by chronic administration of iodide in the presence of "autonomous" thyroid tissue. Acta Endocrinol 70:463, 1972

51. Hales, I, Cowie G, Myhill J, Reeve TS: Autonomous functioning nodules and thyrotoxicosis. Med J Aust 1:198, 1967

52. Jellins J, Kossoff G, Wiseman J, Reeve TS, Hales IB: Ultrasonic grey scale visualization of the thyroid gland. Ultrasound Med Biol 1:405, 1975

53. Nelson NC: Thyrotoxicosis. In Hardy JO (ed): The Thyroid Gland. Rhoads Textbook of Surgery. Philadelphia, Lippincott, 1977, p 689

54. Charkes ND: Scintigraphic evaluation of nodular goiter. Semin Nucl Med 1:316, 1971

55. Wiener JD: A systematic approach to the diagnosis of Plummer's disease (autonomous goiter), with a review of 224 cases. Neth J Med 18:218, 1975

56. Miller JM, Horn RC, Block MA: The evolution of toxic nodular goiter. Arch Intern Med 113:72, 1964

57. Miller JM: Application of scintillation scanning in thyroid disease. In Quinn JL III (ed): Scintillation Scanning in Clinical Medicine. Philadelphia, Saunders, 1964, p 43

58 Selby JB, McClellan JT: Hyperthyroidism: Graves' and Plummer's disease. Clin Med 75/3:21, 1968

59. Rosenbloom AL: Definition of Plummer disease. J Pediatr 92:691, 1978

60. Wiener JD: [Reply to ref. 59.] J Pediatr 92:691, 1978

61. Wiener JD: Autonomously functioning thyroid nodules (Plummer's disease). J Pediatr 91:682, 1977

62. Wiener JD, Frensdorf EL: Thyroid autonomy (Plummer's disease) with contralateral malignancy—mere coincidence? Acta Med Scand 200:509, 1976

63. Guinet P, Tourniaire J, Guillaud M, Briere J, Dalmais J, Chalendar D: Adénome toxique et cancer thyroïdien. Ann Endocrinol (Paris) 32:513, 1971

64. Thijs LG: De koude schildkliernodus. Thesis, Free University, Amsterdam, 1973, p 16

65. Mortensen JD, Woolner LB, Bennett WA: Gross and microscopic findings in clinically normal thyroid glands. J Clin Endocrinol Metab 15:1270, 1955

66. Reinwein D, Gieshoff B, Ufacorro U, Interthal I, Strötges W, Emrich D: The natural course of the autonomous thyroid nodule. Presented at 9th Annual Meeting of European Thyroid Association, Berlin, 1978, Ann Endocrinol (Paris) 39:59A, 1978

67. Coindet JF: Nouvelles recherches sur les effets de l'iode, et sur les précautions à suivre dans le traitement du goître par ce nouveau remède. Ann Chim Phys 16:252, 1821

68. Wiener JD: Über Kropf, Hyperthyreose und Jodbehandlung—Hommage à Jean-François Coindet de Genève. Schweiz Med Wochenschr 110:1784, 1980

69. Livadas DP, Koutras DA, Souvatzoglou A, Beckers C: The toxic effects of small iodine supplements in patients with autonomous thyroid nodules. Clin Endocrinol 7:121, 1977

70. Höfer R, Vetter H: Scanning in Noncancerous Thyroid Disease. Medical Radioisotope Scanning. Vienna, IAEA, 1959, p 213

71. Guinet P, Tourniaire J, Briere J, Pousset G: L'adénome toxique après intervention sur la thyroïde. Lyon Méd 200:459, 1968

Chapter 4

Is Prevention of Hyperthyroidism Complicating Pregnancy Justification for Routine Ablative Therapy for Hyperthyroidism in Women in the Childbearing Years?

Joel I. Hamburger, M.D.
Sheldon S. Stoffer, M.D.

INTRODUCTION

Although hyperthyroidism is a common disease of women in the childbearing years, hyperthyroidism in pregnancy is uncommon. Hyperthyroidism reduces fertility and this is the principal factor limiting the number of pregnant hyperthyroid patients. Reports dealing with hyperthyroidism in pregnancy almost always include less than 50 patients. Since July 1961, 1269 hyperthyroid women between the ages of 19 and 39 years have been treated at Northland Thyroid Laboratory (NTL), but only 50 were pregnant. When the initial treatment of hyperthyroidism is surgery or radioactive iodine this reduces the number of patients who will subsequently have pregnancies complicated by hyperthyroidism.

Pregnant hyperthyroid patients are usually treated with antithyroid drugs.[1-9] Radioactive iodine (^{131}I) is contraindicated since it would cross the placenta to the fetus. Thyroidectomy has been employed with success in later stages of pregnancy,[10,11] but this treatment is not popular because of concern for fetal wastage.[8]

Probably most pregnant hyperthyroid patients are not treated in medical centers, and thus are not included in published reports. Therefore it is impossible to know how many are treated annually nationwide. More important, what the outcome of these complicated pregnancies has been is also unknown. If data in the medical literature[5] reflect what might be expected from treatment by experienced specialists, then it must be concluded that these are high risk pregnancies. When less experienced physicians monitor treatment the results can be disastrous. We have recently reviewed a case (for the plaintiff's attorney) of a child with permanent mental retardation resulting from overdosage of methimazole to the mother. The hyperthyroidism was managed by a family practitioner without appropriate monitoring.

In spite of appreciation of the special maternal and fetal risks of pregnancy complicated by hyperthyroidism, study of the literature indicates a remarkable indifference to the prevention of these complicated pregnancies. Patients treated once for hyperthyroidism during pregnancy have even been permitted to continue antithyroid drugs (ATD) after delivery and experience two or more pregnancies complicated by hyperthyroidism,[2,6,9] even when the initial pregnancy produced a damaged infant.[9]

The treatment of hyperthyroidism most often advised for young women is antithyroid drugs, a treatment which prolongs hyperthyroidism while improving chances of conception. Ironically, ATD are often advised by physicians who consider themselves conservative. They avoid the use of ^{131}I therapy out of concern for genetic effects. Similarly, conservative physicians prefer to avoid the risks of thyroidectomy. This "conservative" treatment exposes women to the risks of pregnancy complicated by hyperthyroidism. These pregnancies terminate unfavorably often enough to permit the argument that ^{131}I therapy or thyroidectomy employed before the patient becomes pregnant is actually the safer approach.

The above considerations have led us to ask the following questions:

(1) Is prevention of hyperthyroidism complicating pregnancy justification for routine ablative therapy for hyperthyroidism in women in the childbearing years?

(2) How often is there an opportunity for ablative (^{131}I or surgical) therapy of hyperthyroidism before the patient becomes pregnant?

EXPERIENCE OF NORTHLAND THYROID LABORATORY

There were 50 patients with both pregnancy and hyperthyroidism. Twenty-six of the 50 patients had recognizable hyperthyroidism from 1 to 12 months before becoming pregnant. Five patients were treated unsuccessfully with [131]I. For three of these patients the poor results were attributed to a small dose of [131]I. The remaining 21 patients were treated with antithyroid drugs (17 patients), Lugol's solution (two patients), kelp (one patient), and no treatment (one patient). Therefore, for at least 24 patients more aggressive initial therapy could have prevented pregnancies complicated by hyperthyroidism.

Two patients required thyroidectomy while pregnant because they developed toxic reactions to both ATD. Nine patients, including four of the five patients who had previously received ^{131}I therapy, experienced remissions in the hyperthyroidism in the third trimester of pregnancy and remained euthyroid subsequently. Five patients were lost to follow-up before or after the pregnancies terminated. Forty-two of the 45 infants were full term and normal. There was one premature birth, one spontaneous abortion at 3 months, and one stillbirth at 6 months. No fetal goiters were observed. The 34 patients who still required propylthiouracil

(PTU) treatment after delivery were advised to have ^{131}I therapy or thyroidectomy. Thirty-three elected ^{131}I; one preferred operation. None of our patients has had a second pregnancy complicated by hyperthyroidism.

DISCUSSION

Pregnancy Complicated by Hyperthyroidism Is Avoidable

Pregnancy complicated by hyperthyroidism is uncommon, but continues to exact a fetal toll in terms of wastage and thyroid abnormalities.[2,6,9] The frequency of these complicated pregnancies could be reduced if definitive (^{131}I or thyroidectomy) rather than suppressive (ATD) therapy were employed for hyperthyroid women for whom the possibility of childbearing can be anticipated in the near future. For most hyperthyroid patients there is time for such a choice before the pregnancy intervenes.[12] This was the case for 26 of our 50 pregnant hyperthyroid patients, and for 83 of 123 patients recently reported.[1,2,5,6,11]

The Risk of Pregnancy Complicated by Hyperthyroidism

To assess the risk of this dual condition, and thus to determine how necessary it might be to prevent it, a review was undertaken of 12 papers published since 1960, dealing with a total of 411 pregnancies in 364 women.[1-11,13] In the first 20 weeks of pregnancy the fetal loss was 5%, not different from that expected for uncomplicated pregnancies. However, in the remaining 392 pregnancies, after the 20th week of gestation, there were 26 (6.6%) fetal or neonatal deaths, compared to an expected incidence of 1.6%. By chi-square analysis this is a highly significant increase ($p < 0.001$). These late gestational losses occurred in all reports with roughly equal frequency. By contrast, fetal thyroid abnormalities which might be attributable to ATD were not evenly distributed. Six of 16 such abnormalities were included in two papers with the same senior author.[9,13] Three reports, including 96 pregnancies, had no fetal thyroid abnormalities.[2,5,8]

Neither a 10.6% incidence of prematurity, nor a 3.5% incidence of nonthyroidal congenital anomalies, differed from that associated with uncomplicated pregnancies. The possibility that ATD treatment may adversely affect the future intellectual capacity of the fetus has been suggested.[4] There are no data to support this suggestion, as long as fetal hypothyroidism is avoided. However, Mann et al.[14] have shown that some of the progeny of hypothyroxinemic mothers have depressed intelligence quotients. Therefore, this is a potential risk of improperly monitored ATD treatment.

Maternal complications in the 12 papers reviewed included two deaths, three episodes of thyroid crisis, six episodes of preeclampsia, and congestive heart failure in two patients.

Even those with considerable success in the management of pregnant hyperthyroid patients can appreciate that antithyroid drugs are an added risk to the fetus which may be beyond the physician's control. Women do not always cooperate either in self-administration of medication or in returning for regular follow-up examinations. However, lack of concern, or lack of foresight for this risk, was demonstrated by the authors of nine of the 12 papers reviewed, since they permitted women to have two and even three successive pregnancies while taking antithyroid drugs, rather than initiating definitive treatment after the first episode.

Advantages of Definitive (^{131}I or Surgery) Therapy for Hyperthyroid Women Planning Childbearing

Definitive treatment of hyperthyroid women who plan childbearing in the near future would seem likely to improve the fetal salvage rate and eliminate antithyroid drug–induced goiter, without any appreciable increase in the risk of other fetal problems. Three recent reports deal with ^{131}I therapy for a total of 190 children with hyperthyroidism.[15–17] These patients subsequently had 193 pregnancies with no increase in fetal loss or anomalies. Indeed, two reports on the subsequent progeny of young patients treated with cancer doses of ^{131}I revealed no increase in these fetal complications.[18,19] These results are consistent with calculations indicating that ovarian radiation from ^{131}I therapy should not materially increase the risk of fetal anomalies.[20]

Some physicians still favor thyroidectomy for young hyperthyroid patients. Operative risks have been greatly reduced in recent years. However, there is no assurance that the enviable records achieved in major medical centers can be duplicated in the average community hospital. In one report,[8] hypocalcemic crisis occurred during delivery in one of seven women treated surgically earlier in the pregnancy. A second woman also developed hypoparathyroidism, and one had persistent hyperthyroidism. When definitive therapy is elected, the choice between ^{131}I and thyroidectomy must take into consideration the relative risks of the two treatments. This may be influenced by the talent available in any given locale.

We no longer see any point in continuing to argue that ^{131}I is a safer form of ablative therapy than thyroidectomy. Those who refuse to pay heed to the safety record of 40 years' experience with ^{131}I therapy, to the scientific data supporting the safety of this treatment, and who prefer that their patients take the established risks of thyroidectomy[21] will not be persuaded otherwise. For the issue under consideration, the form of ablative therapy selected is not crucial.

Risks of Definitive Therapy

Neither method of definitive therapy is risk free. Hypothyroidism is a potential problem with serious reproductive implications. This may be avoided by the use of thyroid hormone, but patients may fail to cooperate. Still, the treatment of hypothyroidism is a less formidable undertaking than monitoring of ATD during pregnancy. In the final analysis, there is no risk-free method of dealing with the implications of hyperthyroidism for women in the childbearing years. Although use of ATD may appeal to the conservative instincts of many physicians, our analysis suggests that definitive alternatives may be safer.

Definitive Therapy of Hyperthyroidism in Young Women is Preferable to ATD

It should not be too difficult to convince most prudent physicians that patients who have experienced one episode of pregnancy complicated by hyperthyroidism should not persist with ATD therapy if further pregnancies are planned and the hyperthyroidism is not in remission after delivery. This advice would be reasonable even if that pregnancy terminated with a normal infant. After all, why tempt fate? The many opportunities for errors (patient as well as physician) with serious consequences make the deliberate exposure to repeat episodes poor judgment, in our opinion. If this point is accepted, then it might be easier to take the next step of advising definitive rather than ATD treatment to prevent even the initial pregnancy complicated by hyperthyroidism. We consider it good judgment to advise women who plan or might plan pregnancy within 2 or 3 years to avoid ATD therapy. Similarly, we warn young women who wish to be treated with ATD that in the event circumstances change and childbearing should be contemplated, ATD should be abandoned in favor of definitive therapy. We suspect that this advice is not given more often simply because physicians do not consider the long-term implications of the treatment they advise. They fail to think ahead.

COMMENTARY

Demetrios A. Koutras, M.D.

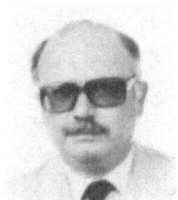

A commentary is supposed to be a criticism, that is, a difference of opinion. Since both the authors of the chapter to be criticized as well as the author writing the criticism are presumably reasonable experts in their field, such a criticism will rarely mean a radical disagreement. Much more often it will consist simply of a relative difference in the emphasis for or against a procedure. This commentary will follow this general rule rather than be an exception to it.

The basic question is whether conservative treatment of hyperthyroidism with antithyroid drugs (ATD) is ever justified. If not, then women of childbearing age should have ablative treatment, for the same reason as every other hyperthyroid patient. If conservative treatment is justified, then it should be considered whether such women present different indications than the general thyrotoxic population.

Advantages of ATD Therapy

All three treatment modalities available have merits and disadvantages. ATD treatment has the merit of leaving the thyroid gland intact, it does not lead to permanent hypothyroidism, and it may restore the pituitary-thyroid axis to normal. After all, ATD reduce the concentration and production of thyroid stimulating autoantibodies.[22,23] So, ATD may be considered a treatment actually directed at the etiology of the disease, whereas ablative treatment simply reduces the amount of hyperfunctioning tissue without removing the cause. Perhaps, for this reason in some cases eye signs may improve after ATD.

Disadvantages of ATD, ^{131}I, and Surgery

On the other hand, drug therapy requires continuous treatment for 1 to 2 years, in spite of some reports to the contrary,[24] and patient compliance is essential. However well the treatment is carried out, a proportion of patients relapse, and this is the main disadvantage. Ablative treatment by surgery or ^{131}I is fast and effective. Nevertheless, these treatments also have undesirable side effects. Surgery by experienced practitioners is associated with a negligible mortality, but other complications are not negligible.[21] Hypoparathyroidism, hoarseness, and hypothyroidism occur quite frequently, more often than many surgeons admit. Although Girling and Murley[25] acknowledged only one case of parathyroid insufficiency in 123 patients operated, Gouillat et al.[26] reported hypoparathyroidism in 2.7% of 1911 thyroidectomies. The proportion increased to 8.3% in the patients operated upon for Graves' disease. Hoarseness is another common complaint, usually attributed to injury of the recurrent laryngeal nerve. Gabriel and Chilla[27] reported permanent paralysis of the recurrent laryngeal nerve in 2.1% of patients and temporary paralysis in another 4.2%. More important, 49.3% of their cases had some hoarseness, even if the recurrent laryngeal nerve was left apparently intact. My experience is consistent with this. Many patients notice a change in the quality of the voice even if there is no paralysis of a major nerve trunk. Undoubtedly, surgery for Graves' disease, when a bilateral subtotal thyroidectomy is performed, results in more complications than operation for a single cold nodule, where one thyroid lobe is usually left alone. Furthermore, reports reviewed in this and other similar papers emanate from specialized centers. What the morbidity rate is for general surgeons doing occasional thyroid surgery is left to the reader's guess.

Radioiodine therapy does not have the undesirable side effects of subtotal thyroidectomy. Hypothyroidism, however, is quite frequent, both following surgery and especially after [131]I. This is so well known that no further documentation is required.

Problems with Hypothyroid Patients After Ablative Therapy

Hypothyroidism can be relieved with one or more thyroxine tablets daily, but substitution treatment may not be as simple as it seems. First of all, patient compliance is important. Since hypothyroidism is permanent, substitution treatment will be needed when the patient grows old, debilitated, uncooperative, and possibly confused. Second, fairly often patients on thyroid substitution complain of practically anything imaginable, attribute the complaints to the thyroxine, and it takes considerable effort to persuade them that thyroxine is not responsible for those symptoms. Some patients with similar complaints simply stop the treatment without consulting an endocrinologist. Third, if the patient acquires a heart problem including tachycardia among its other manifestations, it is very difficult to persuade both the patient and the cardiologist that thyroxine treatment is not responsible.

How Often Does ATD Treatment Lead to Permanent Remission?

This is the crux of the matter. If permanent remission is the rule, then a course in cooperative persons is indicated to avoid the late inconveniences outlined above. If permanent remissions are rare, then there is no point trying ATD. Ablative treatment should be undertaken as soon as possible.

There is no consensus on this matter, even among leading experts in the field. The late pioneer of ATD, E. B. Astwood, and his followers favored ATD treatment of hyperthyroidism, reporting a long-term remission rate of 54%.[28] Many other experts in the United States report lower remission rates, and favor a more radical approach. This low permanent remission rate reported in the United States may be related to the high iodine intake in that country.[29] However, in Greece I have obtained a 60% remission rate in 75 patients treated with carbimazole.[30] Good results have also been reported in other countries,[31,32] whereas Hart in Canada had a success of 33%.[33]

In my series, all 75 patients were treated with carbimazole, starting with 30 mg/day and reducing the dose gradually as indicated.[30] T_3 was given in a daily dose of 30 μg. This dose was so chosen because it prevents severe hypothyroidism without providing full substitution for the hormone output of the gland. Thus, drug-induced hypothyroidism is reduced in degree but not abolished, so that the physician will appreciate when it is necessary to decrease the carbimazole dose. Patients were seen approximately every 6 weeks and the treatment continued for at least 18 months. If at the end of this period the maintenance dose of carbimazole was more than 7.5 mg/day, treatment was continued for an additional number of months with a reduced dose. All patients were followed for at least 6 months after the end of the treatment, usually to 1 to 2 years or more.

Clinical Findings Related to Success or Failure with ATD

Patient thyroid status when last seen was euthyroid in 60% of both sexes. However, 70% of those aged 25 to 45 years remained euthyroid, compared to 30% of the younger and 42% of the older patients ($P < 0.025$). When the goiter was not larger than 50 g (i.e., twice normal), the long-term remission rate was 68%, compared to 46% for patients with larger glands. Surprisingly, a reduction of the gland size during treatment was not itself a reliable sign of a good prognosis. When definite eye signs were present, 43% of the patients remained in remission, whereas the proportion rose to 67% in those without ophthalmopathy. The most important factor was whether the dose of carbimazole could be reduced to 5 mg/ day. If so, the chance of a lasting remission was 75%; if not, 46% ($P < 0.02$). Of course, some patients without a relapse when last seen may have a new thyrotoxic episode several years later, and so a long-term remission (for 1 to 2 years or more) is not synonymous with a permanent remission. Nevertheless, after the first 6 months the recurrence rate falls exponentially. Also, several patients have preferred a course of drug therapy every 5 or 10 years to ablative treatment. Careful patient selection can thus greatly improve the long-term remission rate.

ATD therapy should be tried as permanent treatment only in cases of Graves' disease. It is futile to do the same for toxic nodular goiter, either of the single adenoma type or the multiple autonomous foci variety, where the chances of permanent remission are practically nil. Ablative treatment should be offered to Graves' patients with the HLA antigens B8 or DRW3 and also to those in whom autoantibodies binding to the TSH receptor persist after treatment.[34] Thyroid suppressibility can also be used for predicting the long-term outcome, but is not as reliable as HLA typing and the assay of immunostimulins. A low maintenance dose of the drug is another favorable sign.[28,30,33] On the other hand, a relapse after a full course of ATD should be considered a bad prognostic feature. Furthermore, if a cold nodule is present in a gland with Graves' disease, surgery should be performed. In 65 such patients we have found a malignancy rate of 21.5%, compared to 12.1% in 859 euthyroid patients with cold nodules.[35] This could not be due to patient selection, because Graves' patients are more likely to be operated upon than euthyroid patients with cold thyroid nodules.

Treatment of Hyperthyroidism in the Young Woman Planning Pregnancy

Ablative treatment should be offered to such a patient more liberally than under other circumstances, but this need not be an absolute rule. ATD therapy may be undertaken if the woman does not desire an immediate pregnancy and if clinical findings suggest chances of a lasting remission are good. Ablative treatment is not a panacea. It usually means conversion of the hyperthyroid state to hypothyroidism, and the need for lifelong follow-up is not eliminated. The possibility of long-term or rare complications from ^{131}I therapy is still considered in most European centers, and the liberal administration of radioactive substances is always regarded as undesirable. Some people are reluctant even to order a simple radiograph without a clear indication, let alone administer a therapeutic dose of ^{131}I and irradiate both the patient and his environment.

What Are the Risks of Hyperthyroidism During Pregnancy?

If a young woman becomes thyrotoxic during pregnancy, despite favorable prognostic features (above), this need not lead to a catastrophe. She can be handled with ATD with a fair amount of safety both for her and for the fetus. In the hands of experienced physicians, the subsequent intellectual and physical development of the progeny is normal.[36,37]

The author has personally treated several pregnant thyrotoxic patients without harm to the children born subsequently. The dose of carbimazole given was 15 mg/day for florid cases, decreasing as quickly as possible to a maintenance dose of 2.5 to 7.5 mg/day or stopping it altogether, always preferring undertreatment rather than overtreatment. The patients were followed-up every month. In addition to a meticulous clinical examination, tomography of the Achilles tendon reflex was performed and estimates of serum T_4 and RT_3U (resin uptake of radioactive T_3) were obtained, allowing the calculation of the FTI (free thyroxine index). This should always be done in pregnancy because total serum T_4 alone is not a reliable index: it is increased by the estrogen-mediated increase of the thyroxine-binding globulin which occurs in pregnancy. Of course, if the true free thyroxine concentration is available, it should be preferred to the indirectly calculated FTI.

Most other authors also consider small doses of ATD as the treatment of choice in thyrotoxicosis during pregnancy.[38,39] It may well be that propylthiouracil is safer than carbimazole for the pregnant woman.[36,37] In any case, thyroid hormones should not be given together with the ATD. Thyroid hormones do not cross the placenta in amounts adequate to protect the fetus, whereas they increase the dose of ATD required by the mother.[40] If in the future new thyroid analogs or new modes of administration permit the delivery to the fetus of thyroactive substances, this position may change.

Needless to say, such a treatment should not be undertaken by those without sufficient experience. What may happen under these circumstances is well illustrated in the patients described by Hamburger and Stoffer. Such a deplorable outcome as permanent mental retardation of the child should not happen if the mother is properly treated and excessive doses of ATD are avoided.

In conclusion, childbearing age is a further indication for ablative treatment, but not an absolute one. If the chances of a permanent remission are good, conservative drug treatment may be tried. If a pregnant woman is thyrotoxic, the situation should be handled by an experienced physician; otherwise the results may be disastrous.

COMMENTARY

James C. Sisson, M.D.

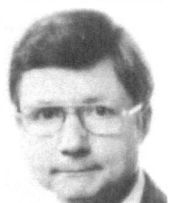

Hamburger and Stoffer make a compelling case for ablative therapy in young women with hyperthyroidism. Without prompt thyroidectomy or expeditious administration of ^{131}I, persistent hyperthyroidism frequently complicates pregnancy, and attempts to control the disease then, too often harm fetus or mother. Generally speaking, physicians would be wise to follow the advice offered in this chapter.

However, a broader and somewhat philosophic view is worthy of our thought and hope, if not of our current practice. The ablative treatments of hyperthyroidism destroy an organ and in so doing they substitute one disease (albeit a more easily treated one) for another. But ideally, therapies should leave no residual of altered homeostasis. This was the goal of treatment with antithyroid drugs. Whereas in the United States permanent remissions after withdrawal of propylthiouracil or methimazole are now uncommon,[40] a year or two of drug administration still eliminates hyperthyroidism in over half the patients found in some areas of the United Kingdom.[41] Similar remission rates following a period of drug usage were also recorded in the United States in previous decades.[42] The causes of the decline in the permanent effectiveness of the drugs have never been satisfactorily defined; the responsible factors could disappear as mysteriously as they came. Furthermore, we are only beginning to comprehend how medications may attack the basic nature (presumed autoimmunity) of the hyperthyroidism of Graves' disease.[43,44] It is then possible, through a good deal of luck and careful scientific inquiry, that high incidences of success will again favor patients who are given antithyroid drugs.

Thus, for a cooperative and fully informed woman suffering from hyperthyroidism, a trial of propylthiouracil or methimazole could be undertaken. Contraception would be mandatory until treatment and hyperthyroidism were ended. The trial would cease after a predetermined period of 1 or 2 years. The criteria for remission would be rigorous and unmistakenly fulfilled before pregnancy is sanctioned: clinical well being, normal thyroid size, normal concentration of serum hormones, and normal responses of thyrotropin to injected thyrotropin-releasing hormone and of radioiodine uptake to suppressive doses of thyroid hormone.[45] Failure to fulfill the criteria would constitute a prescription for ablative therapy.

In summary, ablative therapy should be the rule for women who, in their child-bearing years, develop hyperthyroidism. However, rare exceptions can be envisioned. And we should not lose hope that better treatments will be found.

SUMMARY—CHAPTER 4

It is of interest to note that both Koutras, who has achieved success with antithyroid drugs in 60% of his patients and Sisson, who seems to agree with the American reports of much poorer results, came to virtually identical conclusions with respect to the treatment of hyperthyroid patients in the childbearing years. Ablative therapy should be the rule; however, exceptions may be made for those patients who have clinical findings favorable for antithyroid drug therapy and are willing to postpone childbearing for 1 to 2 years. This advice makes sense. One cannot help but wonder why it is so seldom heeded, even in large teaching centers where patients have been allowed to have two or even three episodes of pregnancy complicated by the need for continued treatment with antithyroid drugs. To this author the responsibility for this attitude lies with some of our leading teachers who still advise against radioactive iodine therapy in younger women. Because most physicians have little enthusiasm for surgical management when an effective nonsurgical alternative is available, antithyroid drug therapy can become the treatment of choice by default. Experts who teach this approach are usually able to deal with the occasional patient who becomes pregnant while on antithyroid drugs without a disaster. However, many hyperthyroid patients are not treated by experts. Nonexperts seldom publish their experiences. Hence one cannot do more than appreciate the potential risk of antithyroid drug therapy in pregnant hyperthyroid patients when managed by nonexperts. Because of this risk, in my opinion, experts who are teachers and molders of the therapeutic habits of the medical profession at large might do well to consider the consequences of their teaching in terms of the relative risk of therapeutic misadventure when treatment is monitored by the average physician, rather than by the physician expert.

Joel I. Hamburger, M.D.

REFERENCES

1. Asper SP, London F: Thyrotoxicosis and pregnancy. Trans Am Clin Climatol Assoc 72:110, 1960
2. Herbst AL, Selenkow HA: Hyperthyroidism during pregnancy. N Engl J Med 273:627, 1965

3. Levy RP, Kopelson M. Ryan KJ: Hyperthyroidism during pregnancy. N Engl J Med 274:165, 1966

4. Werner SC: Hyperthyroidism in the pregnant woman and the neonate. J Clin Endocrinol 27:1637, 1967

5. Bokat MA: Treatment of hyperthyroidism during pregnancy. In Astwood EB, Cassidy C (eds): Clinical Endocrinology II. New York, Grune & Stratton, 1968, pp 236–243

6. Ayromlooi J, Zervoudakis IA, Sadaghat A: Thyrotoxicosis in pregnancy. Am J. Obstet Gynecol 117:818, 1973

7. Goluboff LG, Sisson JC, Hamburger JI: Hyperthyroidism associated with pregnancy. Obstet Gynecol 44:107, 1974

8. Worley RJ, Crosby WM: Hyperthyroidism during pregnancy. Am J Obstet Gynecol 119:150, 1974

9. Majtaba Q, Burrow GN: Treatment of hyperthyroidism in pregnancy with propylthiouracil and methimazole. Obstet Gynecol 46:282, 1975

10. Hawe P: Pregnancy and thyrotoxicosis. Br Med J 2:817, 1962

11. Talbert LM, Thomas CG, Holt WA, Rankin P: Hyperthyroidism during pregnancy. Obstet Gynecol 36:779, 1970

12. Reinfrank RF: Hyperthyroidism and pregnancy. South Med J 64:299, 1971

13. Burrow GN: Neonatal goiter after maternal propylthiouracil therapy. J Clin Endocrinol 25:403, 1965

14. Mann EB, Holden RH, Jones WS: Thyroid function in human pregnancy. Am J Obstet Gynecol 109:12, 1971

15. Starr P, Jaffe HL, Oettinger L: Later results of ^{131}I treatment of hyperthyroidism in 73 children and adolescents: 1967 followup. J Nucl Med 10:586, 1969

16. Hayek A, Chapmen EM, Crawford JD: Long-term results of treatment of thyrotoxicosis in children and adolescents with radioactive iodine. N Engl J Med 283:949, 1970

17. Safa AM, Schumacher OP, Rodriguez-Antunez A: Long-term follow-up results in children and adolescents treated with radioactive iodine (^{131}I) for hyperthyroidism. N Engl J Med 292:167, 1975

18. Sarkar SD, Beierwaltes WH, Gill SP, Cowley BJ: Subsequent fertility and birth histories of children and adolescents treated with ^{131}I for thyroid cancer. J Nucl Med 17:460, 1976

19. Rosvoll RV, Winship T: Thyroid carcinoma and pregnancy. In Cassano C, Andreoli M (eds): Thyroid Research. New York, Academic Press, 1965, pp 1042–1044

20. Robertson JS, Gorman CA: Gonadal radiation dose and its genetic significance in radioiodine therapy of hyperthyroidism. J Nucl Med 17:826, 1976

21. Foster RS Jr: Morbidity and mortality after thyroidectomy. Surg Gynecol Obstet 146:423, 1978

22. Beech K, Nistrup Madsen S, Thomsen M, Svejgaard A: The influence of treatment on thyroid stimulating antibodies in Graves' disease. European Thyroid Association 10th Annual Meeting, Abstract No. 99, Newcastle upon Tyne, July 2–6, 1979

23. McGregor AM, McLachlan SM, Rooke P, Rees Smith B, and Hall R: The influence of methimazole on the thyroidal autoimmune response in vitro. Eighth International Thyroid Congress, Abstract No. 78, Sydney, Australia, February 3–8, 1980

24. Greer MA, Kammer H, Bouma DJ: Short-term antithyroid therapy for the thyrotoxicosis of Graves' disease. N Engl J Med 297:173, 1977

25. Girling JA, Murley RS: Parathyroid insufficiency after thyroidectomy. Br Med J 1:1323, 1963
26. Gouillat C, Bouchet A, Soustelle J: Le risque parathyroidien dans la chirurgie du corps thyroïde. J Chir (Paris) 116:505, 1979
27. Gabriel P, Chilla R: Dysphonie nach Strumektomie. Kehlkopf und Stimmveränderungen als Folge von Schilddrusenoperationen. Chirurg 49:576, 1978
28. Hershman JM, Givens JR, Cassidy CE, Astwood EB: Long-term outcome of hyperthyroidism treated with antithyroid drugs. J Clin Endocrinol Metab 26:803, 1966
29. Wartofsky, L: Low remission after therapy for Graves' disease. Possible relation of dietary iodine with antithyroid therapy results. JAMA 226:1083, 1973
30. Koutras DA: Treatment of Graves' disease with carbimazole. Mater Med Greca 4:569, 1976
31. Hung W, Wilkins L, Blizzard R: Medical therapy of thyrotoxicosis in children. Pediatrics 30:17, 1962
32. Horster FA, Klein E, Oberdisse K, Reinwein D: Ergebnisse der Behandlung von Hyperthyreosen mit antithyreoidalen Substanzen. Dtsch Med Wochenschr 90:377, 1965
33. Hart IR: Predictors of relapse after antithyroid drug therapy for hyperthyroid Graves' disease. Eighth International Thyroid Congress, Abstract No. 79, Sydney, Australia, February 3-8, 1980
34. McGregor AM, Rees Smith B, Hall R, Petersen MM, Miller M, Dewar PJ: Prediction of relapse in hyperthyroid Graves' disease. Lancet 1:1101, 1980
35. Livadas D, Psarras A, Koutras DA: Malignant cold thyroid nodules in hyperthyroidism. Br J Surg 63:726, 1976
36. Burrow GN, Bartsocas C, Klatskin EH, Grunt JA: Children exposed in utero to propylthiouracil. Subsequent intellectual and physical development. Am J Dis Child 116:161, 1968
37. McCarrol AM, Hutchinson M, McAuley R, Montgomery DAD: Long-term assessment of children exposed in utero to carbimazole. Arch Dis Child 51:532, 1976
38. Emrich D, Bay V, Freyschmidt P, Hackenberg K, Herrmann J, von zur Muhlen A, Pickardt CR, Schneider C, Scriba PC, Stubbe P: Therapie der Schilddrüsenüberfunktion. Dtsch Med Wochenschr 102:1261, 1977
39. Burrow GN: Hyperthyroidism during pregnancy. N Engl J Med 298:150, 1978
40. Mestman JH, Manning PR, Hodgman J: Hyperthyroidism and pregnancy. Arch Intern Med 134:434, 1974
41. Alexander WD, McLarty DG, Horton P, Pharmakiotis AD: Sequential assessment during drug treatment of thyrotoxicosis. Clin Endocrinol 2:43, 1973
42. Solomon DH, Beck JC, VanderLaan WP, Astwood EB: Prognosis of hyperthyroidism treated by antithyroid drugs. JAMA 152:201, 1953
43. McGregor AM, Petersen MM, McLochlan JM, et al.: Carbimazole and the autoimmune response in Graves' disease. N Engl J Med 303:302, 1980
44. Hattengren B, Forsgren A, Melander A: Effects of antithyroid drugs on lymphocyte function in vitro. J Clin Endocrinol Metab 51:298, 1980
45. Buerklin EM, Schimmel M, Utiger RD: Pituitary-thyroid regulation in euthyroid patients with Graves' disease previously treated with antithyroid drugs. J Clin Endocrinol Metab 43:419, 1976

Chapter 5

Is Long-Term Antithyroid Drug Therapy for Graves' Disease Cost-Effective?

Joel I. Hamburger, M.D.

INTRODUCTION

Antithyroid drugs (ATD) have been employed for the treatment of hyperthyroidism (principally Graves' disease) since the 1940s. ATD treatment will be followed by remission in the hyperthyroidism for some patients. Initially good results were claimed for 50–70% of patients.[1,2] Recently success has been achieved in 15–30%,[3-5] excepting the unique report of Slingerland and Burrows[6] in which a 76% remission rate is claimed after prolonged treatment. Favorable candidates for ATD are young, have small goiters or goiters which regress during treatment, and have mild hyperthyroidism of short duration.[1,5,7,8]

Although it is common to read reports dealing with more than 1000 radioactive iodine (^{131}I)–treated hyperthyroid patients, most papers on ATD therapy deal with a few hundred or less. This is because ATD treatment generally requires more than 1 year. Even then patients in remission must be followed for several years before concluding that remissions will be maintained. Impediments which prevent completion of a protracted course of treatment and observation include toxic reactions, noncompliance, dissatisfaction with prolonged treatment, persistent or enlarging goiter, inadequate response to the ATD, refusal to return for follow-up during or after completion of treatment, and patient relocation. The availability of ^{131}I, a simple and decisive alternative, may be the most important factor limiting the number of patients who persist with long-term ATD therapy. Nevertheless, some physicians favor ATD therapy, advising a trial for nearly all patients with Graves' disease.[4,6,9] Out of concern for the cost-effectiveness of long-term ATD treatment, short-term treatment has been studied.[4]

The experience from our clinic will be presented because it appears to be so unsatisfactory that it has raised the following question: Is ATD therapy worth the expenditure of time and resources that it entails?

EXPERIENCE OF NORTHLAND THYROID LABORATORY

Methods of Treatment and Follow-Up

Between 1961 and 1978 patients with Graves' disease referred to the author were offered the option of ATD, ^{131}I, or thyroidectomy after discussion of the advantages and disadvantages of these alternatives. In the diagnosis of Graves' disease a radioactive iodine uptake was performed to exclude the temporary hyperthyroidism of silent thyroiditis.[10] Patients less than 20 years old were encouraged to try ATD therapy, as were those up to age 40 years with small goiters and mild hyperthyroidism. Otherwise patients were advised to have ^{131}I therapy, but ATD were administered if the patients preferred. Patients were reevaluated at monthly intervals until the hyperthyroidism was controlled. Thereafter evaluations were performed at 3-month intervals. After the euthyroid state was established (usually by 3 to 6 months after the treatment was started) the ATD dose was progressively reduced, as long as hyperthyroidism did not recur, in the hope that the drug could be discontinued after 18 to 24 months, sooner if possible. After ATD discontinuation patients who remained euthyroid were reevaluated, initially in 1 month, then 6 months, and annually to exclude a relapse.

Age and Sex Distribution

Table 5-1 presents the age and sex distribution for 245 patients given ATD with the objective of achieving a remission in the hyperthyroidism. The age cited is the age at which treatment was begun. Most of the patients (138 [56%]) were less than 20 years old because the majority of older patients preferred ^{131}I therapy. Eight patients, lost to follow-up after only one or two visits, are excluded from further consideration.

Reasons for Abandoning ATD

Table 5-2 shows why ATD therapy was abandoned for 162 patients. The principal reason was patient dissatisfaction with progress. Fourteen patients changed their minds less than 6 months after the treatment was started. This is usually too brief a period to achieve a remission. For 84 patients ATD therapy was continued for

Table 5-1. Age and sex distribution of 245 patients treated with antithyroid drugs.

Age (years)	Male	Female
<10	4	6
10–19	34	94
20–29	6	47
30–39	5	26
40–49	1	13
50+	4	5
Total	54	191

6 months to 8 years (average 1.81 years) without regression of the goiter or success in withdrawing the ATD. Thirty-eight of these patients achieved remission, only to relapse one or more times until alternate treatment was given. Case 1 is exemplary.

CASE 1: **FAILURE OF ANTITHYROID DRUG THERAPY FOR JUVENILE GRAVES' DISEASE**
An 11-year-old boy was treated with methimazole, 12.5 mg t.i.d., for 4 months with poor control. Consultation was requested. The heart rate was 120/min and the thyroid gland was diffusely enlarged, 2.5 times normal size. The serum T_4 concentration was 16 μg/dl (NR 5.5–11.5) and the serum T_3(RIA) was 360 ng/dl (NR 80–220). The dose of methimazole was increased to 15 mg q.i.d. In 1 month he was euthyroid. Treatment was continued for 2 years

Table 5-2. Reasons for abandoning antithyroid drug treatment.

Reason	< 6 months	6 months to 1 year	> 1 year to 2 years	> 2 years to 3 years	> 3 years to 4 years	> 4 years	Total
Patient dissatisfaction with progress[a]	14	26	31	12	8	7	98
Toxicity	16	8	3	—	—	1	28
Unsightly[b]	3	7	7	—	—	2	19
Hyperthyroidism not controlled	10	5	2	—	—	—	17
Total	43	46	43	12	8	10	162

[a]Two patients objected to the continuing costs.
[b]Three patients developed sudden massive enlargement of the goiter with increasingly severe hyperthyroidism.

with gradual reduction in methimazole dosage. The goiter completely regressed and methimazole was discontinued. Nine months later hyperthyroidism recurred. Methimazole, 5 mg t.i.d., was instituted with a good response. In 15 months another remission was achieved. However, a relapse occurred in 6 months.

Two additional courses of methimazole were given, each for about 1 year, and after each remission a relapse occurred within 6 months. His total duration of methimazole therapy was 6 years and 8 months. After the fourth relapse he had reached the age of 18 years, and he and his family requested ^{131}I therapy.

Two patients were neither poor enough for Medicaid, nor well enough insured to cover most of the costs of the treatment. After 1 and 1.5 years without a remission they requested less costly treatment.

For 28 patients ATD were abandoned for toxicity or suspected toxicity. These reactions will be discussed in conjunction with Table 5-3.

Unsightly goiters were a problem for 19 patients, 15 of whom were teenage girls, the rest young women. For 16 patients the goiters either failed to regress or gradually enlarged. None were hypothyroid from overdoses of ATD. Three patients had sudden massive increases in goiter size associated with marked increase in hyperthyroidism. Case 2 illustrates this problem.

CASE 2: MASSIVE GOITER DEVELOPING DURING ANTITHYROID DRUG THERAPY OF GRAVES' DISEASE

A 12-year-old girl was referred for evaluation of hyperthyroidism after treatment with methimazole 5 to 10 mg daily for 4 years with little if any improvement. The heart rate was 120; the skin was moist, warm, and fine in texture. The reflexes were hyperactive and there was a moderate tremor. The thyroid gland was diffusely enlarged, about three times normal size (Fig. 5-1A). The free thyroxine index (FTI) was 5.6 (NR 1.4–4.0) and the 24-h radioactive iodine uptake was 52%. Our plan was to control the hyperthyroidism until a remission (very unlikely because of the goiter size) or until she was well through puberty (age 15 or 16) when radioactive iodine would be given. Methimazole was increased to 10 mg q.i.d. She was followed at 3-month intervals during the next 4 years, with good control of her hyperthyroidism. Then the goiter enlarged dramatically within a few weeks to fill the entire neck (Fig. 5-1B). The face was swollen, suggesting moderate thoracic inlet compression. She had lost 2 lb. The FTI was 5.2 and the T_3(RIA) value had increased to 516. She was then 16 years old. Thy-

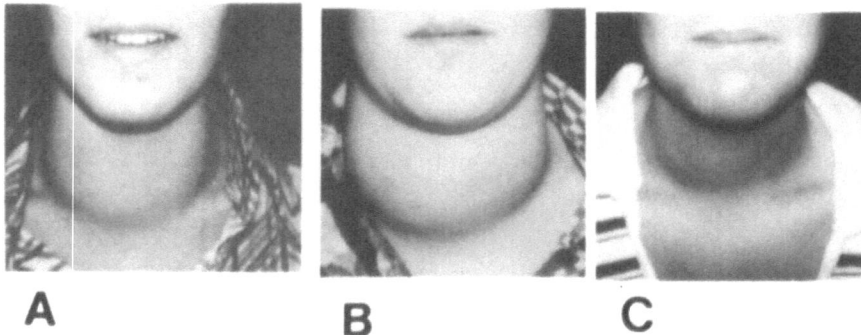

A   **B**   **C**

Figure 5-1. A The patient when first seen. **B** After sudden exacerbation in hyperthyroidism and massive enlargement of the goiter. **C** After successful ^{131}I therapy.

roidectomy was advised because of the gross disfiguration and compression. However, the patient's brother had undergone thyroidectomy and developed an unsightly keloid. Therefore the patient and parents requested ^{131}I therapy. This treatment was successful (Fig. 5-1C).

For 17 patients hyperthyroidism was never adequately controlled, even with PTU doses as high as 300 mg q.i.d. Eight of these patients admitted not taking their medication regularly (not at all in one instance); four others denied dereliction, but did not seem truthful; for the remaining five patients the disease seemed truly unresponsive. Regardless of reason, these patients were treated by other methods.

Toxicity of ATD

Table 5-3 lists the 62 "reactions" reported by 50 patients, the drug presumably responsible, and the actions taken. Skin eruptions varied from a localized mild evanescent erythematous macular pattern to a disseminated urticarial form with intense pruritus. For less severe eruptions patients were reassured and treatment continued. Otherwise the drug was changed, or if the patient was unwilling to chance another reaction ATD therapy was abandoned for an alternative treatment.

Rheumatologic reactions usually took the form of acute swelling involving several joints. One patient had full-blown serum sickness. Most of these patients requested another form of treatment.

Table 5-3. Types of toxic reactions and action taken.[a]

| Type of reaction | No. of episodes | Drug | | Action taken | | |
		PTU	M	ATD discontinued	Continued same drug	Alternate drug
Cutaneous	28	21	7	13	7	8
Rheumatologic	7	5	2	5	—	2
Pharyngitis with or without fever or fever alone, blood count normal	17	14	3	4	12	1
Granulocytopenia or agranulocytosis	6	3	3	5	—	1
Hepatocellular	3	3	—	3	—	—
Nausea	1	1	—	1	—	—
Total	62	47	15	31	19	12

[a]There were 62 reactions in 50 patients: 40 patients had 1 reaction, 8 patients had 2 reactions, and 2 patients had 3 reactions.
PTU, propylthiouracil; M, methimazole.

In the absence of leukopenia we could not be certain whether the drugs were responsible for episodes of pharyngitis with or without fever, or fever alone. In most instances we assumed the complaints were not drug related and continued the ATD. For severe, persistent, or repeated episodes a change was made to the alternate drug, or if the patients preferred, ATD therapy was discontinued and another treatment employed.

There were two episodes of agranulocytosis and four of granulocytopenia. Four of these patients had blood counts performed for acute febrile throat infections, but for the other two patients granulocytopenia was detected on routine blood counts performed at the time of scheduled examinations. All patients recovered spontaneously after withdrawal of the drug. Five patients were treated with [131]I. The sixth patient preferred a trial of the alternate ATD. She later went into a remission, but relapsed 2 months later and was finally treated with [131]I.

Hepatocellular toxicity manifested by cholestatic jaundice and abnormal liver function tests occurred in three patients. They were treated with ^{131}I when the jaundice cleared.

The last patient had persistent nausea for which ATD therapy was discontinued in favor of [131]I.

Of the 31 patients for whom ATD were discontinued for alternate treatment after toxic reactions, in three patients the reaction was only a secondary reason for abandoning ATD therapy. The principal reason was patient dissatisfaction with progress.

Remission After ATD Therapy

Table 5-4 shows that 82 patients achieved one or more remissions: 72, once; seven, twice; two, three times; and one, four times. Fifty-two remissions in 38 patients

Table 5-4. Correlation of duration of treatment with duration of remission.

Duration of treatment before remission[a]	No. of patients who achieved remission	No. still in remission[b]			No. relapsed[b]		
		< 6 months	6 months– 2 years	> 2 years	< 6 months	6 months– 2 years	> 2 years
< 6 months	7	1	2	1	3	0	0
6 months–1 year	16	0	6	2	4	4	0
> 1 year–2 years	38	4	4	9	6	13	2
> 2 years–3 years	12	7	2	0	1	2	0
> 3 years–4 years	4	3	0	0	0	1	0
> 4 years	5	1	0	2	2	0	0
Total	82	16	14	14	16	20	2

[a]Before last remission if more than one.

[b]After last remission if more than one; 72 patients experienced 1 remission; 7, 2 remissions; 2, 3 remissions; and 1, 4 remissions.

failed to persist. Twenty-nine patients subsequently were treated with ^{131}I, one surgically, one with Lugol's solution (a remission was obtained after 1 year of treatment), one resumed ATD and is still being treated, and one is still considering the options. Five patients refused further treatment and were lost to follow-up.

Forty-four patients are in remission, but 16 have been euthyroid for less than 6 months, and 14 for from 6 months to 2 years. Of those who relapsed, 36 of 38 did so within 2 years of entering a remission. Therefore it is certain that a number of the 44 patients in remission will relapse in time.

None of 16 patients with goiter 4 times normal size or larger achieved a remission, and none of 11 patients treated the longest (5–8 years) achieved a remission. Patients still in remission more than 6 months after discontinuation of ATD include 20 of 100 patients less than 20 years old, six of 47 patients between 20 and 29 years old, and only two of 44 patients 30 years old or older.

Summary of Results of ATD Therapy

Table 5-5 summarizes the current status of the 237 ATD-treated patients. Excluding the 20 patients who refused further treatment, the 11 patients still on treatment, one patient lost to follow-up after ATD therapy was abandoned

Table 5-5. Results of antithyroid drug treatment in 237 patients.

		No. of patients
Further treatment refused		20
After 2–6 months	6	
> 6 months–2 years	8	
> 2 years	6	
Still on treatment		11
After 1–2 years	5	
> 2–3 years	3	
> 3 years	3	
Treatment abandoned		162
For ^{131}I	147	
Thyroidectomy	10	
Lugol's solution	3	
Uncertain	1	
Lost	1	
In remission		44
For < 6 months	16	
6 months–2 years	14	
> 2 years	14	
Total		237

because of toxicity, and one patient who relapsed and is uncertain as to what treatment she will now take, we are left with 204 patients treated and followed. Of these 157 (77%) were eventually treated with ^{131}I or thyroidectomy. Only 44 (22%) are in remission, and of these 30 (15%) have been in remission less than 2 years. One of the patients achieved a remission after treatment for 4 years, but 4 years later, without intervening treatment, she was hypothyroid. A second patient was treated for 6 months and achieved a remission, although there was a persistent firm goiter and high antithyroid antibodies. Two years later, at age 18, she had a thyroidectomy for cosmetic purposes.

DISCUSSION

Reasons for Failure with ATD

ATD therapy for hyperthyroidism has only one advantage over ^{131}I or thyroidectomy, i.e., it does not destroy thyroid tissue. However, substantial disadvantages include a relatively high failure rate, a protracted treatment period, and risk of drug reactions. Success rates of 50% or better for treatment with ATD have been reported.[1,2] Recently, substantially poorer results have been experienced.[3–5] It has been suggested that the proportion of failures is reduced if treatment is extended for many years.[6,9] In theory there might be validity to this concept. In practice it is exceedingly difficult to maintain patient compliance for the many years required for a high remission rate. Even the patient who objects to destructive therapy may reconsider as the year pass by without success. The simplicity and decisiveness of ^{131}I therapy or thyroidectomy becomes increasingly attractive. Dissatisfaction with progress in eliminating either hyperthyroidism or a sizable goiter prompted a demand for alternative treatment by 117 (49%) ATD-treated patients in this series. For two patients the economic burden of repeated examinations presented a deterrent to continued treatment.

Reactions to the drugs were the principal reasons for which 28 (12%) patients abandoned ATD, and contributing reasons for three additional patients. It is not always possible to know whether a given manifestation is ATD related. Absence of leukopenia might suggest that pharyngitis or fever was not caused by ATD. Nevertheless, these problems, when recurrent in a patient taking ATD, raise the possibility of a drug-related qualitative defect in leukocyte function. This concern, whether expressed by patient or physician, led to discontinuation of ATD for several patients. Even when ATD were continued each possible toxic event led to an extra physician evaluation thus adding to the economic burden of the treatment. Hence, we have listed all the "reactions" reported. Although deaths have been attributed to ATD toxicity on rare occasions,[11] our patients avoided such serious consequences.

For 17 patients treatment was abandoned for poor control of hyperthyroidism. For more than half of these patients the problem was noncompliance by teenage patients. Six of them were Medicaid patients. There were four additional Medicaid patients, none of whom reliably kept appointments or achieved remissions. Compliance problems in juveniles are common.[12]

In all, 162 (68%) patients abandoned ATD before a determination could be made as to whether a remission might have been obtained had treatment been continued for many years. However, 30 of these patients were treated for more than 2 years without a remission, a reasonable trial in conventional terms. About half the patients given a trial of ATD did not comply with the treatment for 2 years.

Remissions After ATD Therapy

Forty-four patients remained in remission for from less than 6 months to more than 2 years. If it is assumed that all of those who have sustained remissions for longer than 2 years and half the remissions of lesser duration will persist, this would mean that about 29 (12%) sustained remissions will have been achieved. Therefore, for about 88% of the patients ATD therapy will have been unsuccessful. All of these patients could have been treated with ^{131}I or thyroidectomy initially at a considerable saving in time and expense.

Cost-Benefit Considerations Referrable to ATD Therapy

The cost directly attributable to ATD treatment, exclusive of the initial diagnostic workup, for the 208 patients who were unsuccessful was about $130,000. In addition, they still had to bear the additional cost of the alternative treatment. Consideration of the cost-benefit ratio for a therapy with this potential for failure, even after years of treatment, raises serious questions as to its reasonableness. Destructive treatments have been criticized because of the cost for lifelong replacement therapy and annual evaluations. However, lifelong annual evaluation is needed also for those successfully treated with ATD. Some will relapse and others eventually develop hypothyroidism.[13,14] Therefore, the cost differential unfavorable to destructive therapy relates only to the cost of replacement thyroid hormone. However, immediate routine destructive therapy would save the far greater amounts expended for medication and testing for years of therapy for the 88% ATD failures. These savings would pay for replacement thyroid hormone for about 6500 patient years at the rate of $20 per year.

Short-Term ATD Therapy

From the economic point of view short-term therapy advocated by Greer et al.[4] may be a reasonable compromise between abandoning ATD therapy and its undue prolongation. Treatment with 30 to 60 mg of methimazole in a single daily dose for up to 8 months produced remissions in 12 of 31 patients, sustained 6 to 47 months (mean of 29.9 ± 35 months). If success or failure can be predicted after short-term treatment this would reduce concern relative to costs of ATD therapy. Unfortunately, one recent report correlating remission rates with duration of treatment suggests that short-term treatment is not as effective, and that a minimum of 1 year of ATD therapy is advisable.[15] Another study of short-term therapy achieved only 12% sustained remissions.[16]

ATD Therapy Indefinitely

Slingerland and Burrows have suggested that the reason for poor results with ATD is failure to treat long enough.[6] They claimed 76% remissions in patients treated up to 14 years. Experienced thyroidologists who read this report of a series of remarkably cooperative hyperthyroid patients who faithfully took ATD for many years without complaint, misadventure, or defection must wonder how they can eliminate annoying habits exhibited by their patients, including noncompliance, occasional nonresponsiveness, demands for alternative treatment after one or more years without a remission, and a tendency from time to time to develop toxic reactions varying in severity from unpleasant to downright frightening. The age distribution of Slingerland and Burrows' patients is different from ours in that they had no patients younger than 22, whereas 56% of our patients were less than 20 years old. Poor cooperation is common with adolescents, but this led to failure for no more than 12 of our teenage patients. Also, our clinic serves as a referral center, and undoubtedly our patient population is biased in favor of problem cases. Those more amenable to treatment may be managed by family physicians. Finally, some patients with very mild hyperthyroidism and small goiters were treated with Lugol's solution. These patients would have been especially favorable candidates for ATD therapy, and their elimination from our series may have reduced the number of good results.

Whatever the impact of differences in patient composition, a longer period of treatment is not likely to improve our poor results with ATD. None of the 11 patients treated for the longest period of time, 5–8 years, achieved a remission. Also, patients who exhibit relapses in spite of two courses of ATD therapy, covering a total period of 2–3 years, seldom achieve a sustained remission after addtional treatment.[17,18] The report of Tamai et al.[15] suggests that treatment for 1 to 2 years produces more sustained remission than treatment for 6 months. However, these data do not contradict reports indicating negligible benefit from therapy beyond 2 years.

Examination of the data of Slingerland and Burrows reveals that although patients were treated for 1–14 years, the average duration was 4.4 years. Only 17 of 61 patients were treated for more than 4 years. The 14% success rate reported by Wartofsky[3] was achieved by treatment for an average of 1.5 years (longest period 44 months). Our patients were treated for 3 months to 8 years (average 1.9 ± 1.39 years). Is the dramatically higher remission rate of Slingerland and

Burrows the result of "tenaciously continuing therapy until remission is attained, even if this means continuing it for as long as 15 years or more"?

This report curiously reveals that no patients abandoned the treatment because of toxicity, dissatisfaction with progress, enlarging goiter, or poor cooperation. Nor were any lost to follow-up. Of course no patients were included in the analysis of results unless they had completed 1 year of treatment and were followed for at least 1 year after remission. Application of these criteria to our series would exclude most patients with unsatisfactory results. The majority of toxic reactions occurred within the first year. Patients who defected from the study would not be counted and neither would those who never achieved a remission (they would not have been followed at least 1 year afterward). We would have only 29 patients left, and 20 (69%) would be in remission.

This observation led us to examine the earlier report of Hershman et al.[2] with a 54% sustained remission rate. Again, that calculation considered only patients who completed the treatment course. Those for whom treatment was abandoned for any reason were excluded. Even though it is possible that longer ATD therapy will increase the proportion of patients who achieve remission, the very high remission rate claimed by Slingerland and Burrows may relate more to either exclusion from consideration of bad results, or a unique population of patients. Because it seems improbable that many physicians will be so fortunate, we suggest that our data provide a more realistic reflection of what can be expected in terms of ATD results from onset of treatment until termination successfully or otherwise.

Relation of Health Care Delivery System to Cost-Consciousness

Since Slingerland and Burrows practice in a Veterans Administration Hospital, they may encounter a patient population whose options are not as broad as is generally the case in the United States. Also, institutions within the federal government do not have a tradition of concern for cost-effectiveness. This point is exemplified dramatically by the report of Bowers,[19] who claimed that surgical treatment of hyperthyroidism was more efficient than ^{131}I therapy. His surgically treated patients only required an average of 1.6 hospital admissions, an average hospital stay of 42 days and a longest stay of "only" 169 days; compared to ^{131}I-treated patients who required an average of five hospitalizations (up to 15 hospitalizations) and an average hospital stay of 452 days (longest stay 658 days, i.e., almost 2 years). If the reader has trouble believing these numbers, so did Dr. George Crile, Jr., who offered this comment on Bowers' report: " . . . we have to accept that everything Dr. Bowers has said is true in the world that he lives in, but it bears absolutely no relationship to the world I live in." The average hospital stay at the Cleveland Clinic for thyroidectomy was 4 days, for ^{131}I therapy zero days.

Lack of concern for cost-effectiveness may have made it possible for Slingerland and Burrows to pursue ATD treatment so tenaciously. However, most American physicians work in an environment in which they are legally obliged to provide a full and fair discussion of the advantages and disadvantages of therapeutic alternatives, and patients exercise informed consent for treatment and withdraw that consent and seek care elsewhere if they are dissatisfied. In a private consultation clinic there is a powerful incentive to please both patient and referring physician. Indecisive, excessively prolonged, and expensive treatment does not serve this objective. Most of our patients wish to pursue active productive lives without the frequent intrusion of visits to a physician.

We welcome current emphasis on full disclosure of therapeutic alternatives to ensure informed consent. This protects the patient from being treated by a method which he would not have accepted had he been aware of other options. It also protects the physician from responsibility for consequences, medical and economic, of a treatment which is employed at the patient's request. Our patients are provided with a booklet describing in detail the treatments for hyperthyroidism and their limitations.[20] Later a discussion of the options is held. Only then do the patients sign a treatment consent form. We encourage patient participation in the treatment selection because we realize that all three of the major treatments can be employed with success, and that there may be valid differences of opinion as to their relative merits.[21] Nevertheless, after this discussion we do not hesitate to express our opinion that ^{131}I is the most efficient treatment for most patients, and this opinion reduced the number of patients treated with ATD. Patients who elect ATD therapy understand that this choice is not irreversible. Although we will pursue treatment indefinitely if the patient wishes, we also do not dissuade those who are not making progress from resorting to another treatment. A policy of refusing ^{131}I therapy for patients less than 30 or 40 years old would have led many patients to persist with ATD therapy rather than accept the risks and unpleasantness of thyroidectomy. Some would eventually have achieved a remission. However, many would have gone elsewhere to obtain ^{131}I therapy.

Attitudes Outside the United States

Recent travel to thyroid clinics outside the United States has prompted the conclusion that American concern for cost-effectiveness is not always shared abroad. In the United Kingdom, Italy, and Israel, we learned that costs played no part in the decision to treat hyperthyroid patients with ATD or surgically rather than with ^{131}I, because medical care was "free." At the same time physicians complained of lack of funds to upgrade physical plants, for equipment, physicians' salaries, and research. Israel is losing physicians because upon completing their training they have no opportunites to practice. Perhaps it is naive to think that resources not squandered on inefficient medical care might be made available for more useful health-related purposes. Even so, is it necessary that physicians, presumably members of an educational and intellectual elite, participate in irresponsible behavior?

An English thyroidologist assured me that if she had hyperthyroidism she would straightaway visit her surgical colleague. She had yet to experience a single fatality from thyroidectomy. When asked what her attitude might be when sooner or later the inevitable should come to pass, she responded that she would then reconsider. She was then asked why it was necessary for her to experience personally the loss of a patient before reconsidering. Why would she not reconsider before this happened, and thus prevent it? After all, operative death after thyroidectomy is part of the surgical reality.[22] Why should she expect a permanent dispensation from this burden if she continued to supply candidates? Similar claims of freedom from operative mortality were made in Israeli medical centers. However, at one hospital a high incidence of postoperative tetany was a cause of problems because of patient dereliction in follow-up and self-administration of medication. At another center a patient recently subjected to thyroidectomy for hyperthyroidism experienced a prolonged postoperative coma from which he may have permanent neurologic problems. Physicians in both centers maintained that they would still advise operation rather than ^{131}I therapy, because the patients feared the consequences of radiation. This attitude was also expressed in Italy.

Further discussion made it clear that it was actually the physicians who were afraid. Again and again physicians asked how I could be sure that ^{131}I would not cause fetal malformations, if not in the first generation, in the second or beyond. One physician expressed concern for legal action in the event of a fetal malformation, even if no relationship to the treatment could be proved. "After all," he said, "this is not standard treatment for childbearing women in Israel." When asked if he would hesitate to give 10 to 20 times as much ^{131}I to patients in the childbearing age or younger for thyroid carcinoma he responded, "Of course not, but cancer is a life-threatening disease." When then asked how many young patients he had seen die from thyroid cancer he said, "None." When further pressed as to the subsequent progeny of the patients given cancer doses of ^{131}I he was aware of no fetal abnormalities. He and others with the same fears of ^{131}I were aware of the reports[23] indicating no increase in fetal malformations after cancer doses of ^{131}I,[23] and showing again no more risk to the gonads from ^{131}I therapy for hyperthyroidism than from conventional radiographic studies of the gastrointestinal or urinary tracts.[24] In spite of this prevailing attitude, one Israeli thyroidologist had treated 4000 hyperthyroid patients with ^{131}I, many in the childbearing age, without medical or legal mishap. We share the opinion that there has never been any scientific basis upon which to preclude use of ^{131}I at any age (excluding, of course, pregnant or lactating women).[23,25-27]

Risks of Indefinite ATD Therapy Compared to Destructive Therapy

Indefinite ATD treatment, when a remission is not achieved, exposes the patient to the risk of recurrent hyperthyroidism if treatment is abandoned. Those who employ distructive therapy face the risk of hypothyroidism in patients who fail to take thyroid hormone. The manifestations of hyperthyroidism are overt and likely to bring the patient to a physician before cardiovascular decompensation or thyroid crisis proves lethal. Hypothyroidism may be more insidious and therefore more easily overlooked. However, there is a far longer period of time for diagnosis before the disease is lethal. Who can say which situation presents the greater risk to the defecting patient? Since either risk is created by patient noncompliance, physicians can do no more than warn of the consequences of dereliction. Reports of hypothyroidism in ATD-treated patients followed for long periods of time indicate that this complication is not limited to those who received destructive therapy.[13,14]

CONCLUSION

Our data reflect our attitude of flexibility. We did not achieve the best possible results with ATD simply because many patients were unwilling to persist with the treatment for the years which might have been necessary. To have forced them to do so would have required coercion or misrepresentation of the risks or availability of other treatments. We conclude that ATD therapy is inefficient and wasteful of economic and human resources to a degree sufficient to question its continued employment for hyperthyroid patients, other than those who insist upon it regardless of cost-effectiveness considerations.

COMMENTARY

John J. Canary, M.D.

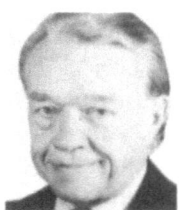

ATD Therapy Is Not an Efficient Way to Treat Hyperthyroidism

The preceding review by Hamburger constitutes a penetrating analysis of a very significant area in clinical thyroidology. The recent data suggesting a substantial decline in the incidence of remissions of thyrotoxicosis with antithyroid drugs (ATD) appear to be not really a change, because the methods utilized by the earlier workers weighted their results in favor of a higher frequency of remissions. Close agreement between the data of Wartofsky[3] and Greer et al.[4] regarding a much lower occurrence of permanent remissions with both long-term ATD therapy and with much shorter periods of ATD treatment, and Hamburger's reanalysis of the data of Soloman et al.,[1] Hershman et al.,[2] and Slingerland and Burrows,[6] demonstrate that there has not been any change in the rate of such remission.

More importantly, as Hamburger points out (and data from my service support his position), if patients with thyrotoxicosis developing before 20 years of age are followed for more than 5 years, less than 5% remain in remission. When those with onset of the disease after age 20 who achieve a remission with ATD therapy are followed for a similar period, less than 11% remain in remission. When follow-up of the latter group is extended beyond 10 years, less than 6% continue in remission. These data are based on a referral consultation practice. Hence, the data are not strictly comparable to those based on an unscreened patient population. It is most likely that I am not asked to see a population of patients who have done well with ATD. These very low percentages of permanent remissions might, most probably, be higher if I were seeing patients without referral.

Thyroidectomy May Be Safer than Either ^{131}I or ATD

In contradistinction to the presentation by Hamburger, who emphasizes the safety of both ATD and ^{131}I, while pointing out that fatal outcomes flow from the surgical treatment, in my laboratory, the only fatalities we have had have been related to either ^{131}I or ATD treatment of hyperthyroidism. We have had no fatalities related to subtotal thyroidectomy for thyrotoxicosis in more than 400 patients. In our most recent experience, now totaling over 150 patients prepared for subtotal thyroidectomy with propranolol alone, there were no fatalities. I have participated in postmortem evaluation of three patients who died of thyroid crisis which developed within 6 to 10 days of ^{131}I treatment. I had seen one of these three patients in consultation. She was 39 years old with a multinodular goiter and paroxysmal atrial fibrillation which responded favorably to propranolol. I advised ^{131}I therapy, with maintenance of propranolol for 6–8 weeks, but this was not done. She remained without treatment for about 1 year, and then was given ^{131}I therapy without ATD preparation or propranolol. Nine days later she was hospitalized in thyroid crisis with flutter-fibrillation and rapidly died. She did not receive ATD, propranolol, or adrenal steroids. The other two episodes occurred about 20 years ago in women in the mid-30s. I did not participate in the treatment of either patient, and details of the treatment are not available. One of the two had received two courses of ATD which induced remissions, only to relapse later. In both instances death was related to cardiac arrhythmia (in one there was congestive heart failure). Neither patient received reserpine. Recently I participated in the treatment of a 34-year-old woman who died of severe hepatic necrosis secondary to propylthiouracil. The clinical course and the autopsy findings on that patient were very similar to those reported by others.[28−31]

My experience is thus diametrically opposite to that of Hamburger. In my experience, ^{131}I and propylthiouracil have fatal potential not shared by the surgical therapy of thyrotoxic patients when performed by experienced thyroid surgeons.

In passing, I am in complete agreement with Greer et al.,[36] that when ATD are used to treat thyrotoxicosis, a once-a-day dose schedule is very effective, and that short-term treatment is as effective in producing remissions as is long-term administration.

Relative Costs of ATD, ^{131}I, and Surgical Treatment of Hyperthyroidism

In an early review favorable to ^{131}I treatment of hyperthyroidism, Chapman[32] estimated the cost of treatment with these three basic therapeutic forms: ATD, surgical, and ^{131}I therapy cost $150, $600, and $300, respectively. His figures were stated to cover the treatment cost for about a 1-year period. Currently in this center, the respective costs for a similar time course are $2800 for ATD, $3000 for ^{131}I, and $2900 for surgery. These costs were developed utilizing not only the estimated costs of initial consultation, but also all laboratory costs such as the frequently measured white blood counts, radioiodine studies, physician office visits, etc., as well as the costs of time off work, parking costs, and so on. The surgical figure includes cost for the operation, operating room, anesthesia, recovery room, and days away from work. The few days of preparation, 4 to 5 days of hospitalization, and the determination of functional status 3 to 4 weeks postoperative make subtotal thyroidectomy by far the most appealing method.

The use of the catecholamine receptor blocking agent, propranolol, or the catecholamine depleting agent, reserpine, permits surgery to be done safely with no more than a few hours of preoperative treatment. The postoperative follow-up is minimal in patients treated in that fashion. These figures, while allowing for the obvious inflation since the publication of the Chapman figures in 1960, indicate that at least in this area of the country, subtotal thyroidectomy is not only the most cost-effective method, it is also the safest.

COMMENTARY

Francis S. Greenspan, M.D.

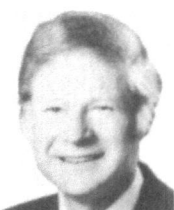

The title "Is Long-Term Antithyroid Drug Therapy for Graves' Disease Cost-Effective?" is provocative. Obviously, if a therapeutic modality has no benefit, then it is not "cost-effective," regardless of how little it costs. On the other hand, if a therapeutic modality is successful even for a selected group of patients, then the relative cost of the treatment is a reasonable factor to consider in selecting an appropriate therapy.

Relative Costs of ATD, ^{131}I, and Surgical Treatment of Hyperthyroidism

It is interesting to examine the actual cost of each therapeutic modality discussed. Table 5-6 presents an approximation of the relative costs for the treatment of Graves' disease. These approximations were made utilizing September 1980

Table 5-6. Approximate costs for various treatments of Graves' disease.

A. Two years of ATD therapy		
Initial workup including consultation, FT₄I,[a] T₃(RIA), ¹²³I uptake and scan		$ 400.00
Follow-up visits at 1, 3, 6, 12, 18, and 24 months, including FT₄I at each visit		440.00
Cost of medication for 2 years		60.00
	Total	$ 900.00
B. ¹³¹I therapy and 2 years of follow-up		
Initial workup including consultation, FT₄I, T₃(RIA), ¹²³I uptake and scan		$ 400.00
¹³¹I therapy		300.00
Follow-up at 1. 5, 3, 6, 12, 18, and 24 months, including FT₄I, TSH at each visit, and one repeat ¹²³I uptake at 3 months		600.00
T₄ replacement therapy for 18 months		50.00
	Total	$1350.00
C. Subtotal thyroidectomy		
Initial workup including consultation, FT₄I, T₃(RIA), and ¹²³I uptake and scan		$ 400.00
6 weeks ATD therapy prior to surgery including two visits, medication, and FT₄I prior to surgery		100.00
4 days hospitalization including OR and anesthesia		2500.00
Surgical fee		1500.00
Follow-up at 3, 6, 12, and 24 months including FT₄I and TSH		400.00
T₄ replacement therapy for 18 months		50.00
	Total	$4950.00

[a]FT₄I, free thyroxine index, or T₄·RT₃U product.

prices in a metropolitan area in northern California, and cover a 2-year treatment period. They also assume no unusual complications such as severe progressive ophthalmopathy, thyroid storm, drug reaction, or other complicating illness. From Table 5-6 it is noted that antithyroid drug (ATD) therapy is certainly the least expensive. It would cost about $900 for a 2-year treatment period. Radioactive iodine is quite comparable, costing about $1350 for the same follow-up period. Surgical therapy, involving hospitalization, operating rooms, anesthesiologists' fees, and surgical fees, is considerably higher, approximately $4950. Thus, if ATD therapy were effective it certainly would be the least expensive method of treatment.

Is ATD Therapy Effective?

Hamburger has reviewed the literature on the incidence of remission after ATD therapy, and has noted the variability in response rate in different clinics. It is fair to say that in selected patients the remission rate, at least for short-term remissions, is about 50%, but the possibility of relapse at a later date is always present. Hamburger's own data are somewhat selective in that there were an unusually large number of patients who were "dissatisfied with the treatment" and requested alternative therapy. This group, plus a large number of patients who had reactions to the drugs (12%), accounted for abandonment or refusal of ATD in 182 out of 230 patients, or 77%. Forty-four patients did achieve a sustained remission. In my experience, patients most likely to achieve a sustained remission are young patients with small glands and mild disease. For this selected group of patients, ATD therapy is certainly cost-effective.

It must be emphasized that patients do have a voice in the selection of therapy for their illness. There are many patients who are unwilling to accept surgery for Graves' disease, and others who are very frightened of radiation in any form. For these patients, ATD therapy is an effective way to control their disease until an unemotional decision can be made. If ATD produce a sustained remission, then a difficult decision (for the patient) has been eliminated; if not, then ATD can be abandoned and an alternative approach, either ^{131}I or surgery, can be utilized.

ATD May Suppress Autoantibodies Which May Maintain Hyperthyroidism in Graves' Disease

Currently Graves' disease is considered an immunologic disorder, occurring in genetically predisposed individuals, in which T-lymphocytes, sensitized to thyroid tissue, stimulate B-lymphocytes to produce thyroid-stimulating immunoglobulin (TSI) which drives the thyroid gland.[33] Neither ^{131}I nor surgery affects the underlying pathogenetic mechanism. Recently, McGregor et al. have suggested that carbimazole inhibits autoantibody synthesis both in vitro and in vivo.[34] If this observation is substantiated it may explain why ATD therapy is effective at all, and may provide a means by which patients could be selected for this type of treatment. Even at the present time, with appropriate selection of patients, ATD therapy can certainly be quite "cost-effective."

COMMENTARY

Monte A. Greer, M.D.

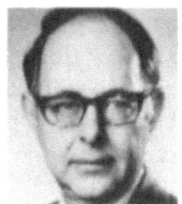

Although my assigned role is to take an adversary position to that of Hamburger, I find it difficult to disagree with the primary arguments of his treatise. Chronic treatment with antithyroid drugs (ATD) is more expensive than ^{131}I therapy and requires more frequent patient contact with the physician. Although almost all patients will go into remission during ATD treatment, prolonged remission once the drugs are stopped is probably maintained only in one-third or fewer of the patients. Toxic reactions, even though these are primarily minor problems, such as skin rash or itching, are considerably more frequent with ATD than with [131]I. I also agree that ^{131}I therapy is a much more reasonable treatment for Graves' disease than is surgery. Not only is it considerably cheaper and easier, it also entails much less risk of morbidity and mortality than does thyroidectomy.

Why I Use ATD

Given my agreement with Hamburger, one might logically ask why I use ATD at all. Perhaps the most important reason is that we are the children of our parents. My training in endocrinology was with Ted Astwood, the originator of ATD therapy for thyrotoxicosis, and I was in his group at the time his protocol for the use of ATD was being formulated in the immediate postwar period. Radioiodine was just becoming available for diagnostic and therapeutic use. At that time, it was clear that essentially all thyrotoxic patients would go into remission while they were receiving ATD and that a significant proportion of them would stay in remission after the drugs were stopped. It was not clear whether the risks of eventual malignancy or hypothyroidism would make [131]I a more dangerous and less appealing choice of therapy than ATD, although the known risks of ^{131}I were obviously much less than those of thyroidectomy. Having been indoctrinated in the logic of using ATD, I have continued to employ them as the primary treatment of choice for patients with "virgin" thyrotoxicosis of Graves' disease, i.e., those with an initial attack who have not relapsed following therapy with ATD or some other modality of treatment. Radioiodine therapy is reserved for the nonvirgins. This is still my basic approach, but I am not convinced it is the correct one.

Modifications of ATD Therapy

Over the years we have learned that certain simplifications of the therapeutic plan are valuable. The standard approach in Astwood's clinic was to treat patients with 100 mg of propylthiouracil or 10 mg of methimazole every 8 h for a period of 1 year. We have made two major changes. In studies being conducted for another purpose,[35] we found that in almost all patients the same total daily dose of ATD is just as effective given in a single daily dose as when given every 8 h.[36] This greatly simplifies therapy and improves patient compliance. Remembering to take medication at specific intervals throughout the day is difficult for most people, especially children. Over the last 5 years we have also been exploring the utility of treating patients with ATD only until they become euthyroid, then stopping the drug, rather than treating them for a full year.[4] Our experience to date is that 25–30% of patients treated with this "short course" of ATD will remain in prolonged remission, thus considerably reducing the total cost and inconvenience to the patient. Patients who relapse can subsequently be treated with [131]I. As Hamburger points out, patients with small goiters and mild thyrotoxicosis are those most likely to remain in lasting remission once ATD are stopped.

Why Not Use ^{131}I Routinely?

Hamburger's question is why not go to ^{131}I therapy immediately in all patients since it is impossible to predict with certainty which patients will stay in remission following ATD and since approximately 75% of all those treated with ATD will require an alternative form of therapy for eventual cure. I agree with his thesis that the overall costs to the nation for medical care would probably be less if all thyrotoxic patients were treated with ^{131}I initially. However, the costs for an individual who was treated with ^{131}I but who would have remained well after a single course of ATD would be greater than if he had been treated with ATD. Continual follow-up is necessary for patients treated either with ^{131}I or ATD, and patients treated with ^{131}I would stand an approximately 50% chance of requiring lifelong therapy with thyroid hormone. Patients treated with ^{131}I may also have a recurrence of their thyrotoxicosis, occasionally even after hypothyroidism lasting several years has been produced by the irradiation.

Patients who remain well after a single course of ATD will save money and will not be subject to a high risk of permanent hypothyroidism and the continual (even if subliminal) underlying concern which would be their fate had they been treated with ^{131}I. At the present writing, I feel that patients likely to remain in remission after a single course of ATD (those with mild thyrotoxicosis and small glands) deserve a trial of drug therapy. If subsequent treatment with ^{131}I is necessary, they have lost little. In patients unlikely to remain in remission following ATD, such as those with large goiters and/or severe thyrotoxicosis or who have relapsed after previous therapy, it may be best to employ ^{131}I as the initial therapy.

COMMENTARY

J. Martin Miller, M.D.

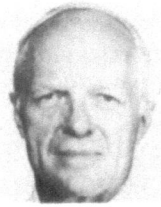

Twenty-five years ago it seemed to me that antithyroid drug (ATD) treatment for Graves' disease, at best 50% effective, was unsuitable for general use since more effective alternatives existed (^{131}I or surgery). To increase the efficacy of ATD therapy we limited our selection to patients with mild hyperthyroidism, small goiters, no congestive oculopathy, and a psychic precipitant (if one was present) that was subject to reversal or nonrecurrence. This last qualification included most juveniles, who could look forward to "growing up." This type of selection gave seemingly permanent remissions in excess of 70%. Many candidates were eliminated because they did not believe they could accept the medical program or the relatively high possibility of failure and change in treatment plans.

We have not been impressed by shrinking "cure" rates and partially attribute this observation of others to decreasing enthusiasm of the prescribing physician for ATD therapy. This feeling is transmitted to the patient and leads to poor compliance, poor control of the hyperthyroidism, and failure. Our philosophy has been that treatment to achieve a remission begins the day the patient becomes euthyroid. We have observed numerous failures in patients treated by others because the euthyroid state was not maintained or indeed not even achieved.

It is virtually impossible to draw scientific conclusions from an experience such as ours with the large number of uncontrolled variables. At the risk of adding anecdotal observations to data which are already unsuitable for scientific interpretation, five patients from our practice are worthy of mention. Four had Graves' disease with goiters of 50 to 75 g, were moderately hyperthyroid, and were males 30 to 35 years of age. All refused ^{131}I therapy, all took methimazole for 9 to 12 months, all had a return of the thyroid to normal size, and all seem to be enjoying a permanent remission of from 5 to 22 years. All were physicians.

The fifth patient was an athletic 16-year-old male with Graves' disease and the largest goiter (over 200 g) we have ever observed with this disease. He was uncontrolled on 80 mg of methimazole daily. He refused surgery and we were loath to recommend [131]I. He insisted on ATD therapy, became allergic to methimazole, and eventually required 3 g of propylthiouracil daily to achieve the euthyroid state. He took 15 pills four times daily for 1.5 years! At the end of this period his thyroid was normal in size, and he has remained euthyroid for 3 years and off all medications.

Patients like these buttress my opinion that physician bias has much to do with the outcome of the therapy, and if the patient is really "sold" on ATD results will be much better than in the experience of Hamburger. Surgical and ^{131}I treatment of Graves' disease are analogous to amputation of an extremity to cure an infection before the days of antibiotics. ATD may be only a moderately more rational therapy than thyroid ablation, but it may be based on the pathophysiology of Graves' disease. At the present time about 10% of our hyperthyroid patients are treated with ATD.

COMMENTARY

Horst P. Schleusener, M.D.

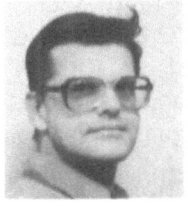

It is widely held that Graves' disease is a genetically determined autoimmune disorder.[37] Some authors believe that antithyroid drugs (ATD) have immunosuppressive effects,[34,38,39] but others maintain that drug therapy only blocks hormone synthesis and does not influence the course of the disease. In this commentary I shall discuss three points of possible importance in ATD management.

Detection of Remission During ATD Treatment

Several methods may be useful to detect a remission during ATD treatment.[40,41] During combined therapy with ATD and T_3, suppression of the early uptake of ^{131}I or ^{99m}Tc pertechnetate suggests a remission, whereas lack of suppression indicates the need for continued treatment. Similar results have been reported for T_4 measurements during combined ATD-T_3 therapy, i.e., patients in remission had significantly lower T_4 levels.[42]

More recently, determinations of TSH-displacing antibodies (TDA) and thyroid adenylcyclase–stimulating antibodies (TsAb) were found useful to indicate remission during treatment.[43-48] (It is unclear whether TDA and TsAb are identical.[47-53]) Figures 5-2-5-4 present our experience with the determination of TDA activity during ATD treatment, an experience which agrees with that of others.[43,45-48] Virtually all patients with persisting TDA activity relapsed, whereas 75% of patients in whom TDA disappeared remained in remission. These data suggest that duration of ATD therapy should be individually determined by performing a suppression test, or in cases of TDA positivity before treatment, by measuring TDA activity during treatment. Theoretically, the measurement of TsAb would be better, but the method is too laborious for routine use.

Prediction of the Long-Term Course of the Disease

Up to now objective methods have not been available to predict prior to treatment whether a patient will have a longstanding remission after ATD treatment. Such a method would make it possible to advise patients to be treated either with ATD or by destructive methods (i.e., surgery or ^{131}I). Several studies have shown that patients with HLA types B8 and DR3 tend to develop autoimmune diseases as Graves' disease.[54-63] Irvine et al.[60] suggested that HLA B8–positive patients be treated primarily with surgery and B8-negative patients with ATD. McGregor et al.[61] concluded that HLA DR3 is of value in predicting poor results from ATD therapy. In our combined Berlin-Vienna study, HLA typing was performed in 122 patients with toxic (scintigraphically) diffuse goiter, 69 of whom had several relapses within 4 to 8 years after treatment with ATD or [131]I. Fifty-three patients had a remission for 2–11 years after ATD therapy.[62,63] In contrast to the encouraging findings previously cited,[60,61] we found that prevalence of HLA DR3 and HLA B8 was not a statistically significant predictor of results (Table 5-7).[63]

When the patients are divided into subgroups, i.e., proved Graves' disease and disseminated suspected thyroid autonomy (see below), there was even less difference in the prevalence of HLA DR3 between the relapse and remission groups. On the basis of the data in Table 5-7 we do not feel that HLA typing will predict

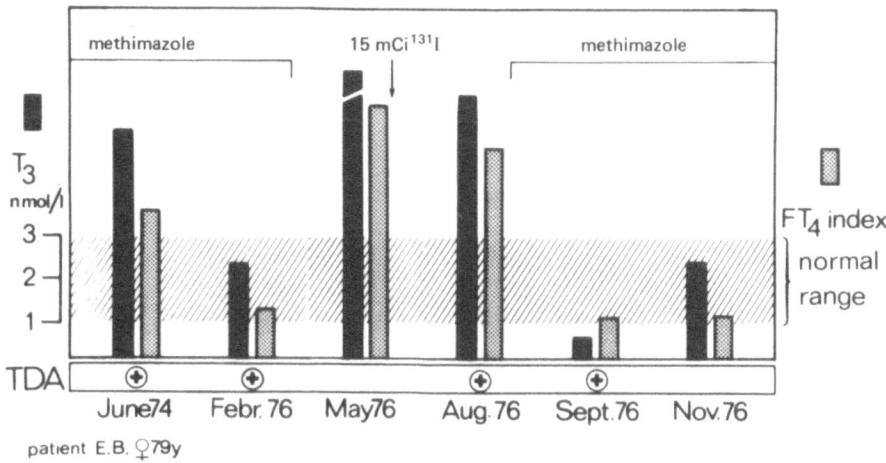

patient E.B. ♀79y

Figure 5-2. TDA activity and thyroid function in a patient with both persistent TDA activity and persistent hyperthyroidism. After the first course of ATD hyperthyroidism relapsed within 8 weeks. [131]I therapy was unsuccessful. Methimazole was reinstituted and thyroid hormone levels fell to normal, but to date the TDA assay remains strongly positive. Data are from Teng and Yeung.[46]

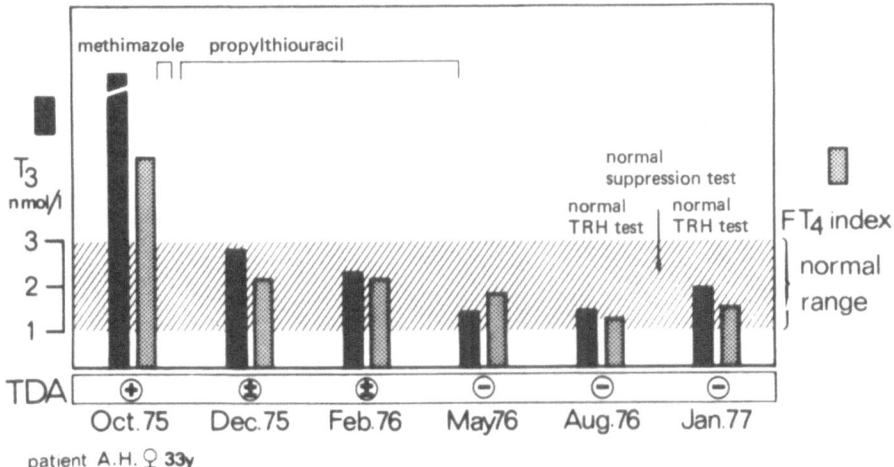

patient A.H. ♀ 33y

Figure 5-3. TDA activity and thyroid function in one patient who went into remission. Before treatment, the TDA assay was strongly positive. In October 1975, treatment was started with methimazole and changed to PTU because of skin eruption. Eight weeks later, the TDA assay was only borderline positive and remained so until February 1976. Since then, TDA assays were negative. During treatment the FT_4 indexes and T_3 levels became normal within 4 weeks and remained so thereafter. After the therapy was stopped, TRH tests were repeatedly normal. The suppression test was performed in September 1976 and ^{99m}Tc pertechnetate uptake fell by 60% after administration of 3 mg T_4. Data are from Teng and Yeung.[46]

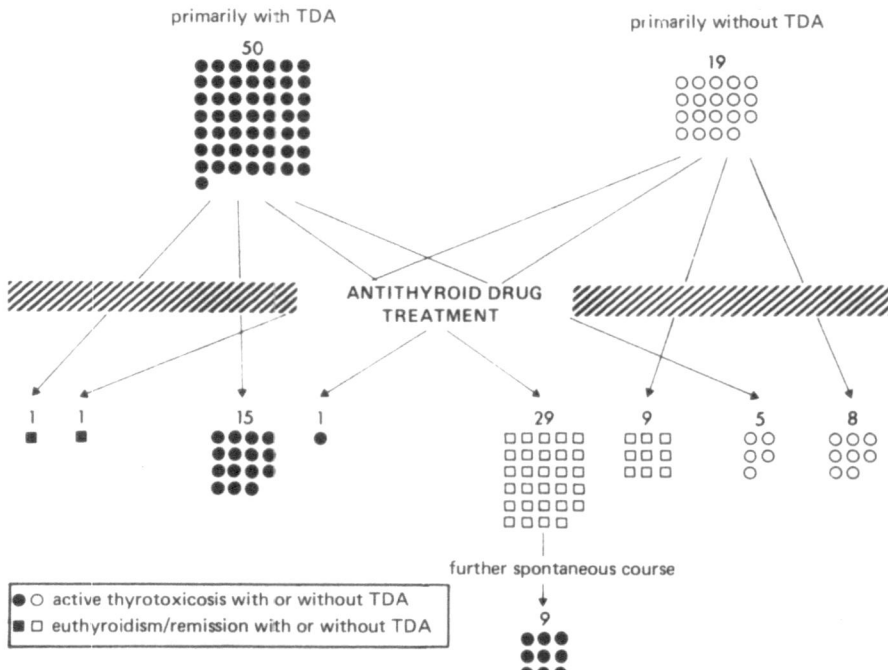

Figure 5-4. Summary of results of follow-up studies in 69 patients. TDA determinations were performed before, at 2-month intervals during, and after ATD treatment. Simultaneously, FT$_4$ indexes were calculated and T$_3$ levels measured. TRH tests were performed before treatment in all patients, and after treatment in 28 of the 40 with normalized T$_4$ and T$_3$ levels; all 28 patients had a normal TSH response to TRH. Normal suppressibility was proved in 8 of 29 patients from the remission group showing disappearance of TDA activity, and in 2 of 9 patients in the remission group which were always TDA negative. *Black symbols,* TDA positivity; *open symbols,* TDA negativity; *circles,* hyperthyroid state; *squares,* euthyroid state. Data are from Irvine et al.[60]

Table 5-7. Prevalence of HLA DR3, HLA B8, and thyroid autoantibodies in patients with repeated relapses of thyrotoxicosis or longstanding remission.

	Relapse group (*n* = 69)	Remission group (*n* = 53)	Controls
HLA DR3 positive	40%[a] ←n.s.→	32%	20%
HLA B8 positive	33%[a] ←n.s.→	28%	18%
TDA positive (before treatment)	71% (p < 0.01)	47%	
Tab: Thyroglobulin antibody	20%	23%	
Mab: Thyroid microsomal antibody	56%	58%	

n.s., no significant difference.
[a]Significant difference from controls.

which patients will respond to ATD. Although the prevalence of TDA activity prior to treatment was significantly higher in the relapse group, the difference was too small to be of predictive value. The differences between our results and those of others[60,61] are unexplained. Possible reasons could be (1) McGregor et al.[61] followed patients only for the relatively short period of 12 months; or (2) the possibility that these workers included not only patients with Graves' disease but also those with disseminated autonomy (see below). A final statement, however, can only be made after examination of a much larger number of patients.

Heterogeneity of Toxic "Diffuse" Goiters

It is unclear whether the 60% prevalence of TDA in hyperthyroid patients with scintigraphically diffuse goiter is explained only by insensitivity of the assay (some authors even doubt the identity of TDA activity and the thyroid stimulator in Graves' disease[49,52,65,66]). However, very recent results from several groups indicate that the patients might suffer from two genetically and pathogenetically different diseases, i.e., Graves' disease (autoimmune thyrotoxicosis) and disseminated thyroid autonomy.[67-76] Disseminated thyroid autonomy may develop in longstanding diffuse or nodular euthyroid goiters, especially in areas of iodine deficiency. It is thought that in these goiters increasing numbers of follicular cells become autonomous so that eventually hyperthyroidism develops. Very often it is exposure to iodine that finally triggers thyrotoxicosis. In contrast to the classical autonomous thyroid adenoma, goiters with disseminated autonomy have autonomous cells scattered throughout.[70] Patients with disseminated autonomy never have Graves' ophthalmopathy, but otherwise the two diseases are indistinguishable by routine procedures such as scintiscan, TRH test, or T_4 or T_3 measurements. The determination of TDA or TsAb activity may possibly help in this differentiation.[73,75,76] In patients with autoradiographically and histologically proved disseminated autonomy, the prevalence of TDA was at most 8%, whereas patients with proved immune thyrotoxicosis (with concomitant ophthalmopathy) had a prevalence of 70 to 80%.[75,76] Furthermore, patients with toxic and scintigraphically diffuse goiter, but without ophthalmopathy and without TDA activity, had a normal prevalence of HLA B8 and HLA DR3.[64] These findings indicate a genetic heterogeneity in toxic diffuse goiter patients. It is unknown whether both disorders have similar long-term courses. Therefore, these newer findings should be considered in reports on the long-term results of ATD therapy.

COMMENTARY

D. Ward Slingerland, M.D.

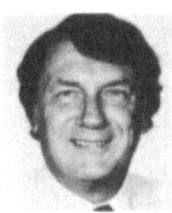

For over 30 years physicians have chosen one of two medical treatments for hyperthyroidism. Each has had a drawback. To ^{131}I the drawback has been and is a high incidence of resulting hypothyroidism. To antithyroid drug (ATD) therapy, it has been but now seems no longer to be a low cure rate.

Disadvantages of [131]I Therapy

In my experience, the incidence of hypothyroidism after ^{131}I therapy of hyperthyroidism is at least 54%, and 75% of patients euthyroid after treatment fail to respond to TSH with the usual stimulation of uptake of radioiodine by the thyroid.[77] Eventually, over half the hyperthyroid patients treated with ^{131}I have to take pills. The thyroid medication, which these patients take by mouth in fixed quantities, attempts to replace the defunct thyroid gland. The normal thyroid, which responds to physiologic stimuli by varying the function of its biosynthetic pathways to change the production and release of thyroid hormone, has been eliminated and in its stead the patient ingests a fixed amount of thyroid hormone. That this substitution does indeed lead to the same overall clinical state provided by an effective, responsive, functioning gland has been queried by some thyroidologists.

Response to ATD

In my experience,[78] the rate of lasting remission after ATD, usually propylthiouracil (PTU), is 84%. Seventy-nine patients were treated for 1 to 16 (average 4.6) years and followed for 2 to 25 years. The average age of patients at the beginning of therapy was 42 years, with a range from 22 to 66 years. They were treated with ATD only, for at least 1 year, and followed for at least 1 year after remission. The usual regimen of 100 mg of PTU every 8 h was modified according to the functional response. Thyroid supplement was added to the regimen on occasion, but rarely on a long-term basis. About once a year a suppression test was usually done: propylthiouracil was stopped, and either 195 mg or 260 mg of thyroid per day for 3 weeks or 75 or 100 μg of liothyronine sodium for 1 week was given. If the uptake on suppression was more than 20%, propylthiouracil therapy was immediately reinstituted. Therapy, in 1-year periods, was usually continued until the uptake on suppression was at or less than 20%.

Why My Experience May Differ From Others

Various ATD treatment regimens used through the years have achieved remission rates ranging from 14 to 72%.[3-6] Hamburger here reports a remission rate of 22%. But in 162 of 237 patients treatment was abandoned, 98 of these because of "patient dissatisfaction with progress." In 24 years we have had only two such dissatisfied patients. Surely the explanation for this is that Hamburger does "not hesitate to express our opinion that ^{131}I is the most efficient treatment for most patients," whereas I do not hesitate to say that in my opinion ATD therapy is the better treatment for most patients. I too explain in detail the pros and cons of ^{131}I versus drug treatment and end by stating that I favor ATD. I emphasize that both treatments will probably lead to a long course of pill taking. But I point out that ATD pill taking will almost surely end, and that when it does, the thyroid will once more be functioning independently and that another disease will not have been produced in the course of curing the first. I explain that the course of the primary thyroid dysfunction seems to be almost always, if not always, self-limited,[7] that my experience is that patients do not have trouble taking the pills as carefully and regularly as they brush their teeth, and that once regulation has been achieved visits twice a year usually suffice. The second visit admittedly involves a 2-day test preceded by 1 week of taking thyroid hormone (triiodothyronine) instead of PTU. Treatment will continue until the suppression test indicates, with a roughly 80% chance of being correct, that the patient will remain well off therapy. It is made clear that therapy will continue indefinitely, on average 4.5 years but possibly 16 or more years. In the event of recurrence, pills will simply be started again. In this way my prejudice is clearly stated, admitted, and justified, hopefully adequately, to the patient. I state that I would treat myself this way. Since my conviction has become this firm, only one patient has refused initial treatment with pills and demanded [131]I.

When I first started treating hyperthyroidism 31 years ago, I did not have this prejudice. Most of my patients were initially treated with [131]I.[8] Many (18) of my earlier PTU patients who experienced recurrences after stopping treatment were retreated with [131]I. As my high indidence of hypothyroidism following ^{131}I gradually became apparent, I began to persist with PTU. I no longer routinely switched to ^{131}I merely on the basis of recurrences. Thus, in some patients treated with PTU, I have had multiple recurrences mostly related to their having stopped treatment on their own. I have also, however, had a recurrence rate of about 20% in patients suppressed below 20%. In these recurrences I doggedly restart PTU therapy. It should be emphasized that Hamburger has a high percentage of young patients. In contrast I do not. Mine is a mature, veteran population presumably somewhat more self-disciplined. I agree that young patients may indeed present a special challenge. I point out, however, that a 20-year-old treated with ^{131}I is not spared the over-50% chance of hypothyroidism for his lifetime—50 years of taking pills.

Reactions to PTU therapy do occur. They have not, in most cases, been of sufficient concern to me or unpleasantness to the patient to warrant discontinuing PTU treatment. I have found that minor reactions can be handled by encouraging patients, antihistamines, or changing from PTU to methimazole. In a total of 106 patients who received PTU as their initial treatment (including the 79 in this study and 27 treated before I became committed to long-term ATD therapy), only five were switched to ^{131}I because of the possibility of a serious reaction such as leukopenia, thrombocytopenia, or granulocytopenia. In two of these five it later became clear that the suspected reaction had not been caused by PTU.

In addition to the maturity of my patient population it is geographically stable. This has surely been a factor in my success. Only six of 106 patients have moved away and all were treated with ^{131}I by others who then managed their therapy. I do not serve in a referral clinic to which a patient comes from afar with the idea of being returned home treated. I fill much more the role of a family physician.

Cost-Effectiveness Considerations

Because PTU treatment has meant, for over 80% of my patients, a final clinical state which may be called normal, I continue to be persuaded that it is, however lengthy, the better treatment. In the best of all possible worlds no more need be said. In the world as it is, the question of the comparative cost of this approach has been vigorously raised. My calculations of the additional cost of PTU treatment assume PTU pills for 5 years, five suppressed uptakes, one and one-third[8] treatment doses of ^{131}I, and thyroxine treatment in 50% for 30 years. A PTU patient need be seen, once clinical euthyroidism is achieved and maintained, twice a year; I consider once-a-year follow-up after ^{131}I essential. Given all the above the total costs are within $100 of each other. A physician, more nervous using PTU, may wish more frequent visits and this difference is what the patient will have paid, when treatment is finished, for a physiologically functioning gland.

Finally, a further comment must be made on the kind of patient I treat. He is usually a male, although the few females we have treated have just as high a rate of lasting remission. He is a mature veteran. He receives free medicine. I personally see each patient on every visit. What I have been pleased to think of as a good doctor/patient relationship has probably been enhanced by gratitude for the absence of cost. The private physician interested in achieving a similar degree of success could, of course, modify his professional charges if his follow-up program makes it necessary, in order to make PTU treatment competitive with [131]I.

Summary

In conclusion, a long experience in treating hyperthyroidism with PTU in an admittedly somewhat unusual patient population has lead to few "failures," few reactions, few "drop-outs," and the high rate of lasting remission of 84%. It would be extraordinary, with this experience, for me to adopt as a primary treatment one which leads in over 50% of treated patients to a permanent second disease calling for perpetual pill taking. A controllable and self-limited disease seems best treated with a controllable and limitable therapy.

COMMENTARY*

Kenneth Sterling, M.D.

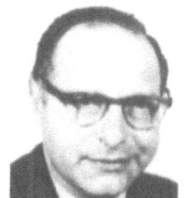

The paper by Hamburger makes some salient points with regard to some of the disadvantages of long-term antithyroid drug therapy for Graves' disease. He has presented his experience with this conventional approach in some detail, including rather careful follow-up data. The 12% "satisfactory" results form a marked contrast with the 76% remission rate reported by Slingerland and Burrows. In view of this marked discrepancy, and the rejoinder by Slingerland, we will not attempt a point by point analysis of all the issues raised by these two antagonistic points of view and philosophies. It is probably sufficient to reemphasize the point made by all parties to this controversy that a great deal depends upon the perspective, objectives, and management philosophy of the physician in charge, as well as on the universe from which the patients are drawn, for example, private patients who may be gainfully employed vs. Veterans Administration (VA) patients.

Combined Antithyroid Drug Regimen for Graves' Disease

Instead of a detailed discussion of the pros and cons of the arguments advanced, it seems far more profitable to present instead an approach I have been employing with rather satisfactory results for almost a decade, which might be termed a "combined antithyroid drug regimen." This consists, in essence, of total blockade of thyroid hormone formation with a single daily dose of methimazole (Tapazole) plus administration of triiodothyronine as Cytomel to maintain approximately euthyroid status—all with a single dose of the medications. This is distinguished from the conventional regimen of antithyroid drugs in divided doses. Many patients who are engaged fully in their work or school activities have had difficulty in adhering to a regimen that requires taking drugs four times a day, even when they are strongly urged to take the medication with each of their three meals and at bedtime. It has, therefore, been particularly advantageous to employ methimazole, because this drug is capable of blocking the thyroid gland completely

*This work was supported in part by the Veterans Administration Medical Research Service and by Grant AM 10739, National Institutes of Health, U.S. Public Health Service.

throughout a 24-h period when given in adequate single doses. With the exception of a very few extremely refractory patients, usually severely neurotic or psychotic, who are unable or unwilling to take medication once a day, we have obtained significantly greater adherence to a regimen consisting of a single daily dose of methimazole, plus supplemental T_3 maintenance, as described below.

The Regimen

The basic concept is to achieve virtually total blockade of thyroid hormone synthesis with a single daily dose of methimazole (Tapazole). In most toxic patients this is usually achieved by ingestion of 80 mg in the form of eight 10-mg tablets; a very small minority (less than one in ten) require 100 mg, and still fewer require 120 mg. The virtue of the single dose is that, in our experience, patients in all socioeconomic levels and linguistic groups adhere better to a regimen that can be followed by performing the required action all at once in the morning. Regimens involving three or four doses a day have, in our experience, a vastly higher incidence of nonadherence. The half-life of [^{35}S]-labeled methimazole in the human circulation is much longer than that of labeled propylthiouracil [W.D. Alexander], making this single-daily-dose regimen possible. These findings have been indicated earlier by thyroidal tracer uptake and clearance procedures by the late Solomon A. Berson and are in general conformity with recent studies on single-daily-dose management at Johns Hopkins Hospital, in which somewhat lesser doses were studied. In contrast to propylthiouracil, which has a duration of action of about 4 h (somewhat reminiscent of sulfadiazine), the effects of methimazole are much more prolonged. In sufficient dosage methimazole will suppress the thyroid gland for a full 24 h. The larger doses required for total blockage of the gland do not appear to have a significantly greater incidence of toxic manifestations (cutaneous, arthritic, or neutropenic) than the more conventional dosages.

The important observation over the course of the first few weeks is rapid clinical improvement associated with falling of the elevated T_4 concentration. If this regimen is conscientiously pursued, the serum T_4(RIA) values will invariably fall to hypothyroid levels, usually about 2 μg/100 ml; therefore, T_3 (Cytomel) is added to the regimen in the form of two or three 25-μg tablets, or else clinical hypothyroidism will supervene. The T_4 level is low because of successful complete thyroid blockade; the T_3 administered is rapidly cleared from the circulation.

The T_3 maintenance can be initiated at the onset, but in any event within 2 weeks of starting blocking therapy. If started initially, the increment of T_3 to an already elevated circulating level is usually proportionally quite slight and no noticeable exacerbation has ever been observed by us. However, in deference to theoretical reservations, we have often been willing to wait, but the T_3 must be initiated without fail within 2 weeks, otherwise serum hormone levels can fall quite precipitously. With T_3 supplementation, the complication of goiter enlargement is avoided altogether. This occasional distressing occurrence during conventional antithyroid drug therapy has never been observed by us in the course of the combined regimen. However, it is important to avoid even transitory hypothyroidism, since even a brief period of hypothyroid status seems, on occasion, to precipitate worsening of eye problems where infiltrative ophthalmopathy exists. Therefore, the addition of T_3 maintenance to the regimen of methimazole in a single blocking dose assures euthyroid status within a matter of weeks as well as preventing the occurrence of enlarging goiter or worsening eye problems, which can be so troublesome with conventional drug management. Consequently, most patients following this regimen will take eight or ten methimazole pills and two or three Cytomel pills every morning for 6 or 9 months, and the T_4 levels, checked periodically, will become extremely low, about 2 $\mu g/100$ ml. The infrequent incidence of nonadherence to the regimen is invariably made evident by failure of adequate depression of the serum T_4 level; the regimen described has proved successful in a wide variety of patients.

Results of Combined Antithyroid Drug Regimen

In many instances palpable goiters will be observed to shrink gradually over the course of several months, which is a favorable prognostic sign. After at least 6 or 9 months of this combined regimen the methimazole is stopped, but the Cytomel is continued. If a patient has achieved long-term remission, including normal thyroid gland suppressibility, the T_4 values will remain low, and after several months of verified low serum T_4 values, all medications are stopped and follow-up of the patient is scheduled at ever-increasing intervals. If, on the other hand, a patient is going to relapse, there will be a gradual rise of the T_4 concentration in the serum, first to the normal range, and eventually to the thyrotoxic range, in spite of continued daily Cytomel. Still later, symptoms would recur unless appropriate measures have been taken. In most instances the chemical evidence of impending relapse in the form of at least two unsuppressed T_4 levels, despite continued T_3 administration, is considered sufficient to warrant ablation therapy, as indicated by the patient's age and by other circumstances. We prefer ^{131}I therapy as the means of ablation, but there remains a group best handled by surgical resection, including those with thyrotoxicosis associated with a hyperfunctioning nodule—so-called "toxic adenoma" or Plummer's disease. The sole instances where we have repeated the above procedures were in patients with a goiter that showed undeniable shrinkage during the course of the regimen. Under these circumstances, a long-term remission often followed a second course of management.

The overall results of the regimen described have not been fully compiled, but they are appreciably better than results with the conventional lower dose therapy with either of the conventional drugs, i.e., methimazole or propylthiouracil. If these observations of a more profound suppressive effect on thyrotoxicosis by blocking doses of methimazole are borne out with further experience and by other clinics, the question will have to be entertained whether total blockade of hormonogenesis may not achieve something more than just a transitory effect during drug therapy—in other words, in many cases a significant reduction of functioning glandular cells. Obviously, this question must be reexplored with an open mind, employing some of the newer adjuncts available for study, including TRH responsiveness.

This regimen has already been published,[79,80] although a definitive statistical study has yet to be compiled. We feel that the results achieved thus far are more encouraging than the rather dismal picture painted by Hamburger and approximate the favorable outcomes claimed by Slingerland and Burrows. Since the approach is both rational and practical and has been in use almost a decade, we recommend it strongly to physicians who manage thyrotoxicosis. The Flowsheet provides abbreviated presentation of the method.

FLOWSHEET
Combined antithyroid drug regimen
for Graves' disease

Monthly tests
Serum T_4 (RIA):
  ∼ 2 μg/100 ml

Methimazole, 80 mg/day
(Tapazole)
and
T_3 (Cytomel), 50 or 75 μg/day.

Continue for 6 to 9 months

Stop methimazole;
continue T_3

Trimonthly tests
Serum T_4 (RIA):
  ∼ 2 μg/100 ml

Serum T_4 (RIA)
rises to mid-normal
range and remains
there several months

Serum T_4 (RIA) rises
above normal on
2 determinations

Remission with
normal suppressibility
by T_3

Impending relapse

Stop all medications
and follow
at ever-increasing
intervals

Long-term remission
or relapse may
ensue

↓

Continue follow-up

Consider ablation
(^{131}I or resection)
unless *marked* shrinkage
of goiter occurs, which may
warrant second course
of combined regimen

SUMMARY—CHAPTER 5

Is antithyroid drug (ATD) therapy for Graves' disease cost-effective? I asked this question because of doubts raised by poor results in my clinic. I shall summarize the responses in three parts:

(1) Considerations of safety, if applicable, should take precedence over costs. Not having invited comment from surgeons I did not expect anyone to advise thyroidectomy to avoid death from radioactive iodine (^{131}I) or ATD.

Canary's surgeons should be commended for more than 400 thyroidectomies without a death. Nevertheless, as already noted, death is an inevitable consequence of the surgical experience; and it is naive for any surgical service to expect an indefinite dispensation from these catastrophes. Those who are impressed with surgical safety should profit from the disasters of others rather than insisting upon reliving them.

That Canary has personally experienced three patients who died of thyroid crisis after ^{131}I should temper the enthusiasm of any prudent physician for that treatment. However, I have not had such deaths after treating more than 3000 patients with ^{131}I in more than 20 years. Canary also had a death from ATD toxicity (see also Miller's commentary after Chapter 7). Deaths in the course of ATD or surgical therapy occur even with highly skilled physicians or surgeons, and these catastrophes can neither be anticipated nor prevented by the exercise of great skill. On the contrary, thyroid crisis after ^{131}I may be attributed to incompetence. As discussed in Chapter 7, this is preventable by appropriate preparation (unless the patient's condition is too severe for any measures to be effective).

Therefore, in terms of immediate patient survival ^{131}I is the treatment of choice.

(2) Cost-effectiveness may impact upon the individual or the entire community. Table 5-8 gives relative cost data for the various treatments.

Upon reading of the "free" medical care which Slingerland provides in a VA hospital, one might not be sure whether to smile or shed a tear. The profligacy

Table 5-8. Relative costs (dollars) of treatments of hyperthyroidism in clinics of various authors.

Treatment	Greenspan[a]	Hamburger[b]	Canary[c]	Greer[d]
ATD	900	450	2800	Highest
^{131}I	1350	1000	3000	Least
Thyroidectomy	4950	3850	2900	Intermediate

[a] 2 years of treatment.
[b] 2 years of treatment; same services as Greenspan.
[c] 1 year of treatment.
[d] Hamburger's interpretation of Greer's comments relative to costs.

inherent in the VA hospital has again recently been emphasized in an exchange of views in the *Annals of Internal Medicine*.[81-83] Although there was some dispute as to whether the average cost for a "free" outpatient visit was merely a shocking $83 or a catastrophic $104, the implications for those who pay taxes are clear.

Patients treated in the private sector have lowest costs when ATD are successful in 6–9 months. Iodine-131 is slightly more costly, whereas thyroidectomy is usually the most expensive treatment (Canary's figures being unusual in that the fees for ^{131}I seem too high while those for surgery seem unrealistically low). Cost estimates for ATD treatment do not include the cost for ^{131}I or surgery for those patients who do not achieve success with ATD. The lower the success rate the more important this consideration becomes.

From the community standpoint, a high failure rate for ATD is a cause of waste which deserves challenge, particularly in an era of concern about escalating costs for medical care. To the community the "free" care of Slingerland is an illusion. Slingerland's suggestion that private physicians should lower their charges so that ATD treatment could be as inexpensive as ^{131}I would be eminently reasonable to a physician who is unconcerned about costs because he renders "free" care.

(3) The cost-effectiveness of ATD therapy depends upon its effectiveness. Sterling suggests that his routine produces results approaching those claimed by Slingerland, but with only 1 year or less of treatment. Unfortunately he has not yet analyzed his data. I agree with Greer, Miller, and Greenspan that younger patients with milder disease and smaller goiters do better with ATD.

Both Slingerland and Miller emphasized the impact of a positive attitude upon results. Physicians can and do influence the choices of their patients by their attitudes, and also by the information they offer. I see many patients who have been sold a thyroidectomy by neglecting to mention surgical risks while misrepresenting the risks of alternative treatments (e.g., "[131]I will make you sterile"). However, when compliance with a treatment must be maintained for many years, as Slingerland advises for ATD, it is more difficult to insulate the patient from more decisive alternative treatments. Also, obtaining informed consent for a method of treatment (i.e., ATD forever) which is so at variance with usual practice that hardly any other authority uses it, in addition to the fact that the method is based upon experience with only about 100 patients, would require a physician to inform his patients that that method was both experimental and not generally accepted. After this introduction most physicians would feel somewhat foolish in attempting to project an attitude of supreme confidence.

After considering the opinions of these experts it seems to me that I should offer more encouragement for a trial of up to 1 year of ATD for younger patients with milder hyperthyroidism and smaller goiters (assuming there are no plans for pregnancy within 2 years). I am especially interested in trying the Sterling regimen. If success is not obtained, ^{131}I could then be given without a great additional economic burden for the individual or the community. Within a few years the large volume of patients seen at my clinic should make it clear what results can be obtained.

Joel I. Hamburger, M.D.

REFERENCES

1. Solomon DH, Beck JC, VanderLaan WP, Astwood EB: Prognosis of hyperthyroidism treated by antithyroid drugs. JAMA 152:201, 1953
2. Hershman JM, Givens JR, Cassidy CE, Astwood EB: Long-term outcome of hyperthyroidism treated with antithyroid drugs. J Clin Endocrinol Metab 26:803, 1966
3. Wartofsky L: Low remission after therapy for Graves' disease. JAMA 226:1083, 1973
4. Greer MA, Kammer H, Bouma DJ: Short-term antithyroid drug therapy for the thyrotoxicosis of Graves's disease. N Engl J Med 297:173, 1977
5. Reynolds LR, Kotchen TA: Antithyroid drugs and radioactive iodine: Fifteen years' experience with Graves' disease. Arch Intern Med 139:651, 1979
6. Slingerland DW, Burrows BA: Long-term antithyroid treatment in hyperthyroidism. JAMA 242:2408, 1979
7. Chevalley J, McGavack TH, Kenigsberg S, Pearson S: A four-year study of the treatment of hyperthyroidism with methimazole. J Clin Endocrinol Metab 14:948, 1954
8. Wool MS: The investigation and treatment of hyperthyroidism. Surg Clin North Am 50:545, 1970
9. Howard JE: Treatment of thyrotoxicosis. JAMA 202:146, 1967
10. Nikolai TF, Brosseau J, Kettrick MA, Roberts R, Beltaos E: Lymphocytic thyroiditis with spontaneously resolving hyperthyroidism (silent thyroiditis). Arch Intern Med 140:478, 1980
11. Rosove MH: Agranulocytosis and antithyroid drugs. West J Med 126:339, 1977
12. Vaidya VA, Bongiovanni AM, Parks JS, Tenore A, Kirkland RT: Twenty-two years' experience in the medical management of juvenile thyrotoxicosis. Pediatrics 54:565, 1974
13. Irvine WJ, Toft AD, Lidgard GP, Gray RS, Seth J, Cameron EHD: Spectrum of thyroid function in patients remaining in remission after antithyroid drug therapy for thyrotoxicosis. Lancet 2:179, 1975
14. Wood LC, Peterson M, Ingbar SH: Hypothyroidism as a late sequela in patients with Graves' disease treated with antithyroid agents. J Clin Invest 64:1429, 1979
15. Tamai H, Nakagawa T, Fukino O, Ohsako N, Shinzato R, Suematsu H, Kuma K, Matsuzuka F, Nagataki S: Thionamide therapy in Graves' disease: Relation of relapse rate to duration of therapy. Ann Intern Med 92:488, 1980
16. Burr WA, Fitzgerald MG, Hoffenberg R: Relapse after short-term antithyroid therapy of Graves' disease. N Engl J Med 297:173, 1977
17. McLarty DG, Alexander WD, Harden R McG, Clark DH: Results of treatment of thyrotoxicosis following relapse after antithyroid drug therapy. Br Med J 3:203, 1969
18. Greer MA: Antithyroid drugs in the treatment of thyrotoxicosis. Thyroid Today 3:1, 1980
19. Bowers RF: Hyperthyroidism: comparative results of medical (^{131}I) and surgical therapy. Ann Surg 162:478, 1965
20. Hamburger JI, Garcia M, Meier DA, Stoffer SS, Taylor CI: The Thyroid Gland. A Book for Thyroid Patients. Southfield, Mich., 1979 (private publication)
21. Utiger RD: Treatment of Graves' disease. N Engl J Med 298:681, 682, 1978
22. Foster RS Jr: Morbidity and mortality after thyroidectomy. Surg Gynecol Obstet 146:423, 1978
23. Sarkar SD, Beierwaltes WH, Gill SP, Cowley BJ: Subsequent fertility and birth histories of children and adolescents treated with ^{131}I for thyroid cancer. J Nucl Med 17:460, 1976

24. Robertson JS, Gorman CA: Gonadal radiation dose and its genetic significance in radioiodine therapy of hyperthyroidism. J Nucl Med 17:826, 1976

25. Freitas JE, Swanson DP, Gross MD, Sisson JC: Iodine-131: Optimal therapy for hyperthyroidism in children and adolescents? J Nucl Med 20:847, 1979

26. Safa AM, Schumacher OP, Rodriguez-Antunez A: Long-term followup results in children and adolescents treated with radioactive iodine (^{131}I) for hyperthyroidism. N Engl J Med 292:167, 1975

27. Stanbury JB, Chapman EM: Nonoperative management of hyperthyroidism. In Varco RL, Delaney JP (eds): Controversy in Surgery. Philadelphia, Saunders, 1976, pp 555–564

28. Eisen MJ: Fulminant hepatitis during treatment with propylthiouracil. N Engl J Med 249:814, 1953

29. Mihas AA, Holley P, Koff RS, Hirschowitz BI: Fulminant hepatitis and lymphocyte sensitization due to propylthiouracil. Gastroenterology 70:770, 1976

30. Colwell AR Jr, Santo D, Land SG: Propylthiouracil-induced agranulocytosis, toxic hepatitis, and death. JAMA 148:639, 1952

31. Weiss M, Hassin D, Bank H: Propylthiouracil-induced hepatic damage. Arch Intern Med 140:1184, 1980

32. Chapman EM: The treatment of hyperthyroidism. N Engl J Med 265:744; 844; 948; 1961

33. Kidd A, Okita N, Row VV, Volpé R: Immunologic aspects of Graves' and Hashimoto's diseases. Metabolism 29:80, 1980

34. McGregor AM, Peterson MM, McLachlan SM, Rooke P, Smith BR, Hall R: Carbimazole and the autoimmune response in Graves' disease. N Engl J Med 303:302, 1980

35. Greer MA, Deeney JM: Antithyroid activity elicited by the ingestion of pure progoitrin, a naturally occurring thioglycoside of the turnip family. J Clin Invest 38:1465, 1959

36. Greer MA, Meihoff W, Studer H: Treatment of hyperthyroidism with a single daily dose of propylthiouracil. N Engl J Med 272:888, 1965

37. Volpé R: The role of autoimmunity in hypoendocrine and hyperendocrine function. Ann Intern Med 87:86, 1977

38. Hallengreen B, Forsgen A, Melander A: Effect of antithyroid drugs on lymphocyte function in vitro. J Clin Endocrinol Metab 51:298, 1980

39. Wall JR, Manwar GL, Greenwood DM, Walters BA: The in vitro suppression of lectin-induced ^{3}H-thymidine incorporation into DNA of peripheral blood lymphocytes after the addition of propylthiouracil. J Clin Endocrinol Metab 43:1406, 1976

40. Alexander WD, McLarty DG, Horton P, Pharmakiotes AD: Sequential assessment during drug treatment of thyrotoxicosis. Clin Endocrinol 2:43, 1973

41. Hackenberg K, Reinwein D: Kontrollierte Hyperthyreose-therapie. Ergeb Inn Med Kinderheilkd 37:20, 1975

42. Romaldini JH, Brombert N, Rodrigues HF, Tanaka LM, Bevilacqua EM, Werner MC, Reis LCF: Management of hyperthyroidism with high dosages of antithyroid drugs (ATD) associated with triiodothyronine (T_3). In Stockigt J, Nagataki S (eds): Thyroid Research VIII. Proceedings of the 8th International Thyroid Conference, Sidney, Australia. Canberra, Griffin Press, Australian Academy of Sciences, 1980, p 633

43. Davies TF, Yeo PPB, Evered DC, Smith BR, Clark F, Hall R: Value of thyroid-stimulating antibody determinations in predicting short-term thyrotoxic relapse in Graves' disease. Lancet 1:1181, 1977

44. Schleusener H, Finke R, Kotulla P, Wenzel KW, Meinhold H, Roedler HD: Determination of thyroid-stimulating immunoglobulins (TSI) during the course of Graves' disease. A reliable indicator for remission and persistence of this disease? J Endocrinol Invest 1:155, 1978

45. Fenzi G, Hashizume K, Rodebush CP, Degroot LJ: Changes in thyroid-stimulating immunoglobulins during antithyroid therapy. J Clin Endocrinol Metab 48:572, 1979

46. Teng, CS, Yeung RTT: Changes in thyroid-stimulating antibody activity in Graves' disease treated with antithyroid drugs and its relationship to relapse: a prospective study. J Clin Endocrinol Metab 50:144, 1980

47. Kuzuya N, Chiu SCH, Ikeda H, Uchimura H, Ito K, Nagataki S: Correlation between thyroid stimulators and 3, 5, 3'-triiodothyronine suppressibility in patients during treatment for hyperthyroidism with thionamide drugs: comparison of assays by thyroid-stimulating and thyrotropin-displacing activities. J Clin Endocrinol Metab 48:706, 1979

48. Zakarija M, McKenzie JM: Clinical significance of assay of thyroid-stimulating antibody in Graves' disease. Ann Intern Med 93:28, 1980

49. McKenzie JM, Zakarija M: Factors and concepts in autoimmune stimulation of the thyroid: autoimmunity in thyroid diseases. In Klein E, Horster FA, Beysel D (eds): Proceedings of the International Thyroid Symposium in Munich, October 1978. Stuttgart, Schattauer Verlag, 1979, p 107

50. Endo K, Kasagi K, Konishi J, Ikekubo K, Okuno T, Takeda Y, Mori T, Torizuka K: Detection and properties of TSH-binding inhibitor immunoglobulins in patients with Graves' disease and Hashimoto's thyroiditis. J Clin Endocrinol Metab 46:734, 1978

51. Ozawa Y, Maciel RMB, Chopra IJ, Solomon DH, Beall GN: Relationship among immunoglobulin markers in Graves' disease. J Endocrinol Metab 48:381, 1979

52. Sugenoya A, Kidd A, Row VV, Volpe R: Correlation between thyrotropin-displacing activity and human thyroid-stimulating activity by immunoglobulins from patients with Graves' disease and other thyroid disorders. J Clin Endocrinol Metab 48:398, 1979

53. Finke R, Kotulla P, Wenzel B, Bogner U, Meinhold H, Schleusener H: Klinische Bedeutung der Bestimmung von schilddresenstimulierenden Antikoerpern (TDA). Dtsch Med Wochenschr (in press)

54. Grumet FC, Payne RO, Konishi J, Kriss JP: HL-A antigens as markers for disease susceptibility and autoimmunity in Graves' disease. J Clin Endocrinol Metab 39:1115, 1974

55. Whittingham S, Morris PJ, Martin FIR: HL-A8: a genetic link with thyrotoxicosis. Tissue Antigens 6:23, 1975

56. Thorsby E, Segaard E, Solem JH, Kornstad L: The frequency of major histocompatibility antigens (SD and LD) in thyrotoxicosis. Tissue Antigens 6:54, 1975

57. Bech K, Lumholtz B, Nerup J, Thomsen M, Platz P, Ryder L, Svejgaard A, Siersboek-Nielsen K, Hansen JM, Larsen JH: HLA antigens in Graves' disease. Acta Endocrinol 86:510, 1977

58. Farid NR, Barnard JM, Marshall WH, Woolfrey I, O'Driscoll RF: Thyroid autoimmune disease in a large Newfoundland family: the influence of HLA. J Clin Endocrinol Metab 45:1166, 1977

59. Schernthaner G, Schleusener H, Finke R, Kotulla P, Ludwig H, Mayr WR: Thyroid stimulating immunoglobulins in HLA-typed patients with ophthalmic Graves' disease, thyrotoxicosis, and Hashimoto's thyroiditis. Acta Endocrinol 87 (Suppl. 215):76, 1978

60. Irvine WJ, Gray RS, Morris PJ, Ting A: Correlation of HLA and thyroid antibodies

with clinical course of thyrotoxicosis treated with antithyroid drugs. Lancet 2:898, 1977

61. McGregor AM, Smith BR, Hall R, Petersen MM, Miller M, Dewar PJ: Prediction of relapse in hyperthyroid Graves' disease. Lancet 1:1101, 1980

62. Schleusener H, Schernthaner G, Mayr WR, Kotulla P, Bogner U, Wenzel B, Koopenhagen K: Evaluation of HLA-typing (A,B,C,DR) and immunological assessment in predicting the long-term course of Graves' disease. In Stockigt J, Nagataki S (eds): Thyroid Research VIII. Proceedings of the 8th International Thyroid Conference. Canberra, Griffin Press, Australian Academy of Sciences, 1980, p 617

63. Schernthaner G, Schleusener H, Kotulla P, Finke R, Wenzel B, Mayr WR: Prediction of relapse or long-term remission in hyperthyroid Graves' disease. Lancet 2:373, 1980

64. Schleusener H, Schernthaner G, Mayr WR, Kotulla P, Bogner U, Wenzel B, Finke R, Meinhold H, Koppenhagen K: Toxic scintigraphically diffuse goiter—two genetically different entities. Evaluation of the assessment of HLA-DR in the distinction of two disorders. (in preparation)

65. Schleusener H, Kotulla P, Fink R, Sorje H, Meinhold H, Adlkofer F, Wenzel KW: Relationship between thyroid status and Graves' disease-specific immunoglobulins. J Clin Endocrinol Metab 47:379, 1978

66. Fenzi GF, Pinchera A, Bartalena L, Monzani F, Macchia E, Mammoli C, Baschieri L: Thyroid plasma membrane antigens and TSH receptor. In Stockigt J, Nagataki S (eds): Thyroid Research VIII. Proceedings of the 8th International Thyroid Congress. Canberra, Griffin Press, Australian Academy of Sciences, 1980, p 703

67. Gemsenjager E, Staub JJ, Girard J, Hetty P: Preclinical hyperthyroidism in multinodular goiter. J Clin Endocrinol Metab 43:810, 1976

68. Dige-Petersen H, Hummer L: Serum-thyrotropin concentrations under basal conditions and after stimulation with thyrotropin-releasing hormone in idiopathic nontoxic goiter. J Clin Endocrinol Metab 44:1115, 1977

69. Emrich D, Bähre M: Autonomy in euthyroid goiter: maladaption to iodine deficiency. Clin Endocrinol 8:257, 1978

70. Studer H, Hunziker HR, Ruchti C: Morphologic and functional substrate of thyrotoxicosis caused by nodular goiters. Am J Med 65:227, 1978

71. Miller JM: Plummer's disease: an overview. J Mol Med 4:3, 1980

72. Elte JWF, Wiarda KS, Bussemaker JK, Froelich M, Bolk JH, Vander-Heide D, Haak A: Autonomously functioning euthyroid multinodular goiter. J Mol Med 4:39, 1980

73. Joseph K, Mahlstedt J, Welcke U: Autonomously functioning thyroid tissue (AFTT) during iodine prophylaxis. J Mol Med 4:87, 1980

74. Joseph K, Mahlstedt J, Gonnermann R, Herbert K, Welcke U: Early recognition and evaluation of the risk of hyperthyroidism in thyroid autonomy in an endemic goiter area. J Mol Med 4:21, 1980

75. Schleusener H, Joseph K, Mahlstedt J, Kotulla P, Bogner U, Wenzel B, Meinhold H: Differences between immunogenic toxic diffuse goiters (Graves' disease) and goiter with disseminated autonomy: preliminary results. J Mol Med 4:129, 1980

76. Schleusener H, Joseph K, Mahlstedt J, Kotulla P, Bogner U, Wenzel B, Meinhold H: Evaluation of thyroid autoantibodies in distinguishing between Graves' disease and disseminated thyroid autonomy. Acta Endocrinol 94 (Suppl. 234):23, 1980

77. Slingerland DW, Dell ES, Burrows BA: The spectrum of thyroid function after radioiodine treatment. In Fellinger K, Hofer R (eds): Further Advances in Thyroid Research. Vienna, Gistel and Cie, 1971, pp 993–1033

78. Burrows BA: Goiter: diagnosis and treatment. Med Clin North Am :1291, 1958
79. Sterling K, Hoffenberg R: Beta blocking agents and antithyroid drugs as adjuncts to radioiodine therapy. Semin Nucl Med 1:422, 1971
80. Sterling K: Diagnosis and Treatment of Thyroid Diseases. Cleveland, CRC Press, 1975
81. Reilly PC Jr, Reilly MC: The cost of outpatient physicians' services at a Veterans Administration hospital. Ann Intern Med 93:128, 1980
82. Jameson JH, Baker CR: Costs in Veterans Administration hospitals. Ann Intern Med 93:782, 1980
83. Reilly PC Jr, Reilly MC: Costs in Veterans Administration hospitals. Ann Intern Med 93:783, 1980

Is There a Place for Long-Term Stable Iodine in the Treatment of Graves' Disease?

Joel I. Hamburger, M.D.

INTRODUCTION

The 1923 report of Henry Plummer established the value of stable iodine for treatment of the hyperthyroidism of Graves' disease.[1] It soon became evident that this effect was only temporary.[2] After a few weeks many patients experienced a relapse or even an exacerbation of their disease. Consequently, stable iodine has been used principally for short-term thyroid suppression, either in the preparation of patients for thyroidectomy, treatment of thyroid crisis, or following radioactive iodine (^{131}I) therapy to hasten the return of the euthyroid state.

Nevertheless, a limited number of reports in the past 50 years showed that long-term administration of stable iodine would produce sustained remission in some hyperthyroid patients.[3-6] The most favorable candidates were patients with mild Graves' disease, especially if the goiters were not large.[3,4,6] Most physicians consider long-term stable iodine not only inadequate, but possibly dangerous.[7-9] In view of the availability of safe and effective alternative treatments, there might seem little reason to consider long-term stable iodine. Nevertheless, there is another point of view worth considering. Stable iodine, Lugol's solution, is cheap, its administration in a single daily dose is all that is required, in the low doses needed for hyperthyroidism it is virtually free of toxicity, and it is a nondestructive form of treatment. If it would be possible to select from the hyperthyroid population those patients for whom this treatment might be effective, it might be a useful alternative. We shall describe our experience with this treatment over the past 19 years to serve as a basis for discussion of the following issues:

(1) Is treatment of selected patients with mild Graves' disease with Lugol's solution worthwhile?

(2) If the results are not substantially better than can be achieved with antithyroid drugs, does this mean that a trial of Lugol's solution has no place?

(3) Would the detection of high antithyroid antibody titers influence the choice between Lugol's solution and antithyroid drugs?

EXPERIENCE OF NORTHLAND THYROID LABORATORY

Selection of Patients

Between 1961 and 1978, 3062 patients were referred to our clinic for treatment of Graves' hyperthyroidism. For 52 of these patients a trial of Lugol's solution was considered reasonable, advised, and accepted by the patients. Follow-up data adequate to assess the effect of the treatment are available for 43 patients. There were 11 males and 32 females ranging in age from 20 to 62 years (mean age 34.6 years). Stable iodine was sometimes employed after radioactive iodine therapy or thyroidectomy, but this report deals only with those for whom iodine solution was the primary treatment. Criteria for selection included the following:

(1) Clinical features of hyperthyroidism were mild (i.e., resting heart rate less than 110 beats/min, weight loss usually less than 5 kg, neither cardiac arrhythmia nor decompensation, no thyrotoxic myopathy, and a thyroid gland no larger than twice normal size (i.e., 40 g estimated weight). There were no additional complicating illnesses (e.g., ischemic heart disease or diabetes) which would place the patient at increased risk in the event of a relapse of the hyperthyroidism.

(2) Serum thyroid hormone concentrations were elevated, but only moderately so (e.g., serum thyroxine concentration no more than 20 to 25% in excess of the upper limit of normal; serum triiodothyronine concentration no more than 50% in excess of the upper limit of normal).

(3) The thyrotoxicosis of silent thyroiditis was excluded by radioactive iodine uptake (RAIU) values of 24 to 52%. Patients with values of less than 35% had nonsuppressibility in response to standard triiodothyronine suppression testing, and more recently blunted responses to thyrotropin-releasing hormone administration.

(4) Only patients for whom good cooperation in a long course of treatment could be anticipated were selected.

Method of Treatment

Stable iodine (Lugol's solution), 3 drops once daily in fruit juice, was given for 8 to 18 months. The shorter treatment periods were employed for patients with unusual sensitivity to the suppressive effects of iodine, such that as little as 1 drop daily produced hypothyroidism or borderline low thyroid hormone levels. Treatment was continued for a longer period if the thyroid gland remained enlarged and blood thyroid hormone levels remained in the mid- or upper normal range. No patients were treated for more than 18 months. If hyperthyroidism failed to respond, escaped from control, or recurred after withdrawal of iodine, an alternative therapy was employed.

After commencing the treatment the patients were seen initially at 1 month to determine that control of hyperthyroidism had been achieved, and then at 3-month intervals to ensure that control was maintained. In some instances an increase in the dose of Lugol's solution 3 to 5 drops daily was followed by an improved response.

After Lugol's solution was discontinued thyroid function was reassessed initially at 1 month to rule out a rapid recrudescence of the hyperthyroidism, then at 6 months and annually thereafter.

Results of Treatment

Lugol's solution was abandoned for six of the 43 patients because of poor control of the hyperthyroidism, and for six because of escape from control. For eight patients a relapse occurred after discontinuation of iodine. These 20 patients were treated with [131]I. The RAIU before Lugol's solution ranged from 20 to 53% (average 35.4%). After discontinuing Lugol's solution the RAIU ranged from 26 to 67% (average 43.8%). These latter values were achieved within 2 to 12 weeks (average 6.3 weeks), except for one patient who relapsed 18 months after discontinuing Lugol's solution. For those patients whose treatment was delayed beyond 4 weeks, the delay was because of failure to return when requested in all but one instance. One patient had a prolonged period of suppression of the uptake lasting 3 months, but during this time she was euthyroid or nearly so. Hyperthyroidism was eliminated with a single treatment of ^{131}I for all patients. None experienced a temporary exacerbation of the hyperthyroidism after administration of the [131]I.

Twenty patients have remained in remission after withdrawal of Lugol's solution from 3 months to 14 years (mean duration 4.6 years). One patient developed hypothyroidism 12 years after treatment.

Three patients are controlled on Lugol's solution from 9 to 15 months.

There were no toxic reactions to the medication. However, one patient, well controlled on Lugol's, had the medication discontinued when she was admitted to a hospital by her gynecologist. A D and C was well tolerated on the second hospital day, but an ovarian wedge resection on the eighth day was followed by thyroid storm. She responded well to conventional therapy for thyroid storm, and was treated with [131]I 2 weeks later.

There were no differences in mean age, sex, or goiter size between the responding group and that for which iodine treatment failed. Antithyroid antibodies were detected with about the same frequency in the two groups.

DISCUSSION

Hyperthyroid patients are usually treated with ^{131}I or thyroidectomy because to most physicians and patients the benefits of prompt and decisive elimination of the disease outweigh the costs of destruction of much (if not all) of the thyroid gland. Long-term antithyroid drug therapy is employed less often as appreciation of the high failure rate grows.[10]

Objections to Long-Term Stable Iodine Therapy

Stable iodine has been useful for the control of persistent mild hyperthyroidism after thyroidectomy or ^{131}I therapy. These patients appear to be sensitive to the suppressant effects of stable iodine. However, long-term administration of stable iodine as the primary treatment of Graves' disease has not been popular. Saxena et al. state that it is ineffective in producing long-term remission.[7] Engbring observes that the euthyroid state can rarely be achieved or maintained after this treatment.[11] Braverman suggests that thyrotoxicosis may be more severe upon withdrawal of iodine.[9] The data presented indicate that these criticisms, although probably applicable to most patients with Graves' disease, might not be appropriate for those with mild hyperthyroidism.

As we have discussed this treatment in various formats, we have been challenged to show that the success we have achieved with stable iodine is better than that which might have been obtained with antithyroid drugs. In our clinic the best results with antithyroid drugs have been achieved in patients with small goiters and mild hyperthyroidism. However, this is not relevant to the issue. Stable iodine has important advantages over antithyroid drugs, including simplicity (once daily administration is suitable for all patients), economy (the cost of medication is negligible), and safety (there is virtually no toxicity in low dosage), while (as with antithyroid drugs) there is no destruction of thyroid tissue. These advantages can be enjoyed by only a small proportion of Graves' hyperthyroid patients, i.e., those preferably younger patients with small goiters and mild toxicity.[3,4,6] For these patients definitive elimination of hyperthyroidism is less urgent and there is something to be said for the preservation of an intact thyroid gland, even if that gland has an increased risk of subsequent functional failure.[12] If the iodine treatment fails to control the disease, or there is escape or relapse, one can easily proceed with ^{131}I therapy.[13] The duration of RAIU blockade by stable iodine is roughly inversely proportional to the severity of the thyrotoxicosis, and always less than that for euthyroid patients. Most of our patients were treated or could have been treated with ^{131}I within 4 weeks after stopping Lugol's solution. At the time of ^{131}I therapy the RAIU values were almost always as high as prior to the institution of Lugol's treatment, and sometimes the values were higher. Thus, the use of stable iodine did not present a barrier to subsequent administration of [131]I.

Another criticism is that treatment with Lugol's solution repletes follicular stores of thyroid hormone, rather than depleting them as is the case with antithyroid drugs. Therefore in the event of an emergency surgical procedure, or an intercurrent infection, the risk of thyroid crisis might be greater in patients taking iodine. None of our patients have had to undergo emergency surgery. Nevertheless this complication may be possible, but as long as the euthyroid state is maintained by the treatment there is no risk. The risk applies to those who escape, and the duration of the risk is only until control is achieved by other means. Since these patients had mild hyperthyroidism the magnitude of the risk would be small except perhaps for the very few who experience a substantial increase in the severity of the hyperthyroidism. The one patient who experienced an episode of thyroid storm following a wedge resection had been well controlled on Lugol's solution previously. The medication had been stopped when she was admitted to the hospital, presumably as part of "hospital routine." The history apparently did not alert the gynecologist to obtain consultation prior to proceeding with the operation. Nevertheless, the possibility of thyroid storm in patients who have hyperthyroidism under control with drugs, and not definitively eliminated by ^{131}I or thyroidectomy, is a legitimate potential concern. Before closing discussion on this point it should be noted that I have seen several patients who experienced sudden marked exacerbation of hyperthyroidism while on antithyroid drugs. Thus this risk is not avoided by their use. Whether all hyperthyroid patients should be treated from the onset by ^{131}I or thyroidectomy at the earliest practical time is a valid question which is addressed in Chapter 5.

Antithyroid Antibodies and Response to Stable Iodine

We expected that high titers of antithyroid antibodies, signifying the probable association of Hashimoto's thyroiditis, might improve the chances of a response to stable iodine, since the sensitivity of patients with Hashimoto's thyroiditis to the suppressant effects of iodine are well known.[9] Our experience does not support this concept. However, not many patients have been treated since improved assays for antithyroid antibodies have been available. Therefore we shall continue to study this point.

Patients Unsuitable for Long-Term Stable Iodine Therapy

Stable iodine is not employed for patients with toxic autonomous nodules. This form of hyperthyroidism does not have the propensity for remission characteristic of Graves' disease. Also, patients with toxic multinodular goiters are unsuitable. They are less likely to respond to iodine,[8] and if not, or if escape or relapse occurs, it takes much longer for the radioactive iodine uptake to recover than in patients with Graves' disease. Furthermore, multinodular goiter is the type of goiter which may be particularly prone to exhibit the jodbasedow phenomenon, and administration of iodine thus may exacerbate the hyperthyroidism. Finally, toxic multinodular goiters occurring in elderly patients are often associated with cardiac complications. These patients are best treated promptly and decisively.

CONCLUSION

For the present I am continuing to suggest use of this simple, safe, and economical treatment for about three or four patients with mild Graves' disease each year. I believe it should not be forgotten.

COMMENTARY

Lewis E. Braverman, M.D.

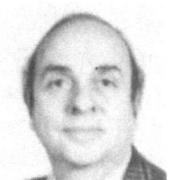

In view of the availability of other methods to treat thyrotoxic Graves' disease, it is perhaps more radical to recommend a "conservative" approach to the long-term treatment of this disorder, i.e., stable iodine administration alone. Prior to the availability of the antithyroid drugs (ATD), and drugs which deplete catecholamines (reserpine) or specifically block the β-adrenergic receptor (propranolol or sotalol), iodides were the only specific therapy for thyrotoxic Graves' disease. Doses as little as 0.25 drop Lugol's solution daily were sometimes sufficient to control the symptoms of active Graves' disease. Hypothyroidism occasionally occurred during treatment, but was reversed after iodide withdrawal.[14] During the 1920s and 1930s, however, the average iodine intake in the United States was far below current estimates. the diagnosis of the self-limited syndrome of low radio-iodine uptake painless thyrotoxicosis (silent thyroiditis) could not be made, and measurements of serum hormone concentrations were not available. Furthermore, during these years, many patients received stable iodine therapy as preparation for definitive surgery, so that few prospective studies are available to determine the short- and long-term results of treatment with stable iodine alone. Finally, thyroid storm was not an uncommon occurrence before the use of ATD and it seems reasonable to assume that if stable iodine therapy was as efficacious as suggested, this complication should have been avoided.

Stable Iodine Even in Carefully Selected Patients Produces Results No Better than ATD

Hamburger has suggested that stable iodine therapy for active Graves' disease be restricted to those patients with mild symptoms who will cooperate in a long course of treatment, with goiters no larger than twice normal size, with no complicating illnesses, and with only a 20 to 25% elevation of serum T_4 concentration and less than a 50% elevation in serum T_3 concentration. If such therapy is so efficacious, why restrict stable iodine to so few patients? This becomes evident from Hamburger's experience. In their studies of 3062 patients referred for treatment of thyrotoxic Graves' disease, only 52 patients were selected for treatment with Lugol's solution alone for 8 to 18 months (1.7%). Of these 52 patients, 43 were available for sufficient follow-up data to be included in the series. Treatment with Lugol's solution was abandoned in 12 of these 43 patients because of poor control of the hyperthyroidism or escape from control and eight others relapsed after iodine withdrawal, resulting in a 47% failure rate. In the 23 patients "successfully" treated with stable iodine, three are now on Lugol's solution; remission in the remaining 20 patients after iodine withdrawal ranged from 3 months to 14 years, but it is not stated how may patients are in remission for less than 2 years. These statistics strongly suggest that the remission rate following long-term treatment with Lugol's solution in this highly selected group of patients with thyrotoxic Graves' disease is similar to that observed in some recent series following long-term ATD therapy in unselected patients with Graves' disease.[15-17] Indeed, it is generally agreed that the remission rate following ATD therapy in patients with mild disease and small goiters (as in Hamburger's series) is even higher.

Disadvantages of Stable Iodine Therapy

Treatment of even a selected group of patients with thyrotoxic Graves' disease with stable iodine has sufficient problems to markedly restrict its use. The major antithyroid effect of iodine on thyroid gland function in patients with hyperthyroidism is a partial inhibition of thyroid hormone release and a transient partial inhibition of hormone synthesis (acute Wolff-Chaikoff effect). The thyroid usually escapes from this latter inhibitory effect on hormone synthesis, and synthesis of hormone rapidly returns. This results in a gland rich with stored hormone. ATD, on the other hand, act by inhibiting hormone synthesis. When a quantity of drug had been administered which sufficiently blocks hormone synthesis, euthyroidism ensues and escape does not occur. In contrast to stable iodine therapy alone, the thyroid is depleted of stored hormone during and after ATD therapy. Furthermore propylthiouracil, but not methimazole, also partially inhibits the peripheral outer ring deiodination of thyroxine resulting in a decreased peripheral generation of the more active iodothyronine, triiodothyronine. This brief discussion of the mechanism of action of iodine and ATD emphasizes the major problems with stable iodine. These include the following:

Escape from Stable Iodine Suppression of Hormone Synthesis and Release
Emerson et al. carefully studied patients with thyrotoxic Graves' disease treated with stable iodine alone and their results demonstrated that thyroid function tests in most of these unselected patients do not return to normal and that escape from the effects of stable iodine frequently occurs within 2 to 3 weeks.[8] An even greater threat to the patient is an abrupt cessation of stable iodine therapy leaving a gland rich in hormone stores whose release from the thyroid is no longer blocked by

iodine. A marked worsening of thyroid function and even thyroid storm could then rapidly occur, a complication rarely if ever seen following cessation of ATD therapy. These problems were seen in Hamburger's patients since hyperthyroidism was not controlled in six patients, six patients escaped from control of their thyrotoxicosis while on Lugol's solution, and eight patients rapidly relapsed after iodine was discontinued. It was not stated whether the thyrotoxicosis was more severe in the patients who escaped or relapsed, although at least one patient (number 3) became far more hyperthyroid while receiving Lugol's solution. Finally, the worst complication of stable iodine therapy was observed even in this very selected group of patients, i.e., the occurrence of thyroid storm shortly after the withdrawal of iodine therapy. Indeed, Hamburger admits that even in this highly selected group, a few patients may experience a substantial increase in the severity of their hyperthyroidism. It is also suggested that the sudden withdrawal of iodine therapy is ill-advised and that such a problem is not common, and is initiated either inadvertently by other physicians or by the patient herself. This potential problem is far more common than suggested and the risk ever present. In contrast to iodine therapy, the abrupt cessation of ATD therapy in patients whose disease is still active but biochemically controlled is not complicated by the rapid onset of severe thyrotoxicosis since the gland has been depleted of hormone stores. It would be extremely rare for thyroid storm to occur within 1 to 2 weeks following ATD withdrawal in patients well controlled on the drugs. Finally, the statement that "sudden marked exacerbation of hyperthyroidism while on ATD has been observed in several patients" is not documented and suggests that the patients were not under adequate control and discontinued the drugs without informing the physician. The problem of poor patient compliance is less risky with ATD than with stable iodine therapy for reasons emphasized above.

Iodine-Induced Thyrotoxicosis
It is now well recognized that jodbasedow's disease or iodine-induced thyrotoxicosis does occur in the United States, especially in elderly patients with nodular goiter.[18] The advocacy of iodine therapy alone in some patients with Graves' disease also presents the problem of a mistaken diagnosis of Graves' disease in patients with nodular goiter or the presence of functioning nodules in patients with Graves' disease.[19] In these patients, stable iodine is contraindicated in the presence or absence of hyperthyroidism and a marked increase in the severity of hyperthyroidism frequently occurs after iodine withdrawal.[18]

Toxicity of Stable Iodine
Although allergic and toxic reactions to stable iodine are uncommon and iodism only occurs with much larger doses of iodine than recommended in this chapter,

attention has recently been directed toward such complications.[20] A list of iodine-induced reactions (Table 6-1) includes hypocomplementemic vasculitis which can occur in patients with underlying autoimmune diseases with doses not too dissimilar to those recommended in the treatment of thyroid disease.[21]

Table 6-1. Extrathyroidal adverse effects of iodide.

I. Sialadenitis
II. Cutaneous (ioderma)
III. Fever
IV. Allergies
    A. Edema of the face; glossitis
    B. Periarteritis nodosa
    C. Rhinorrhea; nasal polyps
    D. Hypocomplementemic vasculitis
        1. Chronic idiopathic urticaria
        2. Systemic lupus erythematosus
        3. Dermatitis herpetiformis

Long-Term Beta Blockers, an Alternative to Stable Iodine

The aim of nonablative therapy of Graves' disease is to induce euthyroidism until the disease goes into spontaneous remission. Methods to predict remission include a return of thyroid suppression during thyroid hormone administration, a normal TRH test, and the disappearance of thyroid-stimulating immunoglobulins from the serum, especially in patients who do not have the histocompatibility antigen DRw3. The latter appears to have the greatest predictability of remission.[22] Since stable iodine therapy has been recommended in patients with mild hyperthyroidism and small goiters and these patients probably have a greater incidence of spontaneous remission, another method of therapy could be used which does not have the problems noted above with iodine therapy or the uncommon toxic effects of ATD. The chronic administration of beta-blocking drugs rapidly controls many of the signs and symptoms of hyperthyroidism without affecting thyroid hormone synthesis and release, although they do slightly decrease the peripheral conversion of T_4 to T_3. This approach to therapy of mild hyperthyroidism,[23] especially in patients previously treated with radioactive iodine or surgery, does offer an alternative to the stable iodine therapy suggested by Hamburger without the risks of more severe hyperthyroidism or induction of hypothyroidism.

Where Stable Iodine Is Useful

Although we do not recommend stable iodine as sole therapy for Graves' disease, iodine administration is certainly indicated in the management of Graves' disease under certain conditions. Iodine therapy is recommended in the preoperative (subtotal thyroidectomy) management of patients first restored to the euthyroid state by ATD, in patients with thyroid storm, and occasionally following radioactive iodine therapy, although approximately 25% of such patients develop hypothyroidism within 3 months which usually disappears following iodine withdrawal.[24] Recently, it has been suggested that euthyroidism is consistently achieved in 10 days following the institution of iodine therapy in patients receiving 160 mg propranolol daily for weeks prior to and during iodine administration.[25] Such an approach has been recommended to prepare patients with Graves' disease for subtotal thyroidectomy and suggests synergism between iodine and propranolol in decreasing thyroid gland function. Other clinics must confirm these observations. Iodine is also recommended in the treatment of endemic iodine deficiency goiter and to markedly decrease the thyroid uptake of radioactive iodine in the event of accidental exposure. Finally, small doses of iodine might be used chronically in patients with mild hyperthyroidism and a small goiter who develop toxic reactions to ATD, and for whom surgery or radioactive therapy are not recommended or refused.

COMMENTARY

William M. McConahey, M.D.

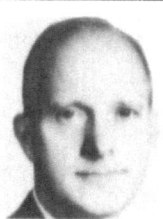

In recent years the use of stable iodine for the long-term treatment of Graves' disease has received little attention, although previously this mode of therapy was employed occasionally and with success. Long-term administration of stable iodine as therapy for Graves' disease should be considered only if the hyperthyroidism is mild and the gland is not greatly enlarged. Before the wide usage of ^{131}I for treatment of the hyperthyroidism of Graves' disease, our group usually employed Lugol's solution for the long-term treatment of patients in whom *mild* recurrent hyperthyroidism developed after subtotal resection of the thyroid for Graves' disease. Such patients usually responded very well to this treatment and remained euthyroid. Occasionally, patients so treated would become hypothyroid when given Lugol's solution. When this occurred, they could be maintained euthyroid by the administration of both Lugol's solution and thyroid hormone. Patients in whom *mild* recurrent Graves' disease develops after ^{131}I therapy also may be controlled by the long-term administration of stable iodine.

At the present time, most patients who have Graves' disease are treated with ^{131}I or antithyroid drugs (ATD), whether the hyperthyroidism is primary or recurrent. Our group usually employs ^{131}I therapy for such patients who are more than 20 years of age. Some workers have considered that the long-term treatment of patients with primary Graves' disease by the use of stable iodine was inadvisable because of either lack of response to treatment or escape from the effects of treatment. However, we agree with Dr. Hamburger and others[3,26] that treatment with stable iodine can be used effectively for a few selected patients who have *mild* hyperthyroidism of Graves' disease and *small* thyroid glands. Such selected patients might include young persons, patients who experience toxic reactions to ATD, and patients who prefer not to have treatment with [131]I.

If the patient with Graves' disease who is being successfully treated with stable iodine becomes a medical or surgical emergency, the physician treating that emergency must know that the patient is receiving stable iodine and continue the therapy. Hamburger's patient who went into thyroid crisis after surgery probably would not have done so had treatment with stable iodine not been inadvertently stopped. Our group has successfully operated on several patients under similar circumstances.

Stable iodine treatment has little, if any, effect and therefore is of no value in hyperthyroidism caused by a nodular goiter (Plummer's disease).

In our opinion, there *is* a place for the long-term administration of stable iodine in the treatment of the patient with Graves' disease who is mildly hyperthyroid, who does not have large goiter, and who is not a suitable candidate for treatment with ^{131}I, ATD, or thyroid surgery. Such treatment is simple, inexpensive, usually effective, and free from any dangerous side effects.

COMMENTARY*

Shigenobu Nagataki, M.D.

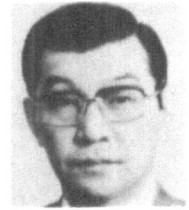

It is generally recognized that iodine ameliorates the symptoms of hyperthyroidism and decreases serum hormone concentrations to the normal range; but this effect usually continues for only a limited time.[1,3-5,7-9,27-29] The majority hold

*The contribution of Hidemasa Uchimura, M.D., to this work is gratefully acknowledged.

Table 6-2. Pertinent clinical data before iodide therapy and thyroid status at the end of treatment for hyperthyroidism.

Patient	Sex	Age	Time of onset	Pulse rate (beats/min)	BMR (%)	Exophthalmos	Goiter	Thyroid status at present
1 M. T	F	29	2m	120	55	−	−	escaped
2 T. S	F	31	1m	140	56	+	++	escaped
3 H. T	F	25	5y 1	96	36	−	+	eumetabolic
4 T. M	M	41	0m	108	19	+	−	escaped
5 H. H	F	30	1m	90	54	−	+	escaped
6 M. H	F	36	2m	102	29	+	+	eumetabolic
7 K. M	F	46	1y2m	96	47	+	−	escaped
8 Y. K	F	55	7m	120	82	+	+	escaped
9 M. T	F	19	2m 1	92	38	−	−	eumetabolic
10 F. S	F	30	0y	132	53	−	+	escaped
11 I. K	F	46	1m	96	47	−	±	eumetabolic
12 T. S	F	42	2m	102	32	−	+	escaped
13 F. N	F	34	7y	90	39	+	+	escaped
14 Y. M	F	32	1m	102	—	−	+	escaped
15 Y. S	F	47	1y2m	96	29	+	±	escaped
16 S. M	M	32	2m	120	65	+	+	eumetabolic
17 K. T	M	61	4m	108	55	−	−	eumetabolic
18 M. I	F	62	3m	84	48	+	+	escaped
19 K. S	F	24	2m	120	62	+	++	escaped
20 F. A	F	30	5y6m	118	37	+	+	eumetabolic
21 T. N	F	53	3m	76	46	−	+	escaped
22 Y. N	M	48	9m	120	42	+	+	escaped
23 T. G	F	22	2m	132	77	++	++	escaped
24 T. K	F	44	2m	108	54	−	±	eumetabolic
25 M. M	M	19	1y	108	35	−	−	escaped
26 Y. S	F	35	2m	120	54	−	+	escaped
27 Y. H	M	42	2y	99	58	+	+	escaped
28 H. F	F	31	1y	100	34	−	+	eumetabolic
29 M. T	F	45	2m	120	46	−	+	escaped
30 S. I	M	25	6m	108	47	+	+	escaped
31 E. K	F	28	1m 2.	96	67	−	+	eumetabolic
32 M. I	M	29	5y	120	59	−	+	escaped
33 M. Y	F	32	3m	92	43	−	+	escaped
34 T. K	F	28	2m	108	65	+	+	eumetabolic
35 S. H	F	20	2m	130	66	±	+	escaped
36 S. N	F	30	2m	120	80	−	+	escaped
37 Y. Y	F	18	2m	120	60	−	−	escaped

Symbols defined in the text.

F, female; M, male; m, months; y, years.

that long-term stable iodine therapy for hyperthyroidism is generally not only inadequate, but possibly dangerous.[7-9] However, a complete or virtually complete remission may be obtained with inorganic iodine therapy alone in 20–30% of patients with Graves' disease.[3,6,27] Therefore, it is important to distinguish patients who may be treated with iodine alone from those who may not. In this commentary, we will describe our experiences with a method to predict the long-term results of iodine therapy for patients with Graves' disease.[30]

Experience of the University of Tokyo, Third Department of Internal Medicine

Almost all untreated patients with Graves' disease who visited our clinic during a period in 1971 were treated only with 3.3 mg of potassium iodide t.i.d. after explaining the advantages and disadvantages of iodine therapy. Table 6-2 shows the clinical data for 37 patients before iodine therapy and thyroid status after 1.5 years of treatment. Patients were asked to visit our clinic at least once every 4 weeks during the course of iodine therapy for clinical and laboratory evaluation of thyroid function. Thyroidal radioactive iodine uptakes (RAIU)[31] were performed before therapy was begun, at 4 weeks of iodine therapy, once every 8 weeks thereafter, and after escape from the iodine effect had occurred. Escape from the iodine effect was confirmed by clinical findings of thyrotoxicosis and elevated serum T_4 levels on two separate occasions. Before beginning iodine therapy, patients were asked to avoid seaweed for 10–14 days prior to measurement of RAIU. During iodine therapy patients were asked to take their drugs even on the day of the measurement of RAIU. Values for the 20-min, 1-h, and 24-h RAIU were determined.

Long-Term Results of Iodine Therapy

Of 37 patients, eight (22%) experienced escape within 4 weeks of iodine treatment and eight (22%) during the following 4 weeks. An additional nine patients (24%) escaped within 6 months of the treatment. The remaining 11 patients (30%) were euthyroid throughout the 1.5 years of iodine therapy, and all of them were euthyroid for a least 6 months after ceasing iodine. No patients escaped after 6 months of control on iodine treatment.

Changes in Thyroid Function during Iodine Therapy

Patients were divided into two groups: group A included those who did not escape from the iodine treatment (11 patients) and group B included those who escaped within 6 months of iodine treatment. Figures 6-1 and 6-2 present the means and standard errors for serum T_4 concentration and RAIU values before and during iodine therapy for the two groups. Values for Group B, shown in these figures, are those obtained 4 or 8 weeks before escape occurred.

During iodine treatment, serum T_4 levels (Fig. 6-1) were within the normal range (5.3–14.5 $\mu g/dl$) in both groups, and differences between the two groups were not significant. In contrast to serum hormone levels, the 20-min RAIU values were significantly higher in group B than in group A at 0, 4, and 12 weeks of treatment (Fig. 6-2). The 1-h RAIU values were higher in group B than in group A only before iodine treatment and differences in values for the RAIU in the two groups were not significant (Fig. 6-2).

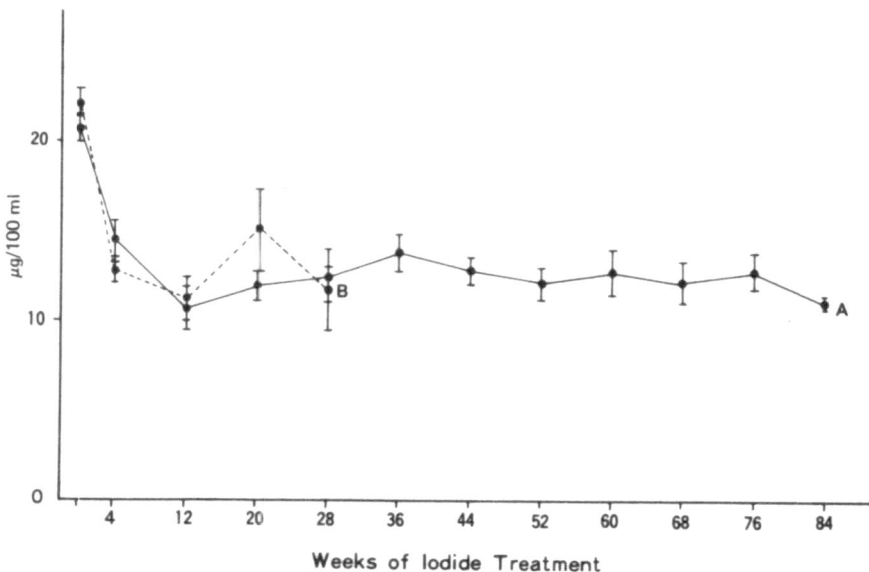

Figure 6-1. Changes in serum T_4 concentration during iodide therapy. *A*, nonescaped; *B*, escaped. Values for escaped patients are those obtained before escape had occurred.

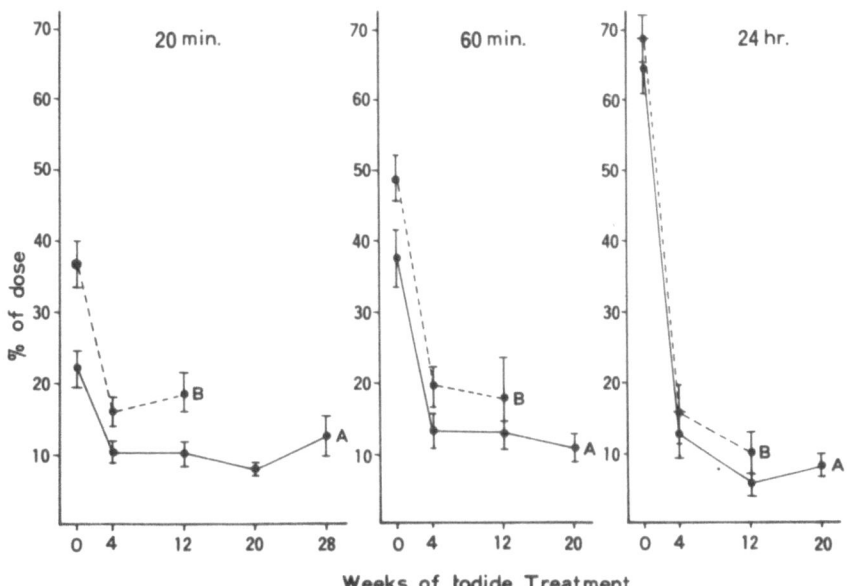

Figure 6-2. Changes in thyroidal ^{131}I uptake during iodide therapy. ●—●, nonescaped; ●- -●, escaped.

Comparison of Thyroid Function before Iodine Treatment in Patients Who Escaped and Those Who Did Not

Figure 6-3 shows values for BMR, T_3 uptake, serum T_4 concentration, RAIU, serum total cholesterol, pulse rate, and degree of exophthalmos and goiter before iodine treatment in 37 patients studied. In this study, degrees of exophthalmos and goiter were defined as follows. Exophthalmos: $(-)$ and $(\pm)$, less than 16.5 mm; $(+)$, 17 mm or more; $(++)$, 20 mm or more. Goiter: $(-)$, palpable but not enlarged; $(\pm)$, not larger than 1.5 times normal size; $(+)$, not larger than three times normal size; $(++)$, larger than three times normal size. There were no significant differences between the two groups.

Figure 6-4 shows values for RAIU before iodine treatment. Open circles represent values for group A patients and solid circles those for group B patients. When values for the 20-min RAIU were divided arbitrarily at 25%, nine patients had values less than 25%, and eight of the nine were in group A. In contrast, of 15 patients whose 20-min RAIU values were greater than 25%, only two were in group A. Similarly, when values for the 1-h uptake were divided at 40%, eight of 14 whose values were less than 40% were in group A, and only three of 22 with values greater than 40% were group A patients. Differences in 24-h RAIU values in the two groups were not significant.

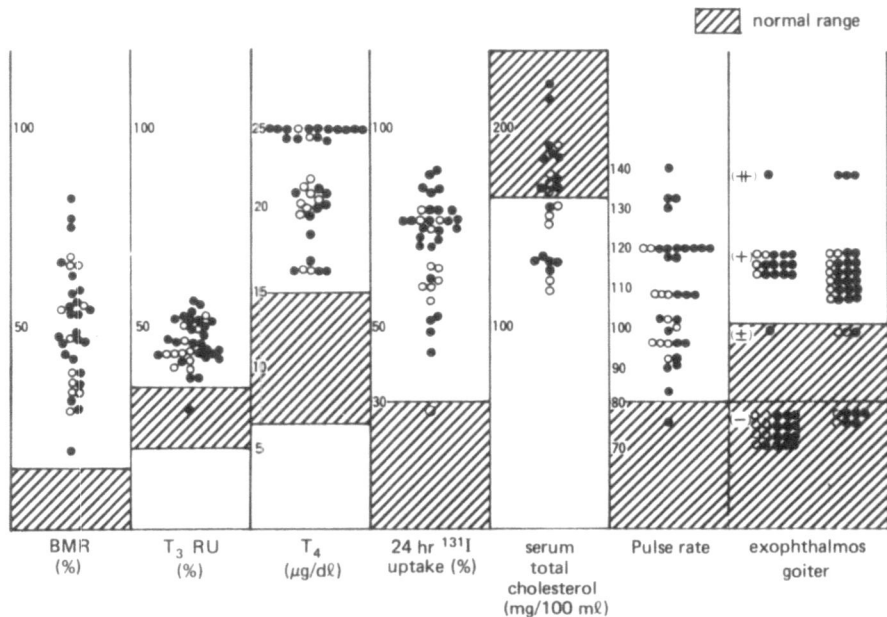

Figure 6-3. Clincal findings and various laboratory data obtained before iodide treatment. ○, nonescaped; ●, escaped.

Changes in RAIU Values at the Time of Escape

RAIU values determined in seven patients at the time of escape were not significantly different from values obtained before escape (Fig. 6-5). Hence, escape is not due to an increase in RAIU.

Discussion

It should be emphasized that the present study deals with patients in Japan, where the average daily iodine intake is approximately 1 mg,[32] and Graves' disease represents 40.1% of thyroid disorders (Hashimoto's disease, 20.5%; adenoma, 15.1%; nontoxic diffuse goiter, 13.1%; carcinoma, 4.0%; myxedema, 3.3%; subacute thyroiditis, 1.8%; other, 2.1%), much higher than the incidence in the United States. Furthermore, the incidence of prolonged remission in hyperthyroidism after thionamide drugs is lower in Japan than in the United States. Remissions are found in about 25% of patients treated for 1 year in Japan,[33,34] in comparison to the remission rate of approximately 50% in the United States[35-38] and Europe.[39-41] However, the remission rate seems to be decreasing recently in the United States.[10]

Although the average daily intake of iodine is 1 mg, the results of the present study have shown that remission may be obtained with daily administration of 10

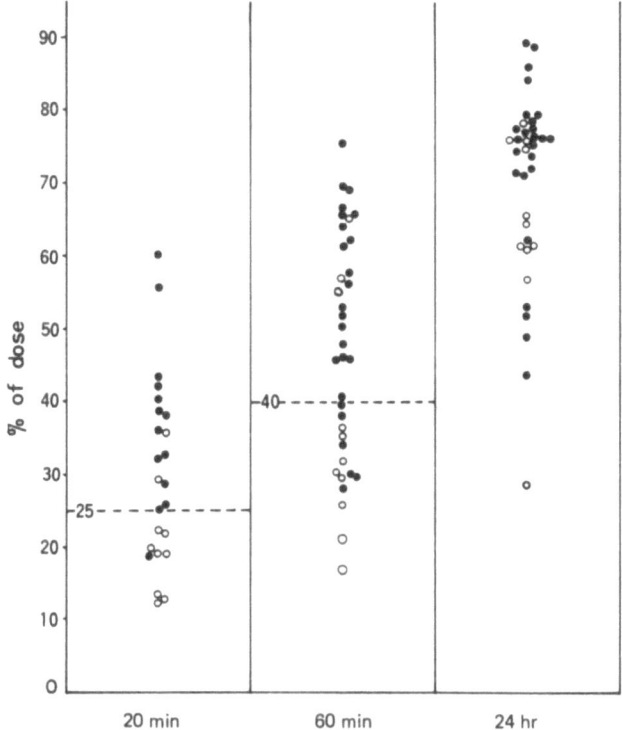

Figure 6-4. Thyroidal ^{131}I uptake before iodide treatment. ○, nonescaped; ●, escaped.

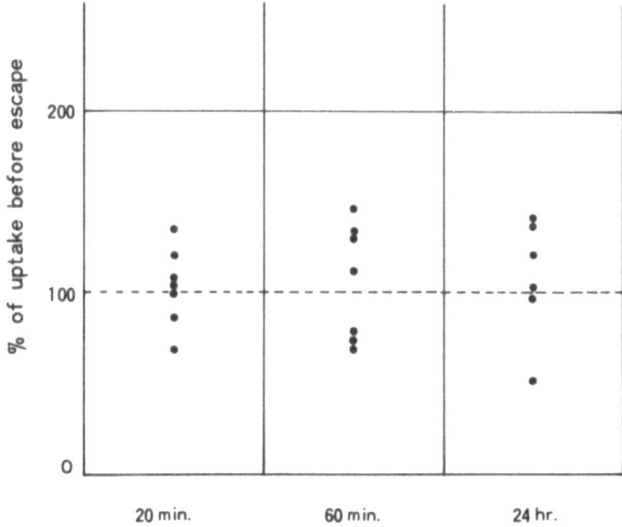

Figure 6-5. Comparison of values for thyroidal ^{131}I uptake before and after escape.

mg of iodine in 30% of unselected untreated patients with Graves' disease. The effectiveness of iodine treatment was comparable to that of thionamide therapy.

The selection of favorable candidates for iodine therapy, therefore, is very important. The present study shows that values for the 20-min RAIU are useful for this purpose.

COMMENTARY

Lawrence C. Wood, M.D.
and Farahe Maloof, M.D.

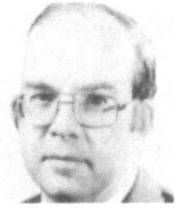 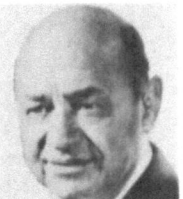

In 1975, the clinical files of the Thyroid Unit of the Massachusetts General Hospital were screened to identify all patients who had received potassium iodide as the primary treatment for Graves' disease. Our purpose was to determine the effectiveness of such treatment as well as the incidence of thyroid failure following potassium iodide therapy.[26]

Selection of Patients

Eighteen patients were found who met the following criteria:

(1) They had good clinical and laboratory confirmation of the original diagnosis of Graves' disease.
(2) They had not had ablative treatment in the form of a subtotal thyroidectomy or radioiodine.
(3) They had good clinical or laboratory follow-up of thyroid function.

All 18 patients were women with an average age of 43 years (range 10–77 years) at the onset of symptoms. Eleven had exophthalmos.

In most instances, potassium iodide was selected as the mode of therapy because of mild hyperthyroidism and the finding of a relatively small goiter. In three patients, potassium iodide was used after a rash appeared during the first 2 weeks of treatment with antithyroid drugs. In other subjects, it was chosen because either the patient or the physician rejected ablative therapy.

In recent years, we have added the iodide-perchlorate discharge test[42] as a screening procedure to help select patients who are likely to respond favorably to potassium iodide. In 1950, Childs et al.[43] used thiocyanate to prove that small quantities of carrier iodide block intrathyroidal organification of radioiodine in hyperthyroid subjects. In contrast, normal individuals require much larger quantities of iodine to suppress thyroid function. But hyperthyroid patients may vary in thyroid gland sensitivity to potassium iodide. Therefore, we now perform an iodide-percholorate discharge test in thyrotoxic patients who are being considered for potassium iodide therapy, and consider a positive response (i.e., discharge of more than 5% of radioiodine from the thyroid following administration of the iodide and perchlorate) as an indication of a likely favorable response to this form of treatment.

Treatment Protocol and Results

Patients were given potassium iodide with an average starting dose of 6 drops (270 mg) daily. Treatment with potassium iodide lasted for 1 to 72 months with an average duration of 26 months.

Seventeen of the 18 patients responded to potassium iodide therapy with symptomatic improvement and normalization of laboratory values. Once a eumetabolic state had been achieved, patients were followed by periodic clinical evaluation and measurements of serum thyroxine (T_4) and thyrotropin (TSH) levels. In several instances, we observed a gradual rise in the serum TSH while the patient was on a stable dose of potassium iodide. When this occurred, reduction of the potassium iodide dosage was followed by a drop in the TSH level to normal (Fig. 6-6).

Five of the 18 patients became overtly hypothyroid from 6 to 24 years after the onset of Graves' disease and an average of 6 years after cessation of iodide

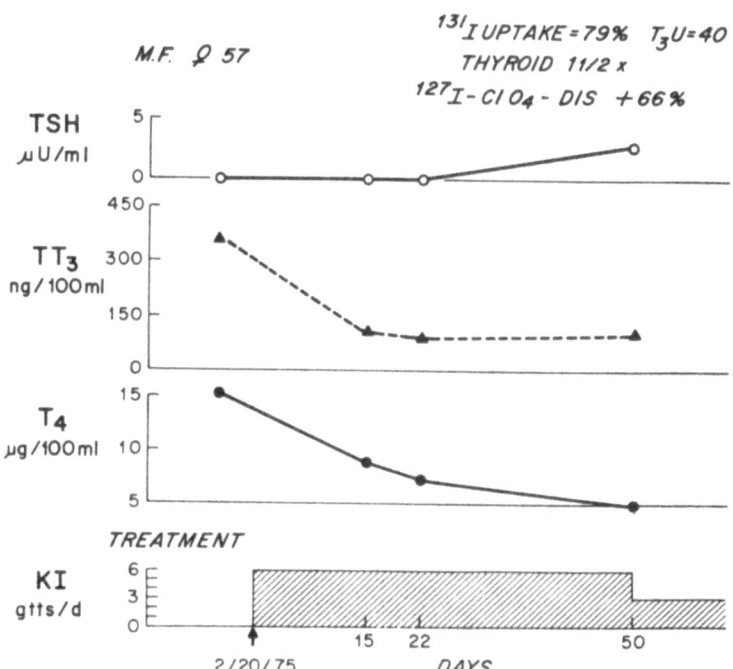

Figure 6-6. The response to potassium iodide in patient M.F., illustrating the recent protocol for the treatment of Graves' disease with potassium iodide.

treatment. Two additional patients appeared "prehypothyroid" at the time their clinical course was reviewed. They felt well, and had normal serum concentrations of T_4 and T_3. However, their serum TSH values were elevated, they had decreased responses to exogenous TSH, and exaggerated responses to TRH. Six of the 18 patients were well without treatment at the time of their last evaluation, while four patients were eumetabolic on iodide treatment.

Our youngest patient, the only patient less than 20 years old, was 10 years old when iodide therapy was begun. Despite an initial improvement on potassium iodide therapy she developed several relapses in her hyperthyroidism later, including a recurrence following her first pregnancy. Eventually a subtotal thyroidectomy was performed.

Discussion

These patients were reviewed primarily to determine how often hypothyroidism developed after a supposedly nonablative method of treatment for diffuse toxic goiter. Although the number of patients in this study is admittedly small, our documentation of thyroid failure in several of these patients suggests that late hypothyroidism occurs in patients with Graves' disease following potassium iodide treatment, as well as after ablative treatment with radioiodine or thyroidectomy. Our selection of patients with firm thyroid glands for potassium iodide therapy may have favored those with a greater degree of associated thyroiditis, patients who might be expected to experience subsequent thyroid failure. Antithyroid antibodies were present in nine of the 11 patients for whom the test was performed.

On the other hand, potassium iodide itself may damage the thyroid gland in Graves' disease. After the introduction of iodine therapy in the 1920s, a greater amount of lymphocytic infiltration was noted in thyroid glands removed surgically.[44] Follis[45] produced the histologic appearance of thyroiditis when he administered iodine to hamsters whose thyroid glands were previously made hyperplastic by thiouracil, potassium thiocyanate, or an iodine-deficient diet. Finally, Belshaw and Becker[46] reported necrosis of follicular epithelial cells following the administration of large doses of iodide to iodine-deficient dogs.

Conclusions

It is our impression that for selected patients with the hyperthyroidism of Graves' disease, potassium iodide can be an effective treatment. Patients most likely to respond to potassium iodide have mild disease, small firm thyroid glands, and positive iodide-perchlorate discharge tests. Long-term potassium iodide treatment probably is not indicated for those with large goiters, marked hyperthyroidism, serious cardiovascular disease, or other associated conditions requiring prompt and certain control of thyroid function. Finally, as for all other patients with Graves' disease, lifelong follow-up is essential if late onset thyroid failure is to be promptly recognized and treated.

SUMMARY—CHAPTER 6

The appreciation of iodine as a two-edged sword in Graves' disease has led to abandoning a therapy that is effective, simple, safe, and cheap. This statement is agreed to by Hamburger and three of the four discussants, who likewise concur in the necessity for a very select approach to the use of iodine therapy. Few physicians in this country have employed iodides as did Nagataki, as most of our patients prefer a treatment with a higher degree of success. Limiting iodine use to glands of small size or with a high degree of autoimmune thyroiditis plus a mild degree of secretory overactivity, as Wood and Maloof suggest, should raise the remission rate to satisfactory level.

An additional indication for this conservative therapy should be considered. With very mild Graves' hyperthyroidism, the patient may consider the symptoms of minor inconvenience or may not be aware of the disease at all. In such instances, in the induction of the hypothyroid state by radioiodine, or long-term treatment with ATD, may be regarded by the patient as something less than beneficial. Aside from medical considerations, in this world of litigation such situations should be avoided.

The major practical limitations of stable iodine therapy for occasional patients with mild Graves' disease are the need for careful selection of candidates for this treatment and the thorough discussion with the patient of the various outcomes possible with this type of therapy.

The arguments against the use of stable iodine are presented forcefully and in depth by Braverman. These include the following:

(1) Even in carefully selected patients the results are no better than with ATD. This conclusion is consistent with the data provided by Hamburger, Nagataki, and Wood and Maloof.

(2) Stable iodine treatment produces a thyroid gland which is rich in stored hormone, rather than hormone depleted as is the case after a period of ATD therapy. Therefore, if a remission is not achieved and iodides are abruptly discontinued, a marked worsening of the hyperthyroidism, even thyroid storm, might occur. This happened to one of Hamburger's patients for whom iodides were discontinued inappropriately by a gynecologist who 1 week later subjected the patient to the stress of general anesthesia and major surgery. However, it seems unrealistic to assume that the use of ATD will preclude the possibility of similar problems in patients who are not in remission from their hyperthyroidism. ATD do not always

control hyperthyroidism, even in large doses. Braverman did not have the opportunity to see Chapter 5 in which Hamburger presented data and an illustrated case report demonstrating sudden marked exacerbation of hyperthyroidism in a patient on propylthiouracil whose dose had been increased progressively to 1200 mg per day.

(3) Iodide escape occurs commonly in patients with Graves' disease, frequently within 2 to 3 weeks. However, in contrast to normal people, some patients with Graves' disease clearly do not escape from the suppressant effects of iodides. These are the ones who respond to this treatment. The higher rate of success achieved by Wood and Maloof may indicate that the iodide-perchlorate discharge test does select favorable candidates for this treatment. Also, the data they cite suggesting that iodides may produce more profound alterations in the thyroid than just suppression are worthy of note.

(4) Long-term beta blockers may be a safer alternative to stable iodine for the treatment of patients with mild hyperthyroidism, especially considering the potential toxicity of iodides. Beta blockers are extremely useful in controlling the tachycardia of hyperthyroidism, and to some lesser degree the tremor. However, those patients with very mild hyperthyroidism for whom stable iodine has been suggested usually have a negligible expression of these clinical features. Therefore it seems unlikely that beta blockers would be very useful. Also, these drugs have their own drawbacks. After discontinuation of beta blockers there is an increase in catecholamine receptors. The sudden discontinuation of these drugs exposes the patient to the risks of hypersensitivity to adrenergic stimulation.[47] In addition, reference to the 1980 edition of *PDR* reveals a litany of such a multitude of possible toxic reactions to propranolol, many of which are life threatening, that one might wonder if the drug should ever be used. By comparison the few potential toxic hazards of iodine would seem to pale to insignificance. Realistically, however, serious toxic reactions for neither drug occur often enough to preclude their use when indicated, as long as reasonable care is employed in patient selection.

Thus there would seem to be a place, albeit limited, for a trial of long-term stable iodine therapy for selected patients with mild Graves' hyperthyroidism.

J. Martin Miller, M.D.

REFERENCES

1. Plummer HS: Results of administering iodine to patients having exophthalmic goiter. JAMA 80:1955, 1923
2. Starr P, Walcott HP, Segall N, Means JH: The effect of iodine in exophthalmic goiter. Arch Intern Med 34:355, 1924
3. Thompson WO, Thompson PK, Brailey AG, Cohen AC: Prolonged treatment of exophthalmic goiter by iodine alone. Arch Intern Med 45:481, 1930
4. Hamolsky MW: Some present day concepts of the therapy of diseases of the thyroid gland. RI Med J 47:336, 1964

5. Nagataki S, Shizume K, Nakao K: Effect of iodide on thyroidal iodine turnover in hyperthyroid subjects. J Clin Endocrinol Metab 30:469, 1970
6. Hamburger JI: Clinical Exercises in Internal Medicine, Vol. I. Thyroid Disease. Philadelphia, Saunders, 1978, pp 71–73
7. Saxena KM, Crawford JD, Talbot NB: Childhood thyrotoxicosis: A long-term perspective. Br Med J 2:1153, 1964
8. Emerson CH, Anderson AJ, Howard WJ, Utiger RD: Serum thyroxine and triiodothyronine concentrations during iodide treatment of hyperthyroidism. J Clin Endocrinol Metab 40:33, 1975
9. Braverman LW: Disorders of iodine excess and deficiency. In Werner SC, Ingbar SH (eds): The Thyroid, 4th ed. Hagerstown, Md., Harper & Row, 1978, pp 528–536
10. Wartofsky L: Low remission after therapy for Graves' disease. JAMA 226:1083, 1973
11. Engbring NH: Current treatment of hyperthyroidism. Wis Med J 67:265, 1968
12. Wood LC, Ingbar SH: Hypothyroidism as a late sequela in patients with Graves' disease treated with antithyroid agents. J Clin Invest 64:1429, 1979
13. Volpé R, Johnston MW: The effect of small doses of stable iodine in patients with hyperthyroidism. Ann Interm Med 56:577, 1962
14. Thompson WO, Thompson PK: Low basal metabolism following thyrotoxicosis. I. Temporary type without myxedema with special reference to role of iodine therapy. J Clin Invest 5:441, 1928
15. Slingerland DW, Burrows BA: Long-term antithyroid treatment in hyperthyroidism. JAMA 242:2408, 1979
16. Yamamoto M, Igarshi T, Kimura S, Tsukamoto S, Togawa K, Ogata A: Thyroid suppression test and outcome of hyperthyroidism treated with antithyroid drugs and triiodothyronine. J Clin Endocrinol Metab 48:72, 1979
17. Tamai H, Nakagawa T, Fukino O, et al.: Thionamide therapy in Graves' disease: Relation of relapse rate to duration of therapy. Ann Interm Med 92:488, 1980
18. Vagenakis AG, Wang CA, Burger A, Maloof F, Braverman L, Ingbar SH: Iodide-induced thyrotoxicosis in Boston. N Engl J Med 287:523, 1972
19. Dobyns BM, Sheline GE, Workman JB, Tompkins EA, McConahey WM, Becker DV: Malignant and benign neoplasms of the thyroid in patients treated for hyperthyroidism: A report of the Cooperative Thyrotoxicosis Therapy Follow-up Study. J Clin Endocrinol Metab 38:976, 1974
20. Wolff J: Physiological aspects of iodide excess in relation to radiation protection. J Mol Med 4:151, 1980
21. Curd JG, Milgrom H, Stevenson DD, Mathison DA, Vaughan JH: Potassium iodide sensitivity in four patients with hypocomplementemic vasculitis. Ann Interm Med 91:853, 1979
22. McGregor AM, Smith BR, Hall R: Prediction of relapse in hyperthyroid Graves' disease. Lancet 1:1101, 1980
23. Pimstone B, Joffe B, Pimstone N, Bonnici F, Jackson WPU: Clinical response to long-term propranolol therapy in hyperthyroidism. S Afr Med J 43:1203, 1978
24. Hagen GA, Ouellette RP, Chapman EM: Comparison of high and low dosage levels of ^{131}I in the treatment of thyrotoxicosis. N Engl J Med 277:559, 1967
25. Feek CM, Sawers JS, Irvine WJ, Beckett GJ, Ratcliffe WA, Toft AD: Combination of potassium iodide and propranolol in preparation of patients with Graves' disease for thyroid surgery. N Engl J Med 302:883, 1980

26. Wood LC, Maloof F: Thyroid failure after potassium iodide treatment of diffuse toxic goiter. Trans Assoc Am Physicians 88:235, 1975

27. Winkler AW, Man EB, Danowski TS: Minimum dosage of thiourea, given together with iodine medication, necessary for the production and maintenance of a remission in hyperthyroidism. J Clin Invest 26:446, 1947

28. Harden RM, Koutras DA, Alexander WD, Wayne EJ: Quantitative studies of iodine metabolism in iodide-treated thyrotoxicosis. Clin Sci 27:399, 1964

29. Nagataki S: Effect of excess quantities of iodide. Handb Physiol Endocrinol 3:329, 1974

30. Nagataki S, Uchimura H: Treatment of Graves' disease with inorganic iodide. Clin Endocrinol 22:231, 1974 (in Japanese)

31. Nagataki S, Uchimura H, Matsuzaki F, Masuyama Y: Comparison of the triiodothyronine suppression test by the 20-minute and the 24-hour thyroidal ^{131}I uptake in patients receiving thionamide drugs. J Clin Endocrinol Metab 38:255, 1974

32. The Report of the Ministry of Health and Welfare, Japan, on "Hashimoto's Disease," 1975

33. Shizume K, Irie M, Nagataki S, Matsuzaki F, Shishiba Y, Suematsu H, Tsushima T: Long-term result of antithyroid drug therapy for Graves' disease: Follow-up after more than 5 years. Endocrinol Jpn 17:327, 1970

34. Niitani H, Iino S, Hayashi K, Watanabe T, Igaya K, Yuri H, Ohno T, Miyamoto M, Ban Y: Treatment of Graves' disease. J Jpn Soc Intern Med 62:164, 1969 (in Japanese)

35. Solomon DH, Beck JC, VanderLaan WP, Astwood EB: Prognosis of hyperthyroidism treated by antithyroid drugs. JAMA 152:201, 1953

36. Reveno WS, Rosenbaum H: Observations on the use of antithyroid drugs. Ann Intern Med 60:982, 1964

37. Hershman JE, Givens JR, Cassidy CE, Astwood EB: Long-term outcome of hyperthyroidism treated with antithyroid drugs. J Clin Endocrinol Metab 26:803, 1966

38. McCullagh EP, Cassidy CE: Propylthiouracil: 4- to 6-year follow-up of selected patients with Graves' disease. J Clin Endocrinol Metab 13:1507, 1953

39. Trotter WR: Nonsurgical treatment thyrotoxicosis Proc R Soc Med 54:869, 1961

40. Alexander WD, McLarty DG, Horton P, Phyrmakiotis AD: Sequential assessment during drug treatment of thyrotoxicosis. Clin Endocrinol 2:43, 1973

41. Alexander WD, McLarty DG, Robertson J, Shimmins J, Brownlie BEW, Harden RMcG, Patel AR: Prediction of the long-term results of antithyroid drug therapy for thyrotoxicosis. J Clin Endocrinol Metab 30:540, 1970

42. Stewart RDH, Murray IPC: Effect of small doses of carrier iodide upon the organic binding of radioactive iodine by the human thyroid gland. J Clin Endocrinol Metab 27:500, 1967

43. Childs DS Jr, Keating FR Jr, Rall JE, Williams MMD, Power MH: Effect of varying quantities of inorganic iodide "carrier" on urinary excretion and thyroidal accumulation of radioiodine in exophthalmic goiter. J Clin Invest 29:726, 1950

44. Weaver DK, Batsakis JG, Nishiyama RH: Relationship of iodine to "lymphocytic goiters." Arch Surg 98:183, 1969

45. Follis RH Jr: Further observations on thyroiditis and colloid accumulation in hyperplastic thyroid glands of hamsters receiving excess iodine. Lab Invest 13:1590, 1964

46. Belshaw BE, Becker DV: Necrosis of follicular cells and discharge of thyroidal iodine

induced by administering iodide to iodine-deficient dogs. J Clin Endocrinol Metab 36:466, 1973

47. Boudoulas H, Lewis RP, Kates RE, Dalamangas G: Hypersensitivity to adrenergic stimulation after propranolol withdrawal in normal subjects. Ann Intern Med 87:433, 1977

Chapter 7

When and How Often Is It Necessary to Prepare Hyperthyroid Patients for [131]I Therapy with Antithyroid Drugs?

Donald A. Meier, M.D.
Joel I. Hamburger, M.D.

INTRODUCTION

The safety and efficacy of ^{131}I therapy for hyperthyroidism is well established. In more and more centers it is the treatment of choice for nearly all hyperthyroid patients. However, no treatment is safe in all circumstances and in all hands. A review of the literature, which dates mostly from the 1950s and 1960s, reveals approximately 50 deaths that occurred within the first month after ^{131}I therapy and were related either to a worsening of the hyperthyroidism or to cardiovascular complications.[1-19] These reports and others[20-24] also describe nonlethal episodes of thyroid crisis, myocardial infarction, heart failure, and cerebral and pulmonary embolization. These catastrophic events were seen primarily in elderly patients with severe longstanding hyperthyroidism, toxic multinodular goiters, and especially if there were congestive heart failure and atrial fibrillation prior to the administration of [131]I.

In 1948, increases in the PBI were reported after ^{131}I therapy.[25,26] It was presumed that the radiation caused disruption of thyroid follicles, releasing preformed hormone into the circulation, as with subacute thyroiditis. To avoid these complications, pretreatment of hyperthyroid patients with antithyroid drugs (ATD) until the euthyroid state is restored has been recommended, after which ^{131}I therapy can be initiated.[27] This can be accomplished rapidly with large doses of ATD.[27] However, ATD pretreatment increases the requirement for ^{131}I therapy, and therefore may reduce the single dose cure rate.[28-31]

Some workers doubt that ATD preparation is necessary, even for thyrocardiacs.[31-33] Eller et al.[32] treated 215 thyrocardiac patients without ATD preparation with no problems. Most patients treated with ^{131}I have a steady decline in the PBI.[33] Only two patients had elevated PBI levels, and neither experienced worsening of their hyperthyroidism.[33] Increases in the PBI might only reflect discharge of noncalorigenic iodinated material.[33]

The development of modern assays for both T_3 and T_4 has prompted a reconsideration of the issue of the possible discharge of thyroid hormone following ^{131}I therapy.[19,34-37] Although these reports are not in complete agreement, it does seem clear that for some patients, perhaps as many as one-third,[37] there may be a rise in both T_3 and T_4 levels about 10 days after ^{131}I therapy. Also, there may be a corresponding worsening of the hyperthyroidism. This may be obscured by the administration of propranolol.

Our interest in this matter was prompted by a recent patient who experienced a substantial exacerbation in his hyperthyroidism after ^{131}I therapy in spite of ATD pretreatment, which improved, but did not completely correct, his hyperthyroidism.

CASE 1: EXACERBATION OF HYPERTHYROIDISM AFTER ^{131}I THERAPY

A 66-year-old man had been hyperthyroid for 6 months. Recently he was given digitalis and diuretics for congestive heart failure and atrial fibrillation. The thyroid was diffusely enlarged, 2.5 times normal size. The serum FTI value was 12.9 (NR 1.4–4.0) and the serum T_3(RIA) level was 609 ng/dl (NR 80–220). Propylthiouracil (PTU), 300 mg q.i.d., was given along with propranolol, 20 mg q.i.d, for 5 weeks after which he felt much better and had gained 9 lb. His heart rate was controlled at 84 beats/min, but atrial fibrillation was still present. The FTI and T_3(RIA) had dropped to 6.4 and 435 ng/dl, respectively. PTU was discontinued for 48 h, 30 mCi of ^{131}I were given (the 24-h radioactive iodine uptake was 48%), and PTU was reinstituted in a dose of 200 mg q.i.d., 48 h later. Propranolol 20 mg q.i.d. had been continued.

Three weeks later the FTI had increased to 9.5 and the T_3(RIA) to 470 ng/dl. However the patient felt well.

Six weeks after ^{131}I therapy the patient was clearly worse, complaining of heat intolerance, weakness, palpitation, and a 6-lb weight loss. The FTI and T_3(RIA) values had increased to 11.5 and 550 ng/dl. The PTU dose was increased to 300 mg q.i.d. Nevertheless he did poorly for an additional 6 weeks, in spite of an increase in PTU dosage to 400 mg q.i.d. Thereafter improvement was progressive, and by 8 months later the PTU and propranolol were discontinued. One month later he was hypothyroid, and has done well on replacement thyroid hormone subsequently.

In this review, the following issues will be addressed:

(1) How great is the risk that ^{131}I therapy will either precipitate thyroid crisis or produce or aggravate cardiovascular complications?

(2) Is preparation of high risk hyperthyroid patients with ATD necessary prior to the administration of ^{131}I, or will the use of propranolol alone provide adequate protection?

(3) If ATD pretreatment is employed, is it necessary to restore the euthyroid state prior to ^{131}I therapy, or may a lesser degree of improvement be adequate?

EXPERIENCE OF NORTHLAND THYROID LABORATORY

The records of Northland Thyroid Laboratory (NTL) patients who were pre-treated with antithyroid drugs in preparation for ^{131}I therapy were reviewed to determine the indications for pretreatment and the outcome of this treatment.

Patients were pretreated with propylthiouracil (PTU) in a dose of 300 mg q.i.d. until the monitoring physician was satisfied that ^{131}I therapy could safely be given. Most patients were treated until they were clinically and biochemically euthyroid, but some were given ^{131}I while still mildly toxic, although considerably improved. The relatively large dose of PTU was employed in the hope of producing more rapid improvement in the hyperthyroidism. Whether patients had toxic diffuse goiter (Graves' disease) or toxic multinodular goiter was not a factor in the decision to prepare for ^{131}I with PTU pretreatment.

Prior to the administration of ^{131}I, PTU was discontinued for 24 h for a 24-h radioactive iodine uptake. This was done to be certain drugs interfering with the uptake of ^{131}I had not inadvertently been taken by the patients. After ^{131}I therapy was administered, PTU was reinstituted, usually in a dose of 150 mg q.i.d., and tapered to discontinuation in 2 to 3 months, assuming a satisfactory response to ^{131}I therapy. Case 2 illustrates this method.

CASE 2:   PREPARATION OF AN ELDERLY HYPERTHYROID PATIENT FOR ^{131}I THERAPY WITH PROPYLTHIOURACIL

A 90-year-old woman was referred for treatment of hyperthyroidism. She had had a goiter for many years, without treatment. Three weeks earlier she was hospitalized for congestive heart failure and atrial fibrillation, and received digitalis and diuretics. A diagnosis of hyper-thyroidism was also established. There was a large multinodular goiter (Fig. 7-1). Her height

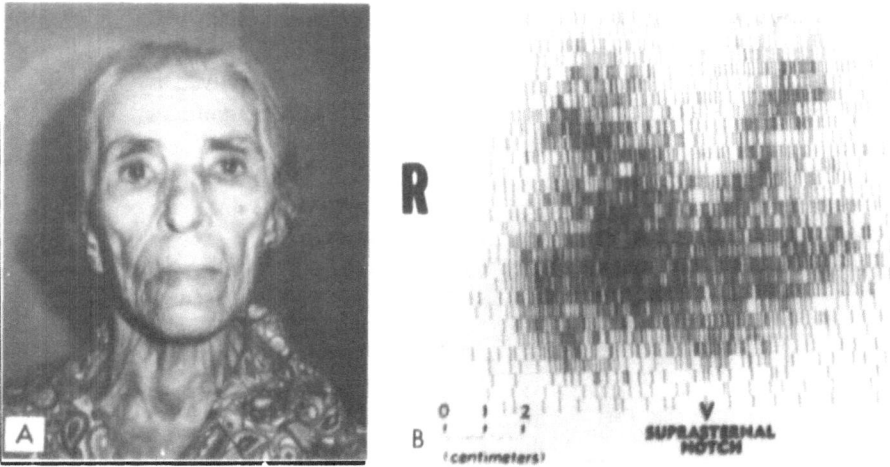

Figure 7-1. A A 90-year-old hyperthyroid woman. **B** The thyroid scan, showing a toxic multinodular goiter.

was 60 inches and her weight was 70 lb. The serum free thyroxine index (FTI) was 10.2 and the serum T_3(RIA) level was 254 ng/dl. The 24-h radioactive iodine uptake was 52%. PTU 300 mg q.i.d. was started.

In 4 weeks the FTI and T_3(RIA) values dropped to 4.1 and 110 ng/dl, respectively. The patient was asked to discontinue PTU and was given 30 mCi of [131]I 2 days later. PTU was resumed 2 days after the ^{131}I, in a dose of 150 mg q.i.d.

Improvement thereafter was progressive. PTU was gradually withdrawn over a period of 6 weeks. Although a large multinodular goiter persisted, the patient remained euthyroid and active until age 93, when she died in her sleep.

Indications for ATD Pretreatment at NTL

Currently 10.6% of patients who receive ^{131}I therapy for hyperthyroidism at NTL are prepared with antithyroid drugs. Review of the records from 1970 through 1980 revealed 135 patients who were treated in this fashion. Table 7-1 gives the age and sex distribution for these patients. Twenty-seven percent of the patients were 70 years old or older.

Table 7-2 gives the indications for pretreatment. Many patients had more than a single indication, hence the total number of indications is greater than the number of patients. Advanced age alone was the most frequent indication. However, in sum the cardiovascular indications were present more often. Sixty-nine (51%) of these patients had evidence of cardiovascular disease. Atrial fibrillation was most common. Congestive heart failure would have been cited more often had this problem not been treated prior to referral of a number of these patients.

Dosage of [131]I Employed

After hyperthyroidism had been controlled to the satisfaction of the monitoring physician, ^{131}I was administered. The initial dosage ranged from 10 to 30 mCi (average 23.5 mCi). Initial doses of 25–30 mCi were received by 61% of the patients. Smaller doses were given to patients with smaller goiters.

Table 7-1. Age and sex distribution of patients prepared for ^{131}I therapy with antithyroid drugs.

Age (years)	Males	Females	Total
<50	4	10	14
50–59	15	34	49
60–69	9	30	39
70–79	4	20	24
80+	2	7	9
Total	34	101	135

Table 7-2. Indications for pretreatment with antithyroid drugs.

	No. of patients
Advanced age	64
Severe thyrotoxicosis	39
Atrial fibrillation	31
Congestive heart failure	10
Coronary artery disease	9
Cardiovascular disease, type unspecified	8
General debility	8
Hypertension	6
Abnormal cardiac rhythm other than atrial fibrillation	5
Uncontrolled diabetes mellitus	3

Results of Treatment

Follow-up data are available for 128 patients (Table 7-3), of whom 118 (92.2%) had the hyperthyroidism eliminated with a single dose of ^{131}I. This is slightly less than the 96% single dose cure rate for hyperthyroid patients in general, which we achieve with our current method of treatment with higher doses of ^{131}I. The difference is attributable to a relatively large proportion of patients with large goiters, often multinodular. Case 3 is instructive in this regard.

CASE 3: "RESISTANCE" TO THERAPY WITH RADIOACTIVE IODINE
A 62-year-old woman was referred for management of hyperthyroidism of 3 months' duration with suspected mild congestive heart failure. The heart rate was 128 beats/min. The blood pressure was 180/78. The lungs were clear and there was only a trace of pedal edema. The ECG revealed sinus tachycardia. The thyroid gland was about 5 times normal size and hyperlobulated. The FTI was 24.2, and the T_3(RIA) level was greater than 800 ng/dl. She was placed on PTU 300 mg q.i.d. After 3 weeks she was much improved. The FTI had dropped to 1.7 and the T_3(RIA) to 389 ng/dl. PTU was discontinued. A 24-h radioactive

Table 7-3. Results of ^{131}I therapy.

	No. of patients
Euthyroid on replacement thyroid hormone	
After 1 dose of ^{131}I	98
After 2 doses of ^{131}I	7
After 4 doses of ^{131}I	1
Euthyroid without replacement thyroid hormone	
After 1 dose of ^{131}I	20
After 2 doses of ^{131}I	2
Lost to follow-up	7
Total	135

iodine uptake (RAIU) was 50%. She was treated with 30 mCi of [131]I. Seventy-two hours later PTU, 150 mg q.i.d., was resumed for 3 weeks, then discontinued.

Six weeks after ^{131}I therapy she was severely toxic. The FTI was 14.4 and the T_3(RIA) was greater than 800 ng/dl. PTU, 100 mg q.i.d., was resumed. Although she responded promptly, she relapsed after withdrawal of PTU, and a second 30-mCi dose of ^{131}I was given 14 weeks after the first treatment. PTU, 100 mg b.i.d., was reinstituted 4 days later and continued for 3 months, during which the patient maintained T_4 levels at the upper level of normal, with intermittently elevated T_3 levels. There were no clinical problems. Shortly after stopping PTU the hyperthyroidism recurred. The FTI was 14.1 and the T_3(RIA) was greater than 800 ng/dl. The RAIU was 51%. A third 30-mCi dose of ^{131}I was given, and PTU, 100 mg b.i.d., was resumed 48 h later maintained for 3 months, and then gradually withdrawn. Once more there was a relapse in her hyperthyroidism. The FTI was 4.9 and the T_3(RIA) was 257 ng/dl. The RAIU was 53%. At this time the patient was hospitalized and treated with 100 mCi of [131]I. To this dose she finally responded, requiring thyroid hormone replacement for hypothyroidism 6 months later. Her large goiter persisted throughout the course of treatment.

In spite of the large doses of ^{131}I given, doses which were selected in the hope of producing virtually complete thyroid ablation, 22 (17.2%) patients have remained euthyroid. These were mostly patients with large multinodular goiters, the type of goiter which is relatively resistant to ^{131}I therapy.

Eleven patients required more than a single dose of [131]I. One patient was lost to follow-up after the second treatment. Nine patients were successfully treated with two doses of [131]I. The single patient who required four doses of ^{131}I has been described above (Case 3).

No patients experienced exacerbation of either their hyperthyroidism or associated cardiovascular problems in the first few weeks after ^{131}I therapy. However, biochemical assays for thyroid hormone levels were not performed routinely, nor were patients examined routinely sooner than 1 month after the treatment.

DISCUSSION

Catastrophic Events After [131]I Therapy

Observations by a sizable number of workers have indicated that the administration of ^{131}I therapy to hyperthyroid patients, especially the elderly with toxic multinodular goiter, longstanding severe hyperthyroidism, and associated congestive heart failure and atrial fibrillation, may be followed by serious complications, even death.[1-24] It has been assumed that these complications could be attributed, at least in part, to exacerbation of the hyperthyroidism by discharge of stored thyroid hormone. It would be inappropriate to accept this explanation in all instances. Radioactive iodine therapy does not work instantly. Its effects are delayed for 4 to 6 weeks or longer in most cases. This allows time for the hyperthyroidism itself to worsen, or for a breakdown in compensation of the cardiovascular system due to the added strain of the hyperthyroidism. For many of the patients included in reports describing serious problems, the dose of ^{131}I given was too small to influence materially the course of the hyperthyroidism. Hence the persistence of the disease, due to inadequate treatment, may have been of more importance than the ^{131}I therapy itself. The following case is instructive in this regard.

CASE 4: SUDDEN DEATH IN HYPERTHYROIDISM

A 44-year-old woman was referred for treatment of hyperthyroidism on a Friday afternoon. She had been sick for 4 years and lost 30 lb. Intermittently she had received antithyroid drugs, in small doses, with poor compliance. She was 63 inches tall and weighed 102 lb. The heart rate was 128 beat/min and regular. The blood pressure was 160/80. The thyroid was diffusely enlarged, 3 times normal size. Blood was obtained for thyroid function tests and the patient asked to return Monday for institution of treatment. When she did not return a phone call was placed to her husband, who informed us that she had died Saturday of a pulmonary embolism.

Had this patient presented one day earlier, on Thursday, she might have been treated with ^{131}I on Friday, and her death on Saturday would surely have been attributed to ^{131}I therapy.

Possible Methods to Avoid Catastrophes After ^{131}I

It cannot be denied that the potential exists for a temporary worsening of hyperthyroidism after ^{131}I therapy. This has prompted suggestions for the avoidance of catastrophic results, including the following:

(1) Prompt and proper treatment of any worsening of the patient's condition.[13]

(2) Hospitalization for close observation of thyrocardiacs and severely toxic patients,[30,38] and the administration of high doses of cortisone in the event of a deterioration in the patient's condition.[14]

(3) Fractionation of the therapy, or a small initial dose.[6,15]

(4) Surgical rather than ^{131}I therapy for thyrocardiacs[39] or large toxic multinodular goiters.[16]

(5) Preparation with ATD, and post-^{131}I, ATD.[6,10,18,24,27,40,41]

(6) Close monitoring for the first 2 weeks after therapy, along with the administration of propranolol.[37]

The first two suggestions imply the inevitablility of reactions, and that nothing can be done other than to be prepared to take corrective action as best one can after the fact. Most workers prefer to prevent the complications. If the discharge of thyroid hormone causes the trouble, and this results from the ^{131}I therapy, it might seem logical to give a smaller dose, and perhaps repeat that dose at intervals until the disease is eliminated. However, too small a dose of ^{131}I permits undue prolongation of the hyperthyroidism, something which might well increase the chance for a serious complication, rather than reduce that chance. This is a lesson painfully learned by Staffurth and Young.[13,39] Similarly, abandoning the field to the surgeons is not an attractive option, especially since many of these fragile patients would be turned down by surgeons prior to being treated with [131]I. Even if operation were contemplated, ATD preparation would be needed. If that were done, and the patients then treated with large doses of ^{131}I, as we did, perhaps unsatisfactory results could have been avoided.[10,41]

Whether propranolol alone will do the job is unclear at this time. It seems well established that many hyperthoid patients can undergo thyroidectomy after preparation with proranolol alone.[42,45] However some episodes of crisis have been reported,[46] although the dosage of propranolol might not have been high enough.[47] Preparing toxic patients for thyroidectomy with propranolol alone, essentially just to see if one could get away with it, makes little sense, and raises serious ethical problems. We would view the preparation of hyperthyroid patients for ^{131}I with propranolol alone, when such preparation is indicated, in the same light. Why take chances when it is not necessary? The savings in time and costs do not justify the risks in our judgment.

For the same reason we advocate pursuing ATD preparation until the patient is euthyroid, barring any toxic reaction which precludes the treatment. Large doses of ATD should be used so as to accomplish the job in a reasonably short period of time.[27]

Since this has always been our practice we cannot say whether we might have done just as well without preparing our patients with ATD. Also it is possible that our clinic, serving exclusively outpatients, may not see as many high risk hyperthyroid patients as some other centers, but we doubt it. Our large body of referring physicians have come to follow our teaching and when severely thyrotoxic or thyrocardiac patients are seen on the inpatient services of most of the hospitals in our area they are treated with ATD and appropriate cardiac drugs, and sent to us as soon as possible for definitive care after discharge. Therefore we have not lacked the opportunity to treat thyrocardiac patients, or severely toxic patients either.

COMMENTARY

David Barzilai, M.D.

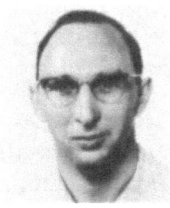

My comments will be based upon experience with 499 patients treated between October 1972 and October 1980 with radioactive iodine (^{131}I) after pretreatment with antithyroid drugs (ATD). Review of the presentation by Meier and Hamburger and other reports[41,48–51] has convinced me that ATD are essential in the preparation of patients for ^{131}I therapy. They suggest that ^{131}I-induced hormonal surge is a latent occurrence, but the work of Shafer and Nuttal[36] shows that changes in T_3 and T_4 levels may occur within 1 day. Nevertheless, critical review of the literature since the 1950s leads one not to a conviction of right or wrong, but rather that the therapeutic policies followed may relate more to the mode of health care delivery system specific to a given country, city, and I dare say, even to given clinics within the same city.[29,51-54]

It is true that the authors of large scale studies may draw definite conclusions, but these are subject to a margin of error. I refer specifically to the paper by Beierwaltes in which he states, "Patients with Graves' disease rarely require pretreatment."[41] I have no doubt that from the economic standpoint in a private system of medical care delivery one might be inclined to abide by the rule that if ^{131}I is to be administered eventually, why bother with prior ATD administration? But we may be forgetting the many reports (with which our experience is in accord) that 40–60% of patients with Graves' disease may go into lasting remission in response to ATD alone (ten of our patients have remained euthyroid for 10 years after a course of ATD therapy). Therefore, it is our strong belief and practice to administer ATD (and since 1967 also beta blockers) first, and reserve ^{131}I therapy for the few who fail to respond to ATD.

The questions left to be answered after these opening comments are as follows:

(1) Will pretreatment with ATD prevent the immediate risk of thyroid crisis after ^{131}I? The 18 references cited by Meier and Hamburger, the recent report of Creutzig et al.,[19] and especially the report of Shafer and Nuttal[36] indicate a substantial risk of complications in the absence of ATD. Shafer's study is even more disturbing. I quote: "Three patients not reported here developed thyroid crisis— one even died." The findings in the report of Horn et al.[55] of thyroid crisis after surgery resemble those in a patient of ours who, following 10 mCi of ^{131}I (without ATD pretreatment), developed thyrotoxic crisis with an extreme, myasthenic, life-threatening picture.

The danger of crisis after ^{131}I therapy of unprepared patients is real, and I believe there are many more cases that are not reported. In conclusion there is no doubt that pretreatment will reduce the danger of possibly lethal thyrotoxic crisis. This calls to mind a statement made by Hamburger at a local meeting in Israel about thyroidectomy: "If even one patient dies why use it?"

(2) Will pretreatment with ATD reduce the frequency of ^{131}I-induced hypothyroidism? Several studies suggest that this is the case.[29,49,56,57] Van Hofe et al.[56] showed that 69% of ATD-pretreated patients were hypothyroid 1 year after ^{131}I therapy. Buchanan et al.[57] showed that 73% of ^{131}I-treated patients who were not pretreated developed hypothyroidism, whereas the incidence of hypothyroidism was 55% in ATD-pretreated patients. In our 499 ATD-pretreated patients there was 25% hypothyroidism in a 5-year follow-up. However, the period of ATD treatment was rather prolonged (6–9 months at least), and our system of delivery of health care led us to employ relatively small doses of ^{131}I (6–10 mCi) even though we were well aware of the limitations of this approach.[50]

(3) Are ATD really dangerous? Our own report on the danger of ATD[58] has made this a very sensitive issue in our clinic with respect to all of the antithyroid drugs. Our system of health care delivery enables us to carry out a very intensive

follow-up of ATD-treated patients (professional fees, charges for laboratory tests, and loss of income because of absence from work are not borne by the patients). We have observed very few side effects and no serious consequences from the use of ATD in the last 8 years. Therefore, excepting those patients who develop reactions which preclude their use, we advise ATD pretreatment for all patients prior to ^{131}I therapy. Nearly all patients can be brought into remission,[54] and the prolongation of time for cure is slight.[52]

There is an additional point not raised by Meier and Hamburger which I would like to address. Is it really absolutely safe to give ^{131}I to patients in all age groups, especially to children and women in the 20s to 30s? In spite of the many studies showing statistical safety in high doses or repeated small doses, many physicians all over the world are reluctant to use it. Since there is a considerable percentage of remission with ATD, why not try ATD as the primary treatment[51,54] before rushing into a decision to employ [131]I?

In the last 10 years we have not seen any post-^{131}I exophthalmos development. During my stay at the Mayo Clinic a few years ago I was impressed by the number of patients who developed exophthalmos after [131]I. These patients were not pretreated with ATD and received large doses of ^{131}I for severe thyrotoxicosis. We suggest that the combination of ATD and beta blockers before ^{131}I is the reason that our patients have not developed exophthalmos.

In conclusion, it is our strong conviction that patients should be treated by ATD to the upper limit of euthyroidism before receiving [131]I. We are fully satisfied with our treatment regimen which includes the following:

(1) Treatment with PTU for 9–12 months, starting with 300–450 mg daily, and tapering to the lowest level to maintain the euthyroid state.

(2) Discontinuation of treatment, and follow-up if a remission is achieved (40–60% of our patients).

(3) For patients who relapse, ATD are again employed for 4–6 weeks, the usual period necessary to regain the euthyroid state; ATD are then stopped for 48 h and an ^{131}I uptake is performed. A high value is usually obtained, and this helps lower the ^{131}I dose that is required. ATD are reinstituted after the ^{131}I therapy has been absorbed by the thyroid gland, and the patients are followed.

In my opinion ^{131}I therapy without ATD pretreatment is absolutely contraindicated. Treatment should be judged individually and not per set formula (item 3).

Before closing I would like to call attention to an "epidemic" of thyrotoxicosis in the north of Israel. In the last 8 years we have treated 1600 patients, 499 of whom received ^{131}I, most of the rest were treated with ATD, and a few surgically. In our opinion the specific stress related to war and the constant threat of war have been of etiologic importance in this "epidemic." This matter is under prospective and retrospective study.

COMMENTARY

David V. Becker, M.D.

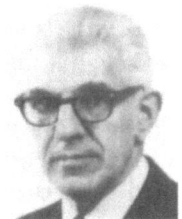

High Risk Hyperthyroid Patients

Older patients with hyperthyroidism, especially those with cardiac disease, are clearly at greater risk from the impact of their increased rate of metabolism than other patients. Prudence suggests that these patients be monitored more closely and controlled more rapidly than younger patients, and generally managed as though they were fragile. Since the potential for complications is relatively high in this group, particular care should be taken to avoid measures that might aggravate underlying disease, especially cardiovascular and metabolic disorders. One important factor that should be minimized is the duration of the thyrotoxic state. For prompt control such patients frequently receive antithyroid drugs (ATD) as initial therapy. When it comes to definitive treatment, radioactive iodine (^{131}I) is preferred for most of these patients. It is general practice today to discontinue ATD for a varying period before ^{131}I administration and then to wait a week before restarting. Such therapy is therefore frequently associated with a period during which the hyperthyroid patient does not receive ATD. That the withdrawal of ATD in preparation for ^{131}I may not be necessary has been suggested,[59] but experience with such a practice has been limited.

It should be noted that for the great majority of patients with uncomplicated hyperthyroidism, preparation with ATD is unnecessary. When symptoms are troublesome, particularly palpitations and tachycardia, adrenergic blocking agents are effective and useful in producing symptomatic relief.

Does ^{131}I Therapy Exacerbate Hyperthyroidism?

A basic question raised in the accompanying article is whether there is a significant risk that ^{131}I will precipitate thyroid crisis ("storm") or aggravate cardiovascular complications. There is little doubt that this can happen, but the question is how often and how great the risk. The observation was made many years ago that an elevation of the protein-bound iodine and an exacerbation of the symptoms of hyperthyroidism can occur in the period immediately following ^{131}I administration.[25] A number of reports of such events have appeared and are cited by Meier and Hamburger, but considering the large number of patients treated with ^{131}I since 1946 (approximately 1 million) the incidence of such complications must be extraordinarily small.

Even rarer are reports of thyroid crisis or death following ^{131}I therapy. Most of these reports were published in the 1950s and 1960s and bear close examination. Although it may be true that approximately 5 deaths have " . . . occurred within the first month after ^{131}I therapy," on review of these cases it seems likely that relatively few were related to the ^{131}I administration. In one series of 17 patients with thyroid crisis,[60] for most of those who received ^{131}I therapy the author attributed the occurrence of crisis to "discontinuation of thyrostatic treatment" as well as to the ^{131}I therapy. One patient died of exacerbation of hyperthyroidism before ^{131}I could be given, but within a few days after ATD were discontinued. The author cautioned that the potential hazardous consequences of withdrawal of ATD should be kept in mind in preparing patients for ^{131}I therapy.

In Waldstein's[61] report of 21 episodes of thyroid storm, two patients received ^{131}I therapy and both treatments were preceded by " . . . withdrawal of propylthiouracil in the belief that the patient was ready for definitive treatment." The author's summary does not include ^{131}I treatment as a precipitating factor but does mention propylthiouracil withdrawal as an important "contributing factor." In another series of 22 episodes of thyroid storm[62] two patients received ^{131}I treatment. For one the storm occurred a month later and in the other patient storm immediately followed subtotal thyroidectomy, ^{131}I having been given many years previously. Thus neither was attributed to [131]I. These authors also implicated ATD withdrawal as a precipitating factor in three other cases of thyroid storm.

In Volpé's series of 542 hyperthyroid patients treated with ^{131}I,[63] clinical exacerbation was uncommon although there were two deaths within 1 week of ^{131}I treatment. These deaths were attributed to congestive heart failure and pneumonia. Neither patient was thought to be in thyroid storm nor " . . . could their clinical state be ascribed to the [131]I."

Review of other reports of deaths after ^{131}I similarly suggest that few could be primarily attributed to that treatment. For some patients, however, the sequence of events is quite convincing in terms of ascribing the deaths to complications of the [131]I. However, such occurrences must be extremely unusual. When they occur they appear primarily in elderly patients with severe cardiac disease, primarily congestive heart failure (perhaps inadequately treated by contemporary standards), and these patients are at great risk even without ^{131}I therapy. There is little doubt that for such patients major efforts should be directed to the control of the hyperthyroidism (and medical disease) as expeditiously as possible, and ^{131}I would not usually be the immediate treatment of choice.

It is of interest that although the presumed mechanism for the exacerbation of hyperthyroidism is radiation thyroiditis with follicular disruption and release of stored hormone or thyroglobulin, most reports of exacerbation of hyperthyroidism following ^{131}I do not describe a painful tender thyroid.[64]

It is relevant to note that the highest incidence of exacerbation after ^{131}I therapy has been reported from Scandinavia and midwestern United States, where a major proportion of hyperthyroid patients have nodular goiter.[65] The distribution of ^{131}I within the thyroid gland is more irregular in nodular hyperthyroid glands than in diffuse goiter.[66] Areas of localized high uptake therefore may receive much larger radiation doses than other areas of the gland as a whole, causing localized severe follicular damage.

Thyroid Hormone Levels After ^{131}I Therapy

One would assume that a symptomatic exacerbation of hyperthyroidism would require that serum levels of thyroid hormone be elevated. Discharge of thyroglobulin into the serum is probably not measured by radioimmunoassays of thyroxine and triiodothyronine, although it might be reflected in protein-bound iodine determinations. Specific measurements of serum thyroglobulin by radioimmunoassay[67] do demonstrate elevation of thyroglobulin levels following ^{131}I treatment. Since thyroglobulin is noncalorigenic, it is probably not responsible for an increase in symptoms of hyperthyroidism.

A number of investigators have examined patients following ^{131}I therapy for evidence of changes in serum thyroid hormone levels. Unfortunately, the data are conflicting and it would appear that factors not yet identified may control the discharge of thyroid hormones under such circumstances. In our experience, the levels of thyroxine and triiodothyronine in the serum do not increase following ^{131}I treatment. However, in the course of treating over 2000 hyperthyroid patients with ^{131}I, we have observed slight exacerbation of symptoms and mimimal neck tenderness on rare occasions. When it does occur, it is usually in patients with toxic nodular goiter who have received very large doses of ^{131}I. Although a direct correlation of radiation thyroiditis with the amount of ^{131}I administered is not usual it is our impression that if tenderness occurs, it is generally more likely after larger doses than after smaller doses.

Disadvantages of ATD Preparation for ^{131}I

The routine use of ATD in preparation for ^{131}I therapy raises another possible problem in addition to the potential for exacerbation of the hyperthyroid state upon their withdrawal. The suggestion has been made that ATD may increase radioresistance, so that unless larger does of ^{131}I are given, the hyperthyroidism may not be eliminated.[29] This is presumably due to the presence of radioprotective SH groups in these agents.

In addition, ATD are known to decrease the iodine pool in the thyroid, increasing the turnover rate of thyroidal ^{131}I and increasing the level of the protein-bound ^{131}I in the blood.[68] The net effect of ATD administration prior to ^{131}I therapy thus may be to decrease the rad dose to the thyroid per millicurie of radioiodine administered. At the same time because of the increased level of serum protein-bound ^{131}I, the radiation dose to the blood under such circumstances may be substantially increased.[68]

Current practice in the United States does not usually entail measurement of the turnover rate of ^{131}I by the thyroid, nor the blood levels of protein-bound radioactivity (and sometimes not even the uptake prior to the therapy, or the uptake of the therapy dose itself). Patients who have received ATD are therefore usually given a "standard" amount of ^{131}I with the result that their thyroid gland may receive a smaller radiation dose than expected. If ATD prepearation for ^{131}I treatment becomes widely used on a routine basis, an increasing number of patients will require multiple doses of [131]I. Alternately, the amount of ^{131}I initially administered could be greatly increased. However, this is accomplished at a price not only of a larger whole body radiation dose (see above), but also of a higher incidence of hypothyroidism, especially in the majority of hyperthyroid patients who have diffuse (nonnodular) goiters.

Variations in Strategy for [131]I Therapy

Although there is wide agreement in the general approach to the management of patients with hyperthyroidism, it is very clear that patient populations differ remarkably in different geographic areas, hospitals, and medical practices for a number of reasons. Thus, therapy strategies must differ depending upon individual experience. In the cases presented from the records of Meier and Hamburger, presumably chosen to illustrate the usefulness of ATD preparation, it would appear that in one case (Case 1), a 1-month period of antithyroid drug pretreatment did not prevent a substantial exacerbation of hyperthyroidism that occurred 6 weeks after [131]I (which may be a little late to attribute to the radioiodine). Other patients (Cases 2 and 3) received huge doses of ^{131}I after varying periods of ATD without exacerbation. In one patient (Case 4) death occurred before ^{131}I could be given. The authors appropriately comment that if ^{131}I had been given it would surely have been blamed for the death.

Their patient population appears to be a very special one with a major proportion of patients with large multinodular goiters. Ninety percent of their patients in this group were over age 50 and their average ^{131}I administered dose was 23.5 mCi, perhaps three times the average given the usual patient with hyperthyroidism. The incidence of hypothyroidism with this regimen was not discussed although 73% of their patients were noted as receiving replacement therapy after a single dose of ^{131}I, and were presumably hypothyroid relatively early after the ^{131}I was administered. Achieving a euthyroid state without supplementary medication is appropriately not a very important consideration in their therapeutic strategy for this group of patients.

Summary

I feel that experience and data indicate that the risk of ^{131}I therapy of hyperthyroidism precipitating thyroid crisis or seriously aggravating cardiovascular complications is extremely low. Nevertheless, in patients with severe hyperthyroidism and with complicating disease it is certainly appropriate and important to treat their "complications" vigorously and to bring their hyperthyroidism under control with ATD as quickly as possible before these patients receive ^{131}I. However, withdrawal of ATD may be of even greater potential danger in this regard than is the ^{131}I.

How long the ATD should be administered before ^{131}I therapy should be individualized, but once started there seems little reason not to continue medication until the patient is as close to euthyroid as feasible. We regard propranolol as an important and useful adjunct to control symptoms, but it does not usually affect the basic pathophysiology of the disease.

I agree with the recommendation of ATD preparation for high risk patients, which is clearly based upon principles of good medical care. However, I feel that the potential for serious complications from ^{131}I treatment has never been demonstrated to be a significant factor in patient management. On the other hand, ATD themselves are not without side effects and possible complications and therefore should be used carefully with awareness of the potential for serious problems.

One concludes by reiterating a basic principle of medical care, that treatment of each patient must always be individualized and should only be instituted with close observation and with full knowledge of the particular patient, as well as thorough familiarity with the proposed and alternative forms of therapy.

COMMENTARY

J. Martin Miller, M.D.

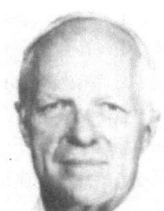

How Dangerous Is ^{131}I Therapy in Unprepared Patients?

The administration of ^{131}I therapy to a patient with hyperthyroidism may produce an elevation of calorigenic hormone in the serum resulting in an exacerbation of the disease, and on rare occasions may seem causally related to the death of the patient. However, the vast majority of hyperthyroid patients treated with ^{131}I in the United States have not been prepared with antithyroid drugs (ATD) and have not had this sequence of events. For them ATD prophylaxis would only have postponed effective therapy.

In my 30-year experience, including treatment of about 2000 patients with Graves' disease with ^{131}I, I have not observed a serious exacerbation of symptoms nor a death. In only three instances did I advise ATD preparation. The first patient had moderately severe angina, did not follow his instructions relative to the complications of ATD (while under care of another doctor), and suffered fatal agranulocytosis. Coincidentally, this was the only fatality from ATD observed during the same 30 years. For two other patients ATD therapy was elected before ^{131}I because of the debility of the patient. Both died anyway 3–4 days after starting the drugs. Had ^{131}I been given, it would most certainly have been blamed.

If the assumption is made that some patients with hyperthyroidism would benefit from ATD prior to the ^{131}I therapy, certain guidelines must be kept in mind. The first of these is: How much hormone is in the gland? If one examines the photomicrographs of patients with Graves' disease operated upon before the use of iodides it is obvious that there is very little stored hormone. Therefore, there is little hormone to be discharged as a consequence of radiation necrosis of the follicular epithelium. The more severe the disease, the less hormone there will be, and presumably the less chance of an exacerbation of symptoms following ^{131}I therapy. If a patient with Graves' disease has been receiving iodides and the hyperthyroidism is fairly severe, consideration should be given to the use of ATD with beta blockers before ^{131}I therapy is given, since hormone stores have been increased.

Toxic Multinodular Goiter May Have Large Thyroid Hormone Stores

On the other hand, the patient with Plummer's disease, the type presenting with a large multinodular goiter, may have a very large amount of colloid present. Although much of the iodine may be in the form of noncalorigenic iodinated amines, the potential for exacerbation of the disease is much greater. We have observed nonfatal exacerbations of the disease in two patients after 50-mCi doses of ^{131}I and fatal thromboembolism within a week after ^{131}I in two other patients, one receiving 50 mCi and the other 100 mCi. The first of the fatalities had been treated unsuccessfully with large doses of propylthiouracil for several months by another physician.

Relationship of [131]I Dose to Possible Exacerbation of Hyperthyroidism

Most of the accumulated experience indicating the safety of ^{131}I administration came from the era when there was some attempt to tailor the size of the dose to the severity of the disease and the size of the thyroid in the hope of avoiding hypothyroidism. Since it has become well recognized that this is usually not possible, there has been an increasing tendency to use large doses of ^{131}I, and this might well increase the number of exacerbations of the hyperthyroidism that would be noted. Certainly the use of doses in the 20- to 30-mCi range increases the number of cases of symptomatic radiation thyroiditis seen after [131]I.

The treatment of Plummer's disease of the multinodular goiter type has usually been accomplished with doses of ^{131}I therapy between 50 and 100 mCi. Often it is impossible to determine the exact volume of tissue that is being treated, as turnover of the iodine in various parts of these large goiters is quite variable. Therefore, the potential for administering an overdose to parts of a large goiter with subsequent undesired effects is very real.

Factors Increasing Susceptibility to Exacerbation After ^{131}I Therapy

We have observed that patients who are capable of the usual hyperkinetic response to hyperthyroidism have tolerated ^{131}I therapy very well. We have treated several patients who seemed to be on the verge of, or were in, actual storm with no ill effect. We agree with others who have exercised caution with patients who seem to be overwhelmed by the disease and exhibit lethargy, often with nausea, vomiting, diarrhea, dehydration, and various cardiovascular problems. These patients often do poorly even with a conservative approach to therapy, and we certainly favor making a maximum effort to restore these patients to a more normal state prior to ^{131}I therapy.

Symptomatic ischemic heart disease is infrequently a complication of hyperthyroidism. For these patients we feel very strongly that the efficacy of the beta blocker must be established before the administration of ^{131}I therapy. One needs to check the life preservers before jumping overboard. Congestive heart failure and various arrhythmias are best dealt with before the administration of ^{131}I therapy.

Before beta blockers became available, we routinely gave stable iodine for a few weeks, beginning 48 h after ^{131}I therapy. If this is done to achieve a more rapid amelioration of the hyperthyroidism, one must avoid preparation of the patient with ATD. ATD preparation produces an iodine-depleted, hyperplastic thyroid gland. The sudden introduction of large amounts of iodine in the regimen of such a patient is about the best way to produce thyroid storm with which I am familiar.

Summary

My overall philosophy on the use of ATD preceding the administration of ^{131}I therapy can be expressed as follows. Most of the deaths I have witnessed from this disease relate to its continued presence rather than to some therapeutic misadventure. Therefore, the prompt institution of definitive therapy is the primary objective. In an individual case, attention must be given to improving hydration, nutrition, and cardiac compensation before the administration of ^{131}I therapy. When a trial of beta blockers is successful in lowering the heart rate and making the patient more comfortable it is very doubtful if anything further is to be gained by prolonging the treatment period with ATD.

COMMENTARY

O. Peter Schumacher, M.D., Ph.D.

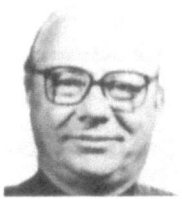

Why Hyperthyroidism May Worsen After ^{131}I Therapy

The debate as to whether antithyroid drugs (ATD) are appropriate to prepare patients for radioactive iodine (^{131}I) therapy continues to be active. In our institution we have treated approximately 5000 patients with ^{131}I without any really serious problems afterward. One of our major concerns about ATD pretreatment is delay in the delivery of ^{131}I therapy. For the few patients who have become ill following ^{131}I therapy, the most common sequence was that ATD were stopped in anticipation of the patient coming to the clinic, following which there was a significant delay between initiation of the studies that led to the delivery of the appropriate ^{131}I therapy and reinstitution of ATD therapy following ^{131}I. It is noted that Meier and Hamburger had the patients stop ATD approximately 48 h before delivery of the therapeutic dose, and ATD were not resumed for 3 or 4 days afterward. Thus, the patients were off ATD for a minimum of 5 to 7 days, which may be sufficiently long to permit escape from ATD therapy.

ATD therapy does not prevent uptake of iodine into the thyroid, only the incorporation of that iodine into thyroid hormone. As soon as one stops ATD therapy the thyroid actively takes up iodine, combines it into hormone, and is then able to deliver that hormone to the peripheral blood for a considerable period afterward. It has been our general impression that most patients who become thyrotoxic after ^{131}I therapy can be included in one of two groups. The first group includes those for whom the hyperthyroidism was becoming more aggressive before ^{131}I therapy was instituted and there was not sufficient time for ^{131}I to control the hyperthyroidism. The second group includes those for whom ATD were stopped long enough to allow the hyperthyroidism to escape, and then after the institution of ^{131}I therapy ATD were not started soon enough to prevent an exacerbation of hyperthyroidism. We conclude, therefore, that ^{131}I does not very often exacerbate hyperthyroidism significantly. Elevations of PBI following ^{131}I therapy may reflect only thyroglobulin release rather than release of T_4.

How to Prevent Exacerbation of Hyperthyroidism After ^{131}I

Obviously a few patients will have an exacerbation of hyperthyroidism following ^{131}I, but we think that these are patients for whom the hyperthyroidism would have become worse regardless of whether ^{131}I were given. Therefore we administer ^{131}I as soon as possible, to minimize the delay after discontinuing any previous

ATD. For example, we stop ATD for only a few hours before performing the ^{131}I uptake, and administer ^{131}I therapy immediately after the 24-h uptake determination. We then reinstitute ATD approximately 24–36 h following ^{131}I therapy. With this approach we have not found that patients have any significant morbidity or mortality following ^{131}I therapy. We often employ propranolol and/or ATD, and in the presence of Graves' disease add Lugol's solution or saturated solution of potassium iodide (SSKI) in order to ameliorate as much as possible the hyperthyroidism that is already present.

Problems of Patient Compliance in ATD Preparation for ^{131}I Therapy

Not mentioned in the report of Meier and Hamburger is the problem of patient compliance. The few times we decided to initiate ATD therapy before treatment with ^{131}I we had considerable difficulty with patients continuing their ATD carefully enough to have an impact on the hyperthyroidism. Consequently, the patients remained thyrotoxic for 2 to 4 months longer than if they had received ^{131}I therapy at the initial evaluation. In view of this, it is our tendency to proceed with definitive therapy as quickly as possible with ^{131}I, and then to follow this rapidly with aggressive ATD and/or propranolol therapy, believing that the critical issue over the long run is the correction of the hyperthyroidism. All other measures have only a temporary effect in the amelioration of the clinical problem.

ATD Preparation for Hyperthyroidism with Lower Radioiodine Uptake Values

Occasionally patients may have hyperthyroidism with low radioactive iodine uptakes entirely aside from those patients who have spontaneously resolving hyperthyroidism. In these patients we often pretreat with ATD for 6 to 8 weeks. This is done not so much to control the hyperthyroidism, but rather to deplete the thyroid of iodine and thus increase the radioiodine uptake to make the therapeutic dose of ^{131}I reasonable and effective in terms of patient management.

Summary

We definitely do not feel that there is any need to delay definitive therapy with ^{131}I because of the severity of the hyperthyroidism and/or advanced age, thyrotoxic heart disease, and so on. The only exception is when the hyperthyroidism seems to be increasing very rapidly, as in thyroid storm, and practical considerations preclude immediate ^{131}I therapy (e.g., radiologist availability). Then we will initiate aggressive ATD therapy first, and at some appropriately well-planned time proceed with ^{131}I treatment. It is in such patients that we have experienced occasional surgical mortality. In view of this minimal but definite mortality, we clearly feel that surgical intervention in such patients is not appropriate because they are so precarious, and ^{131}I therapy is so definitive.

SUMMARY—CHAPTER 7

Becker, Miller, and Schumacher seem to agree that the risk of exacerbation of hyperthyroidism after ^{131}I therapy is very small for patients with Graves' disease, perhaps greater for those with toxic multinodular goiter (Miller). While this volume was in preparation I studied serum thyroid hormone levels 10 days after ^{131}I therapy in 26 patients who were not prepared with ATD and five who were.

Of the unprepared patients, compared to T_3 and T_4 levels obtained just prior to therapy, follow-up values were reduced by one-third or more in 13 patients, reduced or elevated by up to one-third in 11 patients, and elevated by more than one-third in only two patients. No patient experienced any untoward reaction.

Table 7-4 gives data for the five patients prepared with ATD. Patients 1 and 2 were not treated to euthyroidism. However, there was a further drop in T_3 levels and only a modest rise in T_4 levels after ^{131}I therapy. Patients 3 and 4 were treated until euthyroid, and T_3 and T_4 levels were within normal limits 10 days after the therapy. Patient 5 had toxic multinodular goiter. After ATD preparation her T_3 level was normal and her T_4 level was only slightly elevated. Only minor changes in these levels were observed at the 10-day examination. None of the five patients experienced any undesirable reaction to the treatment.

Perhaps blood levels taken sooner after therapy might have shown different results. However, the 10-day period was selected because it seemed probable that not much change would occur in the first few days, and that any discharged hormone would persist (especially T_4) for several days.

Table 7-4. Impact of ATD preparation on post-^{131}I levels of T_3 and T_4 in the blood.

Patient	Goiter type	[131]I Dose (mCi)	Age (years)	Serum hormone levels					
				Baseline		After ATD preparation		10 Days after [131]I	
				T_3[a]	T_4[b]	T_3	T_4	T_3	T_4
1	Diffuse	20	65	485	24	277	16	236	21
2	Diffuse	30	55	682	27	448	18	408	20
3	Diffuse	30	59	710	25	155	9.9	93	6.7
4	Diffuse	20	67	703	23	104	7.3	123	10.4
5	Multinodular	30	66	234	15	124	12	165	13.5

[a]ng/dl, NR 80–82.
[b]ng/dl, NR 5–11.5.

These data provide some support for the contention that substantial discharge of thyroid hormone is uncommon after ^{131}I therapy. However, it does happen in a small proportion of patients. Therefore, it might seem reasonable to employ ATD preparation for hyperthyroid patients in precarious metabolic or cardiovascular balance.

However, Becker, Miller, and Schumacher express concern that ATD preparation may be associated with a worse prognosis than immediate ^{131}I therapy, for the following reasons:

(1) This may delay control of hyperthyroidism.

(2) Interruption of ATD may be followed by a flare-up of the hyperthyroidism.

(3) Noncompliant patients may be exposed to the risk of worsening hyperthyroidism.

(4) ATD may increase radioresistance, and thus the necessity for multiple ^{131}I doses.

Delay in control of hyperthyroidism can be problem whether ^{131}I therapy is given directly or after ATD preparation, if inadequate doses of either agent are given. For this reason we use 1200 mg of PTU daily for preparation of patients for ^{131}I therapy. Smaller doses may be effective, but may take longer. If one is concerned enough about the patient to employ ATD preparation, it makes no sense not to give large doses of ATD. Similarly, we employ large doses of ^{131}I for these patients because we are more concerned about avoiding prolonged hyperthyroidism, or recurrent thyrotoxicosis (in patients with toxic multinodular goiter), than posttherapy hypothyroidism.

Schumacher's warning is well taken that if ATD preparation is employed, the drug should only be interrupted for 24 h prior to administering the ^{131}I, and ATD can be resumed 24 to 48 h later. With the program we have employed we have yet to observe a flare-up in the hyperthyroidism in the ATD-free interval.

Barzilai's argument for routine ATD preparation of all hyperthyroid patients seems based not upon a necessity to prevent reactions from the ^{131}I therapy, but rather in the hope that ^{131}I therapy can be avoided. This issue has been considered in Chapter 5.

Joel I. Hamburger, M. D.

REFERENCES

1. Feitelberg S, Kaunitz PS, Silver S, Simon N, Wasserman LR, Yohalem SB: Hyperthyroidism; treatment with radioactive iodine. Arch Intern Med 85:471, 1950
2. Nelson RB, Cavenagh JB, Bernstein A: Case of fatal thyroid crisis occurring after radioactive iodine therapy. Illinois Med J 101:265, 1952
3. Seed L, Jaffe B: Results of treatment of toxic goiter with radioactive iodine. J Clin Endocrinol 13:107, 1958
4. Nadler SB, Bloch T, Hidalgo JV, Nieset RT: Evaluation of radioactive iodine (131) therapeusis in thyrotoxicosis. J Louisiana Med Soc 106:368, 1954

5. Chapman EM, Maloof F: The use of radioactive iodine in the diagnosis and treatment of hyperthyroidism: Ten years' experience. Medicine (Baltimore) 34:261, 1955

6. Werner SC, Coelho B, Quimby EH: Ten-year results of I-131 therapy of hyperthyroidism. Bull NY Acad Med 33:738, 1957

7. Sheline GE, Miller ER: Radioiodine therapy of hyperthyroidism. Arch Intern Med 103:924, 1959

8. Lamberg BA, Hernberg CA, Wahlberg P, Hakkila R: Treatment of toxic nodular goiter with radioactive iodine. Acta Med Scand 165:245, 1959

9. Rubenfeld S, Lowenthal M, Kohn A, Mitchell N, Brodie SS: Radioiodine in the treatment of hyperthyroidism. Arch Intern Med 104:532, 1959

10. Blomfield GW, Eckert H, Fisher M, Miller H, Munro DS, Wilson GM: Treatment of thyrotoxicosis with ^{131}I. Br Med J 1:63, 1959

11. Volpe R, Schatz DL, Scott A, Peller JA, Vale JM, Ezrin C, Johnston AW: Radioactive iodine in the treatment of hyperthyroidism. Can Med Assoc J 84:37, 1961

12. Monasterio G, Donato L, Saracci R: Presentation of the results of a statistical survey on the treatment of hyperthyroidism with radioactive iodine. Minerva Nucl 8:3, 1964

13. Staffurth JS, Gibberd MC, Hilton PJ: Atrial fibrillation in thyrotoxicosis treated with radioiodine. Postgrad Med J 41:663, 1965

14. Edsmyr F, Einhorn J: Complications in radioiodine treatment of hyperthyroidism. Acta Radiol Ther Phys Biol 4:49, 1966

15. Saterborg NE, Einhorn J: Fractionated ^{131}I therapy in large toxic goiters. Acta Endocrinol 51:7, 1966

16. Miller JM, Weber RE, Block MA: Treatment of hyperthyroidism from the autonomous multinodular goiter. Henry Ford Hosp Med J 15:85, 1967

17. Aach R, Kissane J: Thyroid storm shortly after ^{131}I therapy of a toxic multinodular goiter? Am J Med 52:786, 1972

18. Parker JLW, Lawson DH: Death from thyrotoxicosis. Lancet 2:894, 1973

19. Creutzig H, Kallfelz I, Haindl J, Thiede G, Hundeshagen H: Thyroid storm and iodine-131 treatment. Lancet 2:145, 1976

20. Williams RH, Towery BT, Jaffe H, Rogers WF Jr, Tagnon R: Radioiodotherapeusis. Am J Med 7:702, 1949

21. Beierwaltes WH, Johnson PC: Hyperthyroidism treated with radioiodine. Arch Intern Med 97:393, 1956

22. Caswell HT, Robbins RR, Rosemond GP: Definitive treatment of 536 cases of hyperthyroidism with I-131 or surgery. Ann Surg 164:593, 1966

23. Freeman M, Giuliani M, Schwartz F, et al: Acute thyroiditis, thyroid crisis, and hypocalcemia following radioactive iodine therapy. NY State J Med 69:2036, 1969

24. Shafer RB, Nuttall FQ: Thyroid crisis induced by radioactive iodine. J Nucl Med 12:262, 1971

25. Riggs DS: Elevation of serum protein-bound iodine after large doses of radioactive iodine. Fed Proc 7:251, 1948

26. Soley MH, Miller ER: Treatment of Graves' disease with radioactive iodine. Med Clin North Am 32:3, 1948

27. Bartels EC, Corn LR: Thyroidectomy for hyperthyroidism following unsatisfactory response to radioiodine treatment. Med Clin North Am 44:375, 1960

28. Bauer FK, Blahd WH: Treatment of hyperthyroidism with individually calculated doses of ^{131}I. Arch Intern Med 99:194, 1957

29. Crooks J, Buchanan WW, Wayne EJ, MacDonald E: Effect of pretreatment with methylthiouracil on results of ^{131}I therapy. Br Med J 1:151, 1960

30. Chapman EM: Current concepts in therapy. N Engl J Med 265:948, 1961

31. DeGroot LJ: Treatment of thyrotoxicosis. Mod Treatment 1:176, 1964
32. Eller M, Silver S, Yohalem SB, Segal RL: The treatment of toxic nodualr goiter with radioactive iodine: 10 years' experience with 436 cases. Ann Intern Med 52:976, 1960
33. Maloof F, Chapman EM: Responses to radioactive iodine therapy in hyperthyroidism, with special reference to cardiac provlems. J Clin Endocrinol 11:1296, 1951
34. Wise PH, Burnet RB, Ahmad A, et al.: Intentional radioiodine ablation in Graves' disease. Lancet 2:1231, 1975
35. Schimmel M, Utiger RD: Acute effect of inorganic iodide after ^{131}I therapy for hyperthyroidism. Clin Endocrinol 6:329, 1977
36. Shafer RB, Nuttal FQ: Acute changes in thyroid function in patients treated with radioactive iodine. Lancet 2:635, 1975
37. Tamagna EI, Levine GA, Hershman JM: Thyroid-hormone concentrations after radioiodine therapy for hyperthyroidism. J Nucl Med 20:387, 1980
38. Hales I: Diagnosis and nonoperative treatment of thyrotoxicosis. J Coll Radiol Australasia 8:98, 1964
39. Staffurth JS, Young J: Delay in control of thyrotoxicosis after treatment with radioactive iodine. J Clin Endocrinol 27:1062, 1967
40. McLarty DG, Harden RMcG, Alexander WD: Treatment of thyrotoxic patients with atrial fibrillation. Scot Med J 22:14, 1969
41. Beierwaltes WH: The treatment of hyperthyroidism with iodine-131. Semin Nucl Med 8:95, 1978
42. Lee TC, Coffey RJ, Mackin J, Cobb M, Routon J, Canary JJ: The use of propranolol in the surgical treatment of thyrotoxic patients. Ann Surg 177:643, 1978
43. Michie W, Hamer-Hodges DW, Pegg CAS, Orr FGG, Bewsher PD: Beta-blockade and partial thyroidectomy for thyrotoxicosis. Lancet 1:1009, 1974
44. Caswell HT, Marks AD, Channick BJ: Propranolol for the preoperative preparation of patients with thyrotoxicosis. Surg Gynecol Obstet 146:908, 1978
45. Zonszein J, Santangelo RP, Mackin JF, Lee TC, Coffey RJ, Canary JJ: Propranolol therapy in thyrotoxicosis. Am J Med 66:411, 1979
46. Eriksson M, Rubenfeld S, Garber AJ, Kohler PO: Propranolol does not prevent thyroid storm. N Engl J Med 296:263, 1977
47. Propranolol for thyroid storm [Letter to the editor]. N Engl J Med 296:1120, 1977
48. Enhorn J, Satervorg VE: Antithyroid drugs in RAI therapy of hyperthyroidism. Acta Radiol 58:161, 1962
49. Steinback JJ, Donoghue GD, Goldman JK: Simultaneous treatment of toxic diffuse goiter and ATD: a prospective study. J Nucl Med 20:1263, 1979
50. Kalk WJ, Durbach D, Kanter S, Levin S: Very low doses of RAI for hyperthyroidism—failure to prevent a high incidence of early hypothyroidism. S Afr Med J 57:479, 1980
51. Sugrue D, McEvoy M, Felly J, Drury MI: Hyperthyroidism in the land of Graves'. Result of treatment by surgery, radioiodine, and carbimazole in 837 cases. Q J Med 193:51, 1980
52. Golden AWG, Fraser TR: Effect of pretreatment with carbimazole in patients with thyrotoxicosis treated with ^{131}I. Br Med J 3:443, 1969
53. Hoffman D: Delayed effects of therapeutic levels of ^{131}I: mortality experience in patients treated for hyperthyroidism. Radiol Res 67:556, 1976
54. Greer MA, Kammer H, Bouma DJ: Short-term antithyroid drug therapy for the thyrotoxicosis of Graves' disease. N Engl J Med 297:173, 1977
55. Horn K, Brehm G, Habermann J, Pickardt CR, Scriba PC: Successful treatment of

thyrotoxic crisis by continuous plasmaphoresis with blood cell separation. Klin Wochenschr 54:783, 1976

56. Van Hofe SE, Dorfman SG, Carretta RF, Young RL: The increase of incidence of hypothyroidism within one year after RAI for toxic diffuse goiter. J Nucl Med 19:180, 1979
57. Buchanan WW, Koutras DA, Crooks J: A comparison of pretreatment with potassium perchlorate and methylthiouracil on results of ^{131}I therapy. Br J Radiol 38:536, 1965
58. Barzilai D, Sheinfeld M: Fatal complications following use of potassium perchlorate in thyrotoxicosis. Isr J Med Sci 2:453, 1966
59. Steinbach JJ, Donoghue GD, Goldman JK: Simultaneous treatment of toxic goiter with I-131 and antithyroid drugs: a prospective study. J Nucl Med 20:1263, 1979
60. Lamberg BA: The medical thyroid crisis. Acta Med Scand 164:479, 1956
61. Waldstein SS, Slodki SJ, Kaganiec GI, Bronsky D: A clinical study of thyroid storm. Ann Intern Med 52:626, 1960
62. Mazzaferri EL, Skillman TG: Thyroid storm. Arch Intern Med 124:684, 1969
63. Volpé R, Schatz DL, Scott A, Peller JA, Vale JM, Ezrin C, Johnston AW: Radioactive iodine in the treatment of hyperthyroidism. II. Can Med Assoc J 84:37, 1961
64. Freeman M, Giuliani M, Schwartz F, et al.: Acute thyroiditis, thyroid crisis, and hypocalcemia following radioactive iodine therapy. NY State J Med 69:2036, 1969
65. Becker DV, Hurley JR: Complications of radioiodine treatment of hyperthyroidism. Semin Nucl Med 1:442, 1971
66. Miller JM, Block MA: Functional autonomy in multinodular goiter. JAMA 214:535, 1970
67. Uller RP, VanHerle AJ: Effect of therapy on serum thyroglobulin levels in patients with Graves' disease. J Clin Endocrinol Metab 46:747, 1978
68. Barandes M, Hurley JR, Becker DV: Implications of rapid intrathyroidal iodine turnover for ^{131}I therapy; the small pool syndrome. J Nucl Med 14:379, 1973

Chapter 8

Is Needle Aspiration of the Cystic Thyroid Nodule Effective and Safe Treatment?

J. Martin Miller, M.D.
Joel I. Hamburger, M.D.
Charles I. Taylor, M.D.

INTRODUCTION

In 1955 one of us (JMM) first expressed dissatisfaction with the use of surgical lobectomy for diagnostic purposes in thyroid nodule patients.[1] This attitude was in part related to the observation that some thyroid nodules are cysts, many of which can be eliminated by simple needle puncture.[2-6] In a retrospective study, 88 of 425 surgically excised solitary or dominant nodules proved to be unilocular cysts, 2 cm or more in diameter. The development of techniques utilizing ultrasound to differentiate cystic from solid thyroid nodules has made it simpler to select nodules for aspiration. Nevertheless cyst aspiration is still not widely employed.

Many surgeons prefer to deal with thyroid nodules by lobectomy. Internists and family practitioners hesitate to insert needles into internal bodily structures. Also, there is a lingering doubt about the conclusion that nodules which regress in response to aspiration are necessarily benign.

One of us (JMM) has been performing selective percutaneous aspirations of cystic thyroid nodules since 1965; the others (JIH and CIT) began in 1976. We will present and compare our experiences as a basis for addressing the following issues:

(1) What features of the history, physical examination, or the nodule aspirate are useful in predicting the efficacy of aspiration therapy?

(2) How often will aspiration eliminate a thyroid cyst?

(3) What is the risk that a nodule apparently eliminated by aspiration (therefore assumed benign) will prove to be malignant?

EXPERIENCE AT HENRY FORD HOSPITAL AND NORTHLAND THYROID LABORATORY

Methods of Cyst Identification

Cystic nodules were aspirated at Henry Ford Hospital (HFH) between 1965 and 1974. Initially nodules were selected for aspiration on the basis of history, physical findings, imaging, and ultrasound data. A nodule which appeared suddenly or suddenly enlarged suggested acute hemorrhage. Sometimes this enlargement was painful, more often not. The cystic nodule usually was smooth, round, firm, and resilient. Thyroid imaging revealed a zone of absent function. Occasionally an autonomously functioning thyroid nodule (AFTN) underwent acute hemorrhagic infarction and presented with typical findings of a hemorrhagic cystic lesion. Imaging revealed at least a peripheral rim of tissue with autonomous function. The sequential studies for the diagnosis of AFTN have been described elsewhere.[7] Ultrasound will reveal echo-free zones corresponding to the cystic portion of the lesion.

Cystic nodules were aspirated at the Northland Thyroid Laboratory (NTL) between 1976 and 1980. At NTL, most cysts were discovered when fine needle aspiration biopsies were attempted on hypofunctional nodules, many of which did not have typical physical findings of cysts. Since only hypofunctional nodules were needled, degenerated AFTN were excluded from the NTL series.

Because of the differences in selection methods the two series of cases will be presented separately, and the results compared.

Method of Cyst Aspiration

The aspiration technique is simple. The skin is prepared with alcohol. Local anesthesia is unnecessary for a single puncture. A 20-gauge 1.5-inch needle is used with a 10- or 20-ml syringe (depending upon the cyst size). The nodule is held in a fixed position by the fingers of the opposite hand and the needle inserted perpendicular to the anterior surface of the neck. The operator will experience a sensation of resistance as the capsule is entered, and one of release as the needle penetrates into the cyst.

There were 105 patients in the HFH series, 81 females and 24 males, ranging in age from 14 to 76 years (average 38 years). Eighty-seven nodules were hypofunctional on imaging, 18 were AFTN. The age and sex distribution was similar for the 153 NTL patients, but no AFTN were included.

Results of Aspiration of AFTN

For 16 of the 18 AFTN patients there was a postaspiration residual of 1.5 cm or larger. Seven AFTN were ablated: six with radioactive iodine and one surgically. Two of the patients who received radioactive iodine were treated after their AFTN had progressed from nontoxix to toxic, after 5 and 8 years. Four AFTN treated with radioactive iodine had secreted enough hormone to suppress completely the contralateral lobe. Although the patients were not hyperthyroid, prophylactic ablation was performed. The single AFTN removed surgically was ablated at the patient's request. The remaining nine AFTN patients with residual nodules 1.5 cm or larger and the two patients with AFTN smaller than 1 cm after aspiration have been followed for 6 to 13 years (average 9 years) without discernible change in size or function.

Results of Aspiration of Hypofunctional Cysts

Of the 87 hypofunctional cystic nodules, 69 were successfully managed by aspiration, i.e., the nodule disappeared, or the residual was less than 1 cm and less than 50% of the original size. For 18 patients (21%) aspiration was inadequate, i.e., a residual nodule 1 cm or larger persisted. Table 8-1 summarizes these results.

Table 8-2 provides the corresponding data for the NTL series. Instead of 21% unsuccessful responses, there were 58% (88 of 153 lesions). We attribute this difference to the method of selection. Patients in the HFH series, identified as having cysts by physical findings and ultrasound prior to aspiration, more often had completely cystic lesions. Since those in the NTL series were identified primarily by needle aspiration, more lesions with substantial solid components were included.

Table 8-3 correlates the initial size of the HFH lesions successfully aspirated with the number of aspirations required.

The volume of the aspirate from 66 of the cysts was 2–20 ml, and for three it was 22–55 ml. Seventeen of 26 cysts with an aspirate volume of 5 ml or less were satisfactorily treated by one aspiration. Only 17 of 40 with aspirate volumes of 6–20 ml similarly responded. The larger cystic lesions more often required multiple aspirations. The findings were similar for the NTL series.

In the HFH series no correlation could be made between nodule size and success of aspiration. However, Table 8-4 shows that for the NTL series success was distinctly less likely if the lesion was 4 cm or larger in diameter. Again, this difference is attributed to the inclusion of incompletely degenerated lesions in the NTL series.

Table 8-1. Response to aspiration of cystic hypofunctional thyroid nodules, HFH series.

Response	Number of aspirations				
	1	2	3	4–6	Total
Nodule gone	22	11	7	2	42
Residual <1 cm and <50% of original size	13	7	5	2	27
Residual 1 cm +	2	10	6	0	18
Total	37	28	18	4	87

Table 8-2. Response to aspiration of cystic thyroid nodules, NTL series.

Response	Number of aspirations			
	1	2	3 or more	Total
Nodule gone	34	12	3	49
Residual <1 cm and <50% of original size	11	4	1	16
Residual 1 cm +	36	28	24	88
Total	81	44	28	153

Table 8-3. Correlation of original cyst size and number of aspirations required for successful treatment, HFH series.

Original cyst size (cm)	Number of aspirations				
	1	2	3	4–6	Total
2 or less	7	3	1	0	11
2.5–3.5	19	5	7	3	34
4+	9	10	4	1	24
Total	35	18	12	4	69

Table 8-4. Correlation of response to aspiration with original cyst size, NTL series.

Response to aspiration	Original cyst size (cm)			
	2 or smaller	2.5–3.5	4+	Total
Nodule gone	24	20	5	49
Residual <1 cm and <50% of original size	9	6	1	16
Residual 1 cm +	36	30	22	88
Total	69	56	28	153

Findings on Excised Cysts

Because of unsatisfactory responses to aspiration (in some instances because of patient preference), 39 patients had surgical removal of their lesions. There were 31 benign lesions and eight (23%) malignancies, two follicular and six papillary carcinomas. Case 1 is an example of a cystic cancer.

CASE 1: "CYSTIC" CARCINOMA OF THE THYROID
A 28-year-old euthyroid man detected a painless 4-cm swelling in the right lobe of the thyroid. One year later he sought medical attention. Imaging revealed a "cold" nodule. Needle aspiration produced 10 ml of orange fluid, with a palpable residual mass of about 3 cm. Four

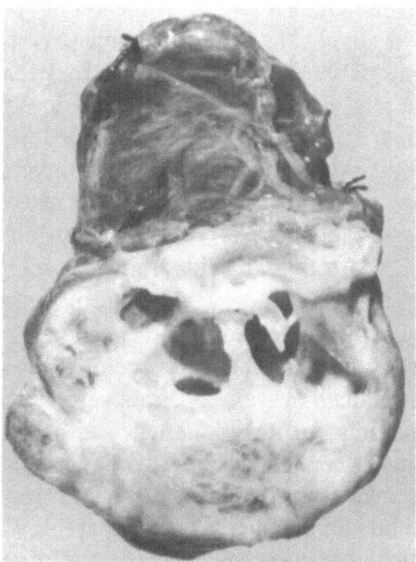

Figure 8-1. Gross surgical specimen showing degenerated cystic carcinoma in the right lobe of the thyroid.

days later the patient returned because the mass had recurred. Repeat aspiration produced 15 ml of old blood. There was again a firm irregular residual. A follicular carcinoma with cystic degeneration was removed. The gross specimen is shown in Figure 8-1. Figure 8-2 is a photomicrograph of the carcinomatous follicles.

This high percentage of cystic carcinoma is not representative of the incidence of malignancy in cystic nodules overall. Rather it reflects the high degree of selectivity employed in advising operation.

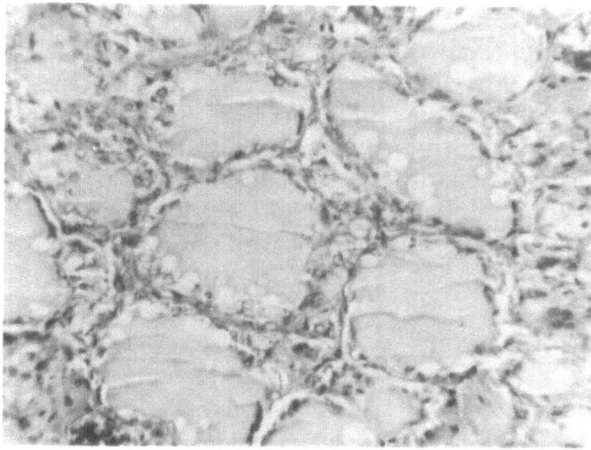

Figure 8-2. Photomicrograph of a section from the surgical specimen seen in Figure 8-1, showing a follicular carcinoma, $\times$ 325

Three of the eight malignancies were in the HFH series, and operation was advised for palpable residual masses (two patients) or prompt recurrence of a large cystic lesion (one patient). One of the five malignant lesions in the NTL series was in a patient who had undergone four previous operations for papillary carcinoma. The sudden appearance of a midline nodule suggested yet another recurrence. A fine needle aspiration biopsy was attempted, expecting that a diagnosis of recurrent papillary carcinoma would be confirmed. However, bloody fluid was obtained followed by collapse of the nodule. Within 3 weeks the nodule recurred. At that time a substantial solid component was evident. Papillary carcinoma was diagnosed by needle biopsy and confirmed at operation. Three of the four remaining malignancies detected in the NTL series proved to be only partially cystic. For one of these patients a preoperative diagnosis of papillary carcinoma was made by needle biopsy. Case 1, above, was the fifth carcinoma.

For the sake of recording our total experience with partially cystic cancers, we note that there were two other such lesions identified at HFH by needle biopsy of the residual when cysts persistently recurred. One was a poorly differentiated follicular carcinoma and one a follicular variant of papillary carcinoma. These cases were part of the HFH biopsy experience between 1976 and 1980.

DISCUSSION

Most but Not All Cysts Are Benign

Much of the literature on thyroid cysts deals primarily with diagnosis,[8-12] rather than results of aspiration. From some reports one might infer that the diagnosis of a thyroid cyst is practically equivalent to a diagnosis of a benign lesion.[11,12] Our retrospective review of 303 thyroid cancers, however, showed that on rare occasions well-differentiated cancers were almost totally cystic, and partial cystic degeneration occurred in 2–4% of thyroid malignancies.[3] Other authors have made supportive observations.[2,4,13] Nevertheless, most cystic thyroid nodules develop after hemorrhage into preexisting benign nodules. The character of the aspirate is a function of the time which has transpired since the bleeding episode. Hemoglobin and its derivatives are more rapidly absorbed than the fluid components of blood. Hence aspiration soon after a hemorrhage will produce a specimen resembling venous blood. Later the aspirate changes from chocolate opaque to olive translucent, and ultimately to a yellow transparent fluid.

Objectives of Cyst Aspiration

The primary objective of cyst aspiration is the nonsurgical elimination of the lesion. This confirms the diagnosis of a cyst and makes the chance of an associated malignancy too small to justify the minimal risks of surgical lobectomy. A second objective is to identify cystic lesions with appreciable solid components, identifiable by palpation after the fluid is withdrawn. This is important because these solid portions have no less risk of being malignant than any other solid nonfunctional thyroid nodule.

Crile[2] reported that 46 of 50 cystic nodules were "cured" by aspiration, and Clark et al.[6] were successful with 21 of 30 cysts. These findings are comparable to those achieved with the HFH series of non-AFTN cystic lesions, i.e., cysts which were identified by physical examination and ultrasound. However, Jensen and Rasmussen[5] found that only 12 of 24 cysts were either totally (five patients) or partially (seven patients) eliminated by aspiration. These results more closely approximate those obtained in the NTL series, where cystic lesions were identified during needle biopsy of hypofunctional nodules.

Does Needle Aspiration Eliminate the Need for Diagnostic Ultrasound?

We believe that the diagnosis of cystic nodules is confirmed accurately and most efficiently as an adjunct to the performance of an aspiration biopsy, without prior diagnostic ultrasound. It is generally appreciated that ultrasound techniques are not completely reliable in the differentiation of cystic from partially cystic and solid nodules.[4,8,14] Since we advise needle insertion for aspiration of fluid in cystic nodules, and for biopsy in solid lesions, and since needle aspiration will reliably discriminate between cystic, mixed, and solid nodules in a simple, convenient, and inexpensive fashion, ultrasound may be considered an unnecessary procedure and a needless expense.[15]

Malignancy in Thyroid Cysts

The finding of malignancy in about one in four cystic nodules selected for operation because of an unsatisfactory response to needle aspiration indicates the need for emphasis of guidelines which may be helpful in the recognition of malignant cysts. If the aspirate appears to be a recent hemorrhage, but there is no history of sudden enlargement, successful aspiration therapy is not likely.[6] These lesions probably recur because of repeated episodes of bleeding, beginning each time after reabsorption of blood lowers the internal nodular pressure. Hence fresh blood at the end of an aspirate suggests that the cyst will recur. Bleeding results from reduction in pressure within the cyst to less than that within an incompletely sealed vessel, or the tip of the needle may traumatize the cyst wall as the cyst collapses around the needle during the aspiration. Partial or complete reappearance of the lesion may occur within 5 min of the aspiration. When this happens, a repeat aspiration will probably be necessary. Recurrent bloody aspirates suggested the possibility of malignancy and led to the diagnosis of most of the cystic cancers that were subsequently excised.

A persistent mass greater than 1 cm is also a matter of concern. However, such a residual, unaccompanied by cyst reformation, is suitable for needle biopsy. Blum et al.[16] emphasized that nodules larger than 4 cm, whether benign or malignant, often have ultrasonic evidence of cystic degeneration. This is why many large cystic lesions in the NTL series failed to respond to aspiration. Needle biopsy confirmed the diagnosis of cancer in four patients with palpable residual masses. For others for whom needle biopsy is impractical or unsuccessful, assuming an acceptable risk, diagnostic lobectomy may be advised.

The possibility cannot be disregarded that a carcinoma which has undergone nearly complete cystic degeneration could respond to aspiration just like a benign nodule. Afterward there may be no palpable residual, or a residual less than 1 cm. Nevertheless, in the absence of any evidence to indicate that carcinomas of this type are more aggressive than other occult carcinomas, it seems safe to advise observation for cysts which respond favorably to aspiration.

Long-Term Results of Aspiration

If a cyst does not recur during 6 months following aspiration, or a residual of less than 1 cm fails to enlarge, a long-term favorable result is probable. A very high success rate for aspiration was achieved for cystic nodules which developed suddenly in the course of an acute hemorrhagic episode. We have also observed spontaneous resolution of nodules of this type, whose cystic character had been indicated by diagnostic ultrasound. This raises the question whether any treatment is necessary for the typical hemorrhagic cyst which suddenly "pops out." Since needle aspiration is so simple, and accomplishes in minutes what might otherwise require weeks, and often relieves discomfort and allays anxiety, we favor its use.

Although the administration of thyroid hormone in a dosage adequate to suppress TSH might seem helpful in preventing recurrences after aspiration of cystic nodules, one of us (JMM) in 1974[3] suggested that this was not the case. Nothing has happened since then to change that opinion. Most recurrences seem related to early hemorrhage, which thyroid hormone is not likely to influence.

Parathyroid Cysts

Lesions which contain clear or opalescent grayish fluid seem to be true cysts. They are usually soft on palpation in contrast to the firm resilient feel of the hemorrhagic cyst. When they recur they do so with fluid of the same appearance. A high level of C-terminal parathyroid hormone permitted the diagnosis of a parathyroid cyst in three patients, and another had the diagnosis confirmed surgically.[17] Similar findings were reported by Clark et al.[6] It may be helpful to remember that the parathyroid cyst may not produce the typical hypofunctional imaging defect associated with cystic thyroid lesions.

Thyroglossal Duct Cysts

We share the view[6] that aspiration of thyroglossal duct cysts is usually unsatisfactory. The amount of fluid tends to be scanty, and the cyst lining seems to promote fluid reaccumulation. Branchial clefts cysts behave similarly.

Cystic AFTN

The tendency for AFTN to undergo central hemorrhagic necrosis is well known, and has been observed in AFTN smaller than 1 mm.[18] This is probably related to the considerable vascularity of these lesions. In four of six patients aged 10 to 16 years the increase in the size of the AFTN resulting from hemorrhage was what brought the nodules to the attention of the patients. Although aspiration was only infrequently successful in reducing the lesion to less than 1 cm, aspiration may produce enough partial reduction in AFTN size to solve a cosmetic problem, so that observation may be pursued in the hope that further spontaneous necrosis will occur in time.

CONCLUSION

Aspiration is a simple, safe, and effective solution to the diagnosis and management of a substantial proportion of cystic thyroid nodules. In centers where needle biopsy is employed on a regular basis, needle aspiration serves to screen patients for whom biopsy may not be necessary. However, even where needle biopsy is not yet available, needle aspiration may reduce the number of unnecessary thyroid operations. The simplicity and safety of introducing a 20-gauge needle into a thyroid nodule makes needle aspiration a procedure which any physician who can palpate a thyroid nodule could undertake. If fluid is obtained and the lesion disappears, the problem may have been solved. If needed, aspiration may be repeated several times, especially if the recurrences become progressively smaller. If the lesion is solid, the patient can be referred for further evaluation. Gaining familiarity with needle aspiration may serve as the first step in the development of a needle biopsy program.

COMMENTARY

Orlo H. Clark, M.D.

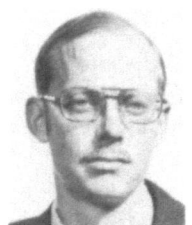

Findings of Miller et al.

Miller et al. ask the question whether percutaneous aspiration of the cystic thyroid nodule is effective and safe. Successful percutaneous aspiration of thyroid nodules was achieved in 69 of 87 (79%) of their patients at Henry Ford Hospital (HFH) and in 65 of 153 (42%) at the Northland Thyroid Laboratory (NTL). These differences were attributed to the inclusion of more patients with partially cystic (mixed solid-cystic) lesions at NTL. Although the success rate of aspiration may vary, at least 42% and as many as 79% of patients with cystic thyroid nodules have avoided unnecessary thyroid resections because of successful aspirations. Since no serious complications were reported and since the procedure is simple to perform, it is difficult to understand why aspiration of thyroid cysts is not recommended for virtually all patients with cystic thyroid nodules.

A critical question from their study is how many of the patients in both series had either partially or purely cystic lesions, either by ultrasonography or by having palpable residual tissue immediately after aspiration. From this information which should be available from their investigation, one might better be able to predict the success rate of aspiration in patients with purely cystic or partially cystic thyroid lesions and the incidence of cancer in these two groups.

Of particular interest are the 39 patients who had cystic lesions removed because of either a failed aspiration or patient preference. Again, it would be interesting to know how many were in each category. Eight of these 39 patients (23%) had malignant thyroid tumors (six papillary and two follicular). This incidence is not dissimilar from that reported for solid or partially cystic lesions, but is higher than that reported for purely cystic lesions.[2,3,13,16,19,20] One of these patients should probably not be included in this series because she developed a cystic lesion after five operations for papillary carcinoma. It is well known that although purely cystic intrathyroidal lesions are rarely malignant, metastatic differentiated thyroid cancer in lymph nodes is frequently cystic.[6]

Value of Ultrasonography in Cyst Diagnosis

We have been interested in the therapeutic effectiveness of thyroid cyst aspiration and in diagnostic techniques or clinical and laboratory tests that might predict whether a thyroid cyst is benign or malignant. Initially, we were not biopsying solid thyroid lesions because of our concern about the reliability of the biopsy or cytologic studies in these lesions and because our pathologists and cytologists had little experience with this technique.[21,22] We therefore used thyroid ultrasonography on all of our patients who had nonfunctioning, or "cold," solitary thyroid nodules to determine whether the lesions were cystic, partially cystic, or solid. It has been shown that ultrasonography was about 90% accurate in predicting whether a thyroid nodule was cystic or solid.[4,13,23] The limitations of thyroid ultrasonography were (1) poor resolution for lesions less than 1 cm; (2) nonfeasibility in the retrosternal area; (3) inconclusive results for lesions larger than 4 cm because of necrosis and hemorrhage in large tumors;[13,16] and (4) inability to differentiate between a purely cystic or partially cystic thyroid nodule. In the last several years considerable progress has been made in the development of ultrasound equipment; resolution for some ultrasound units is currently about 2 mm.[23] Thus, purely cystic lesions can now usually be differentiated from partially cystic lesions. Several questions must be considered before ultrasonography and cyst aspiration should be recommended for all patients with thyroid nodules or thyroid cysts.

What Percentage of Cold Thyroid Nodules Are Cystic?

If only 1% of patients with thyroid nodules have purely cystic lesions then determining whether a lesion was cystic or solid would not be worthwhile since so few patients would benefit even if aspiration therapy were effective.

In response to this question, the incidence of cysts in solitary thyroid lesions removed surgically varies from 6 to 22% (Table 8-5).[2,24–27] Since purely cystic thyroid nodules are "cold" on radioiodine scan and since clinicians frequently cannot distinguish between a cystic or solid thyroid lesion, ultrasonography helps clarify this issue.[4,16,23,26,28] Ultrasonography should therefore be used by clinicians who prefer to perform aspiration biopsy not of solid lesions but only of cystic lesions. If fine needle biopsy of solid thyroid lesions is used, then ultrasonography is not necessary because cyst fluid will be aspirated during biopsy.

Table 8-5. Incidence of cysts in solitary thyroid nodules.

Authors (date)	No. of cysts/ No. of patients	Incidence (%)
Crile (1966)[2]	–	15
Miller and Zafar (1972)[24]	88/425	20
Miskin et al. (1973)[25]	11/50	22
Crockford and Bain (1974)[26]	17/103	16
Clark and Demling (1976)[27]	6/100	6
Walfish et al. (1977)[20]	33/133	25

Should Aspiration Be Performed in All Patients with Thyroid Cysts?

Although cystic thyroid cancers are unusual, we are reluctant to aspirate cystic lesions in patients with a history of radiation exposure because of the multifocal nature of radiation-induced thyroid tumors. Occult thyroid cancers are frequently found (10–25%) in irradiated patients when thyroid resection is performed for larger thyroid nodules found elsewhere within the gland.[22,29,30] Although some authorities consider these occult thyroid cancers to be of no clinical consequence, the natural history of these lesions if untreated is unknown.[30,31] The prognosis after removal is excellent.[32,33] When instituting a program or a new method for evaluating thyroid nodules, the clinician must not miss thyroid cancers. Thus, aspirating a cystic thyroid nodule and missing a smaller cancer elsewhere in the gland must be avoided. In one of my patients with a thyroid cyst, thyroidectomy rather than cyst aspiration was recommended because of a history of radiation exposure. Histologic examination of the thyroid gland determined that the cyst was benign, but a 1.2-cm carcinoma was discovered elsewhere within the gland.

What Is the Incidence of Cancer in Purely Cystic and in Partially Cystic Thyroid Nodules?

Miller et al.,[3] in a retrospective review, found only two instances of cystic carcinoma in 302 consecutively removed thyroid cancers. Blum et al.[16] stated, "The probability of an occult neoplasm in the wall of the cyst is no greater than its probability in the remainder of the thyroid." Thus, purely cystic thyroid cancers less than 4 cm in size are distinctly unusual. Partially cystic thyroid cancers are not uncommon.[20,30] Thus, recurrent cyst formation or partially cystic lesions that leave palpable tissue immediately after aspiration must be viewed with suspicion.

Is Cyst Aspiration Safe?

Yes, and to my knowledge there have been no reports of implantation of malignancy after aspiration of cystic thyroid nodules. In our series of more than 100 aspirations in 70 patients with thyroid cysts there have been no significant complications. Since hemorrhage and vocal cord injury, although rare, have been recorded after percutaneous needle biopsy, these complications should be discussed with the patient.

Is Percutaneous Needle Biopsy Reliable?

Will biopsy miss cystic thyroid cancers? It appears from our experience and that reported in the literature that the chance of missing a cystic thyroid cancer is

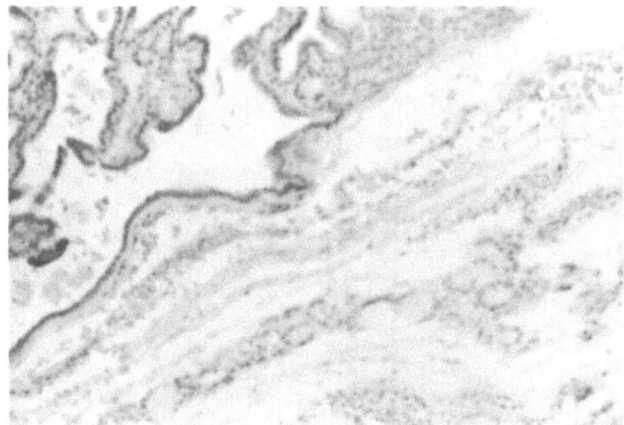

Figure 8-3. Cystic papillary thyroid cancer within a lymph node. Note the papillary projections and columnar cells lining the cyst. (Original magnification, × 250)

small.[2,3,16,22] We would agree with Miller et al. and others[20] that thyroid lobectomy is indicated if a thyroid cyst recurs after three aspirations. I have treated two patients who were referred to me after having cystic thyroid cancers removed by local excision. Because cancer in these lesions was not discovered until the surgical specimens were reviewed, a subsequent operation was required to remove the remaining thyroid lobe (Fig. 8-3). Although there is considerable disagreement as to the extent of surgery indicated for patients with papillary carcinoma, virtually all clinicians agree that excisional biopsy is contraindicated for these tumors.[22]

What Clinical or Laboratory Tests Are Helpful in Determining Whether a Thyroid Cyst Is Benign or Malignant?

Because a few purely cystic nodules are malignant and because it is sometimes difficult, by both ultrasonography and physical examination, to distinguish between partially and purely cystic thyroid lesions, we have been interested in whether cytologic or chemical tests might help determine whether a cyst is benign.

Cyst fluid from all of our patients with purely cystic lesions has been sent for cytologic examination and all of the lesions have been benign (Fig. 8-4). Cytologic examination of cyst fluid from a patient with a cystic metastasis to a large lymph node and from a patient with a partially cystic primary thyroid lesion were positive for papillary carcinoma (Fig. 8-5). If residual tissue persists after aspiration of a cystic thyroid nodule, this tissue should also be biopsied. Needle biopsy of solid lesions has been reported to be more reliable than cytologic study of the cyst fluid because of better cellular preservation.[20]

We have also determined thyroid hormone levels in the cyst fluid.[6] Since thyroid hormone levels are often markedly increased in benign thyroid cysts, and

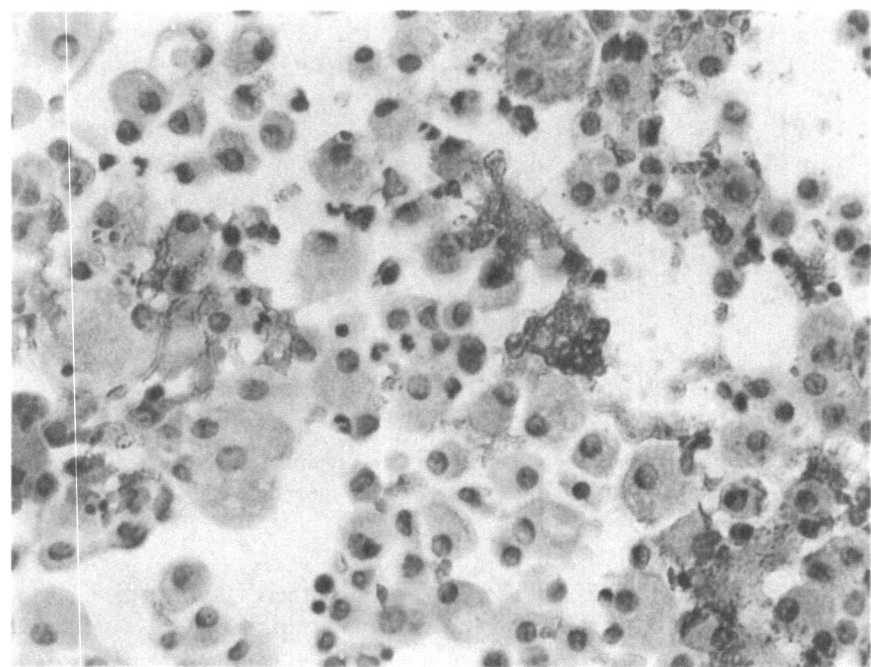

Figure 8-4. Numerous phagocytic cells containing brown coarse pigment and clear vacuoles from a benign cyst. Follicular epithelial cells are absent. (Original magnification, × 400)

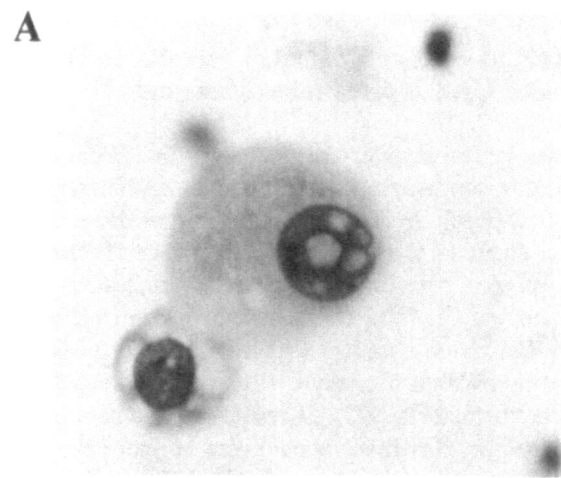

Figure 8-5. A Aspiration biopsy cytology of partially cystic thyroid carcinoma. Intranuclear cytoplasmic inclusions are present. These have smooth perimeters with increased chromatin deposition. Courtesy of John S. Abele, M.D., Department of Pathology, Uni-

since cystic thyroid cancers should not make thyroid hormone, ascertaining the thyroid hormone concentration in the cyst fluid may help determine if a thyroid cyst is malignant. It might also help determine whether a cyst is of thyroid origin, since parathyroid and thymic cysts also occur in the neck (Fig. 8-6).[34,35] We have not aspirated any cystic thyroid cancers, but T_4 levels were slightly increased in cyst fluid aspirated from cystic thyroid metastases in lymph nodes. Table 8-6 lists the clinical and laboratory tests that help predict whether a thyroid cyst is benign or malignant.

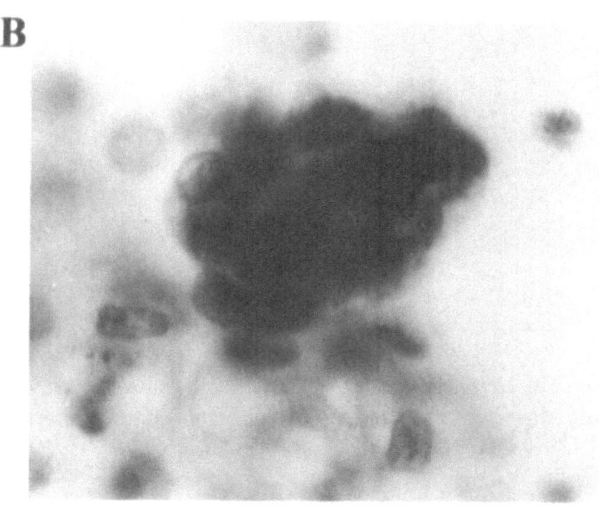

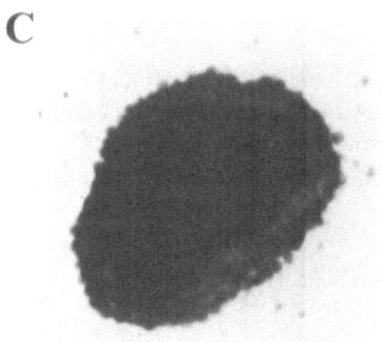

versity of California, San Francisco, CA. **B** A single papillary group shows two central calcifications with fine laminations. Nuclei of the surrounding cells lack intranuclear inclusions but these cells have sharply defined intercellular borders. (Original magnification, × 400) **C** A large calcification without identifiable vascular structures. (Original magnification, × 400)

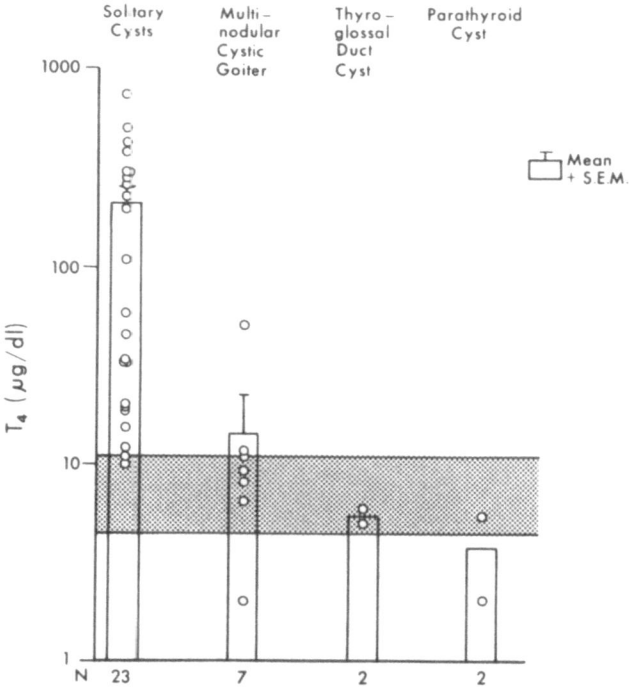

Figure 8-6. T_4 levels (in $\mu g/dl$; log scale) in cystic neck masses. Cyst T_4 levels were higher in the solitary thyroid cysts than in cyst fluid from multinodular goiters ($P <$ 0.025). Courtesy of Clark OH, et al.: J Clin Endocrinol Metab 48:983, 1979.

Is Treatment with Thyroid Hormone Helpful in Preventing Recurrent Cyst Formation After Aspiration?

In contrast to Miller et al., I believe that treatment with thyroid hormone to suppress TSH is worthwhile. Although this treatment is not helpful without aspiration, it does seem to improve results of aspiration.[6,36] Since many thyroid cysts appear to have a functioning cyst wall and are secreting thyroid hormone, it seems

Table 8-6. Malignant potential of thyroid cysts.

Low potential	High potential
Intrathyroidal	Extrathyroidal
Purely cystic	Partially cystic
Negative cytology	(residual tissue after aspiration)
High T_4 level	Radiation history[a]
Hashimoto's thyroiditis	

[a]Cancer present either within the cyst or elsewhere within the thyroid gland.

logical to try to suppress this functioning epithelium.[37] More favorable results for cyst aspiration[2,4,20] may be attributable to the use of larger needles (18 gauge) and in many cases thyroid hormone. Others[5] using smaller needles have not done as well.

Technique of Needle Aspiration

Needle aspiration is performed with the patient in a supine position and the neck hyperextended. The neck is prepared with iodine and a local anesthetic is sometimes used. Aspiration is performed using an 18-gauge needle and 10-ml syringe. After aspiration, gentle pressure is applied to the former cyst site for 5 min. The site of the previous lesion is then repalpated to ascertain whether there is any residual lesion. If there is no residual lesion, aspiration is usually successful.[6]

I agree with the conclusion that aspiration of thyroid cysts is safe and effective. Although most thyroid cysts are benign, determination of thyroid hormone levels and cytologic examination of the cyst fluid are recommended. Aspiration of thyroid cysts is successful in approximately 70% of patients, making operative removal of these lesions unnecessary.

COMMENTARY

George Crile, Jr., M.D.

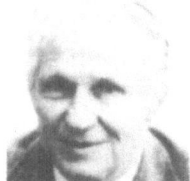

Except in a few unimportant details I agree with everything that Miller et al. have written about needle aspiration of the cystic thyroid nodule. They give an affirmative answer to the question of whether this treatment is effective and safe, and I second the motion.

Cost Implications of Cyst Aspiration

One of my longstanding concerns about the practice of medicine is the continuous escalation of cost. Much of this increase is the result of continuing to use old tests even when new ones are more effective and should have supplanted them. I am referring now to the use of multiple tests of thyroid function and of agglutination and scans and sonograms all done for a simple nodule of the thyroid. Miller et al. speak to this problem eloquently, and I quote, "Since we advise needle insertion for aspiration of fluid in cystic nodules, and for biopsy in solid lesions, and since needle aspiration will reliably discriminate between cystic, mixed, and solid nodules in a simple, convenient, and inexpensive fashion, ultrasound may be considered an unnecessary procedure and a needless expense."

Needle Biopsy May Replace Thyroid Scanning

In my opinion unless there is clinical or laboratory evidence of hyperthyroidism the same can be said of the scan. In patients who are euthyroid, what could the scan tell us that might alter our treatment? Most nodules are cold and therefore would have to be studied by biopsy or, some would say, by excision. A few nodules are warm—they take up some radioactive iodine. So do some cancers. We are no better off than before and we still have to take a biopsy. An occasional nodule will be hot, but unless there is clinical or laboratory evidence of hyperthyroidism, I would not consider removing such a nodule. Many of them either thrombose and leave a harmless shell of active tissue, or never progress to cause hyperthyroidism. I do not believe thyroidectomy is indicated in the prophylactic treatment of such benign and asymptomatic nodules. That is why all I do when I see a new patient with a thyroid nodule is a test of thyroid function and a needle biopsy.

Experience with Needle Aspiration

I was misquoted by the authors when they said I reported, " . . . 46 of 50 cystic nodules were cured by aspiration." The figure was 36 which is much closer to their own. The remaining patients had small residual nodules that gave us no further trouble. In three, larger nodules persisted, were removed, and proved to be benign.

Since 1966, when the above report was made, we have employed needle biopsy routinely in the diagnosis of all thyroid nodules. This, of course, enables us to biopsy any mass remaining after aspiration of the cyst and removes the fear that it could be malignant.

I would like to emphasize the occasional finding of a parathyroid cyst. The authors describe the contents as being clear or opalescent grayish. The only ones that I have recognized have contained absolutely clear waterlike fluid. No thyroid cyst contains that type of fluid.

Technique of Needle Aspiration

We prefer to anesthetize the skin with a drop of local anesthetic and to use an 18-gauge needle to aspirate the cyst. Sometimes the fluid in it is too thick to aspirate through a 20-gauge needle. If one is to rely on cytology the 20-gauge needle will give a good preparation, but I prefer to obtain chunks of tissue by running an 18-gauge needle back and forth through the tissue with suction on the syringe. This is done routinely on any tissue that remains palpable after aspiration of the cyst. Both this material and the contents of the cyst are then expressed into a tiny jar of fixative and sent to the laboratory to be spun down and made into a cell block. This material is comparable to that obtained by a core biopsy but involves much less risk of hemorrhage; in fact, we have had no significant complications following more than 1000 18-gauge biopsies.

I am not certain whether, if cancer were present, examination of the fluid would always reveal malignant cells, but we do always send all the fluid to the pathologists for examination. Occasionally the pathologists will report psammoma bodies associated with fluid from a carcinoma or abnormal cells suspected of being malignant. For instance, I believe that if the fluid in the authors' Case 2 had been examined it might have contained cells that would have aroused suspicion.

Origin of Thyroid Cysts

Finally, I believe that most if not all cysts of the thyroid arise in adenomas or carcinomas. I also believe that feeding suppressive doses of thyroid hormone prevents the growth of most adenomas and well-differentiated carcinomas. For this reason I like to give suppressive doses of thyroid hormone as a lifetime program for all patients who have had thyroid cysts. If this is done it is extremely rare that there is any growth of the nodule in which the cyst arose. Unfortunately, I have no controlled statistics on which to base this opinion, but I know from my experience and from that of Schneider et al.[38] that after lobectomy for papillary cancer, the appearance of new cancers in the contralateral lobe is prevented by thyroid feeding. I believe, therefore, that whenever there are nodules of the thyroid, benign or malignant, the patient will do better if given thyroid hormone.

Conclusion

In conclusion, I agree that the risk of fatal cancer in thyroid cysts has been overestimated, and that cysts, even if they have a malignant component, are apt to be as harmless as other occult cancers of the thyroid.

COMMENTARY

Sten Nørby Rasmussen, M.D.
and Flemming Jensen, M.D.

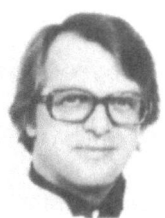 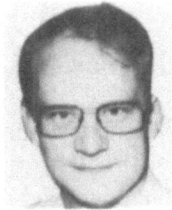

A considerable number of persons sooner or later during their life develop a nodule of the thyroid gland. It is necessary to have some method to select those who will benefit from an operation and those for whom surgery is likely to be superfluous.

Besides clinical examination, which may be fallacious even when performed by

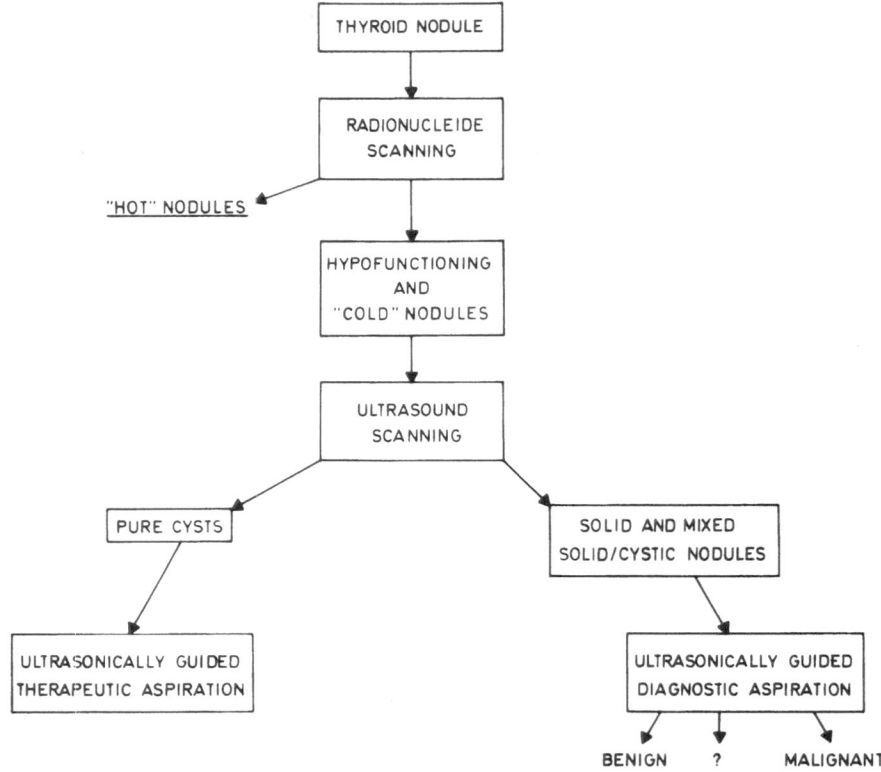

Figure 8-7. Flow chart demonstrating diagnostic and therapeutic approach to solitary thyroid nodules.

experienced examiners, nuclear medicine procedures play an important role. Ultrasonic examination of the thyroid gland and fine needle aspiration of possible malignancies, guided by ultrasound, have become controversial. Our approach to diagnosis and treatment of the thyroid nodule is shown in Figure 8-7, and corresponds to that of Gobien.[39]

Diagnosis of the Thyroid Nodule

Patients who present solitary thyroid nodules are examined by radionuclide scintiscan. "Hot" nodules are not regarded as suspicious of malignancy. Most of the remaining nodules are hypofunctioning or "cold," and they are examined by ultrasound. So are those with no abnormality visualized on the scintiscan. We presuppose that the ultrasonic equipment available is modern, i.e., either contemporary static using 5-MHz short-focused transducers or dynamic linear or sector arrays using at least 5-MHz with optimal focusing at 1–2 cm. By means of such equipment high quality scans are obtained (Fig. 8-8), and high diagnostic sensitivity and specificity are possible in the differentiation of cystic from solid tissues (Fig. 8-9). Fluid-filled cavities of about 2 mm can be detected or excluded. Moreover,

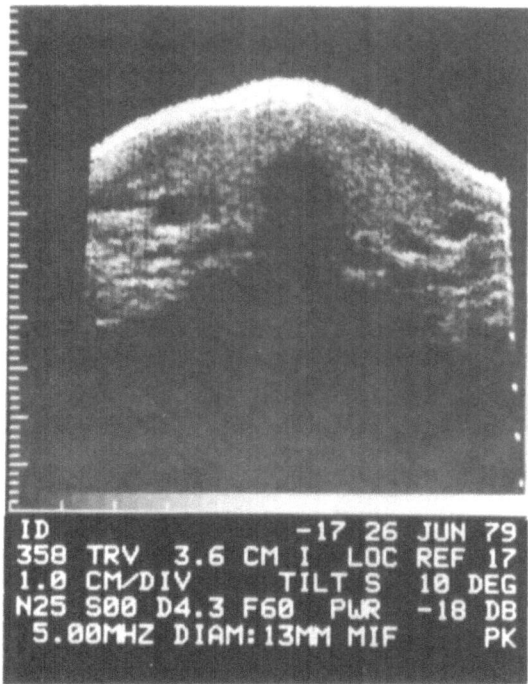

Figure 8-8. Normal transverse scan of the anterior part of the neck with the symmetric thyroid gland containing equally spaced echoes of equally moderate amplitude. The trachea and the large vessels of the neck are seen.

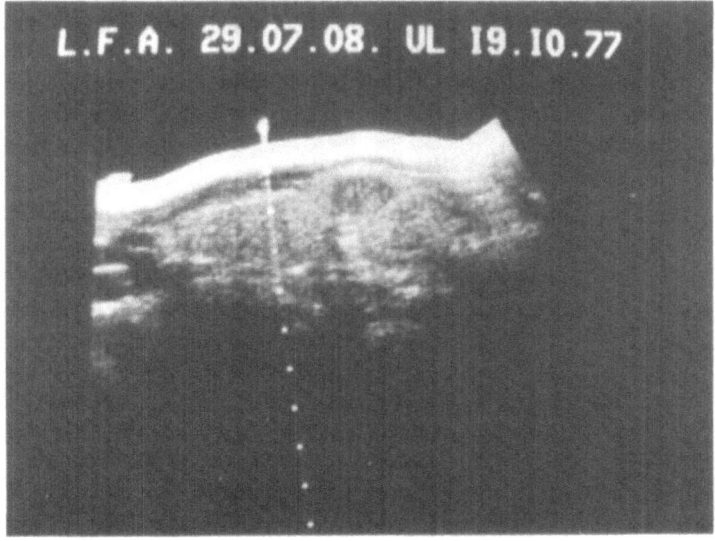

Figure 8-9. Longitudinal scan of a 1-cm, relatively echo-poor, well-circumscribed superficial solid mass—an adenoma.

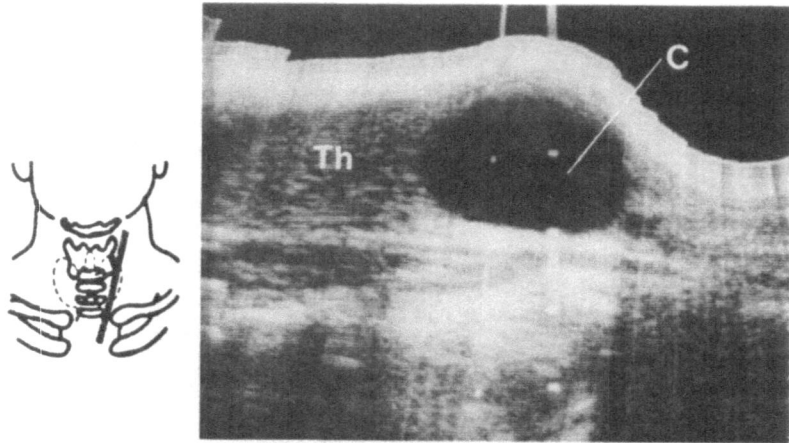

Figure 8-10. A smooth-walled pure cyst, 2 cm in diameter, in the lower part of the left lobe of the thyroid.

in larger cysts, the cyst wall can, by meticulous scanning, be examined to ensure complete smoothness or to detect small projections or irregularities (Fig. 8-10). Secondly, the cyst fluid can be evaluated to some extent, e.g., determine whether it is completely clear and echo free or whether a sediment is present. (The clinical significance of these findings is as yet unclear.) Thirdly, the structures surrounding the nodule may be evaluated, especially the thickness of the wall and its relations to the vessels of the neck. All this information is available with contemporary ultrasonic equipment. Most of the literature cited by Miller et al. relative to ultrasonic diagnostic accuracy is now outdated. Unfortunately, we have not yet seen an original recent series demonstrating the diagnostic precision of high-quality thyroid ultrasonic scanning.

Aspiration of Thyroid Cysts

Based on the ultrasonic examination all nodules are subjected to puncture. An attempt is made to aspirate completely the fluid from pure cysts. This is based on an estimation of the contained volume of fluid. Provided the aspirated volume is equal to the estimated volume, the cyst diagnosis is confirmed. Moreover, repeat ultrasonic scanning of the area should support this impression. Even though the purely cystic lesion is not regarded as suspicious of malignancy, the aspirated fluid is sent for cytologic examination. If the cyst recurs within days or weeks aspiration is repeated up to 5 or 6 times before surgery is considered. Bloody content in the fluid is not an *omen malum* as with other situations, e.g., kidney cysts. When solid or mixed solid-cystic nodules are detected (Figs. 8-11–8-15) fine needle aspiration for cytologic examination is also carried out. Assistance in obtaining representative aspirates is provided by ultrasonic guidance of the needle. Three or more

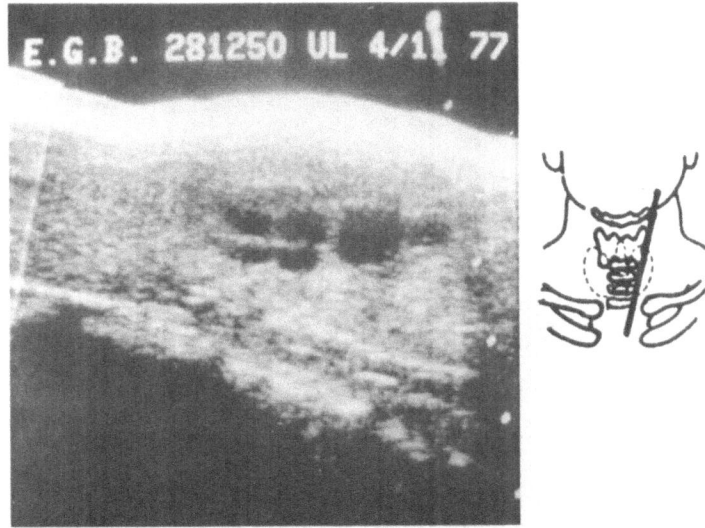

Figure 8-11. An adenoma containing several tiny cystic cavities.

aspirates are taken from different parts of the nodule, including solid as well as cystic areas, and from its center as well as the periphery. We do not find palpation satisfactory to guide the direction and depth of insertion of the needle tip. Without ultrasonic guidance the examiner may hesitate to penetrate deeply, for fear of damaging vessels or other vital structures. Also, he will not be able to obtain

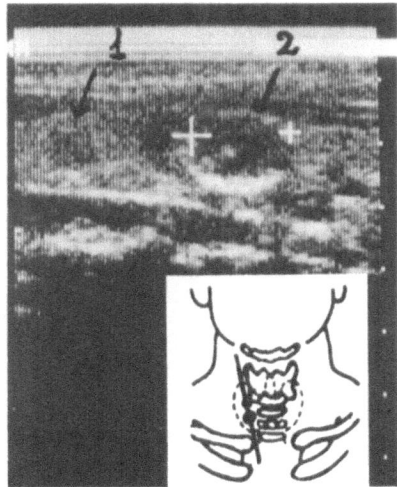

Figure 8-12. A small adenoma (*1*) and the remainder of a spontaneously collapsed cyst (*2*).

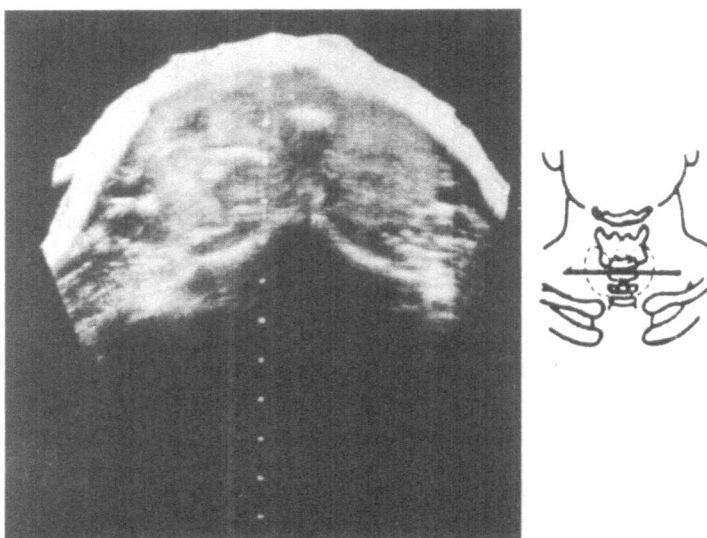

Figure 8-13. Multinodular goiter. The image is nonspecific and may be seen in patients with multiple adenomas, chronic thyroiditis, or cancer. Representative fine needle specimens will elucidate the nature of such a lesion.

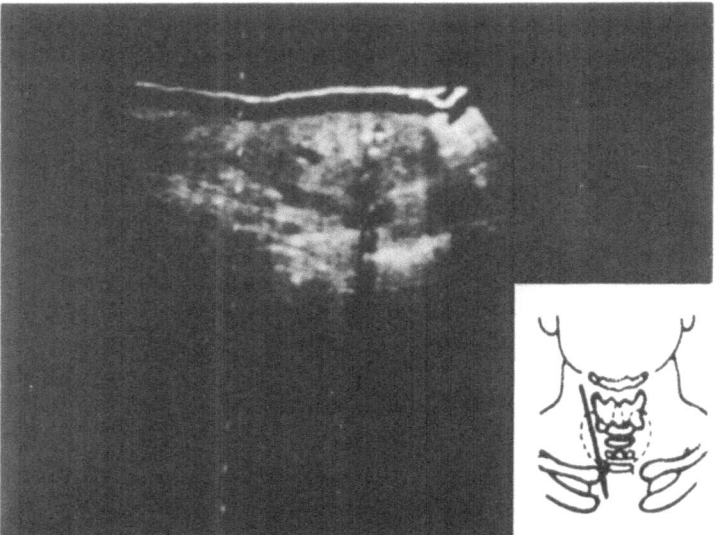

Figure 8-14. Scan from a patient with Hashimoto's thyroiditis. Three distinct deposits of calcification with acoustic shadows are seen. This sign also is nonspecific and demands fine needle aspiration. Cytologic examination revealed Askanazy cells, macrophage infiltration, and clusters of lymphocytes.

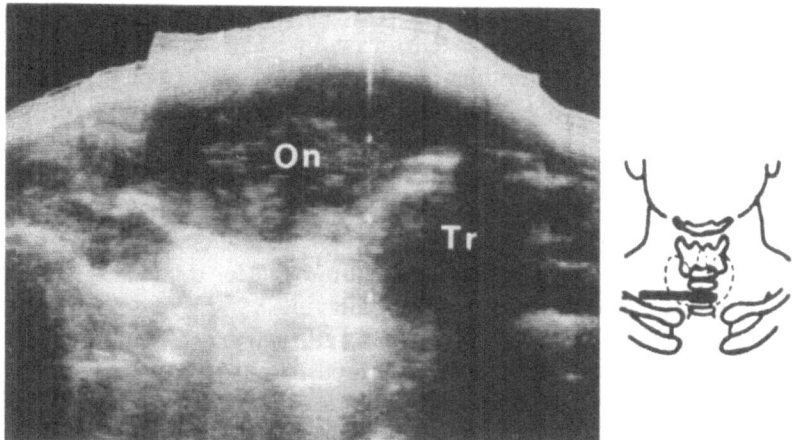

Figure 8-15. Thyroid cancer. Fast growing, solid, nonhomogeneous, rather echo-poor mass with ill-defined borders. Fine needle aspiration contained malignant cells, and final histologic diagnosis confirmed an oncocytoma with focal malignancy. *Tr,* trachea.

aspirates from different parts of the nodule representing different types of tissues, e.g., small necrotic cystic portions in a cancer.

The aspirates should be examined by an experienced pathologist. If there is suspicion of malignancy or the detection of much necrotic material the puncture should be repeated. The patient should also be followed by examination. If the mass enlarges, puncture is repeated.

In conclusion, we find that ultrasonic examination of the thyroid nodule deserves much more attention than given by Miller et al. Ultrasound is valuable in the diagnostic evaluation as well as in the guidance of the needle puncture, whether this be used to empty a pure cyst or to obtain cytologic specimens from a solid or mixed solid-cystic lesion.

SUMMARY—CHAPTER 8

Consideration of the evidence presented by myself and my colleagues as well as the discussants gives the reader a definite affirmative to the question "Is aspiration therapy a reasonable approach to the management of cystic thyroid nodules?"

Although there is general agreement on the question of the value of aspiration therapy, another question requires our attention: "Why is this conclusion not universally accepted and this therapeutic approach routinely used?" Aspiration permits the diagnosis of a thyroid cyst to be made easily and inexpensively. At the same time aspiration provides simple and effective treatment in probably over half the cases. If the cyst disappearance is incomplete and removal is recommended, neither the delay nor the needling has been documented to be of serious consequence. Even the theoretically possible untoward results (as yet unreported) from leaving behind a small undestroyed residual of a differentiated cancer do not vitiate the overall satisfactory results of this form of treatment.

With reference to the use of echography, Drs. Rasmussen and Jensen are quite correct in stating that our observations are based on outdated technology. Although we were pioneers in the use of ultrasound for thyroid evaluation in the Detroit area, we have not ordered such studies in 4 years. We certainly agree that it would at times be helpful to view the exact position of the needle when doing an aspiration or biopsy. (This would be especially true when using a 14-gauge cutting needle.) We feel, however, that ultrasonic guidance would add considerably to the complexity and expense of a procedure that has given us quite satisfactory results as currently performed. Perhaps a limited indication for ultrasonic localization of the biopsy needle would be for the partially degenerated nodule from which previous biopsy attempts produced insufficient cellular material and surgery was contemplated. The needle could possibly be directed to an area of nonnecrotic tissue.

Twenty years ago I was distressed by seeing a cystic thyroid nodule on the surgical pathology table. Eighteen years ago I told a lady, "By taking out your cystic nodule, we will gain experience that will some day make it unnecessary for doctors to operate on similar patients."

That day is here and the patient subjected to surgical lobectomy for an almost totally cystic nodule would have a serious grievance against the responsible physicians unless the therapeutic alternatives had been carefully presented.

J. Martin Miller, M.D.

REFERENCES

1. Miller JM: Carcinoma and thyroid nodules: the problem in an endemic goiter area. N Engl J Med 252:247, 1955
2. Crile G Jr: Treatment of thyroid cysts by aspiration. 59:210, 1966
3. Miller JM, uz Zafar S, Karo JJ: The cystic thyroid nodule. Radiology 110:257, 1974
4. Rosen IB, Walfish PG, Miskin M: The use of B mode ultrasonography in changing indications for thyroid operations. Surgery 139:193, 1974
5. Jensen F, Rasmussen SN: The treatment of thyroid cysts by ultrasonically guided fine needle aspiration. Acta Chir Scand 142:209, 1976
6. Clark OH, Okerlund MD, Cavalieri RR, Greenspan FS: Diagnosis and treatment of thyroid, parathyroid, and thyroglossal duct cysts. J Clin Endocrinol Metab 48:983, 1979
7. Miller JM, Hamburger JI: The thyroid scintigram. I. The hot nodule. Radiology 84:66, 1965

8. Rasmussen SN, Christiansen NJB, Jorgensen JS, Holm HH: Differentiation between cystic and solid thyroid nodules by ultrasonic examination. Acta Chir Scand 137:331, 1971
9. Miskin M, Rosen IB, Walfish PG: Ultrasonography of the thyroid gland. Radiol Clin North Am 13:479, 1975
10. Damascelli B, Cascinelli N, Livraghi T, Veronesi U: Preoperative approach to thyroid tumours by a two-dimensional pulsed echo technique. Ultrasonics 6:242, 1968
11. Thijs LG, Wiener JD: Ultrasonic examination of the thyroid gland. Am J Med 60:96, 1976
12. Fujimoto AO, Omoto R, Hirose M: Ultrasound scanning of the thyroid gland as a new diagnostic approach. Ultrasonics 5:177, 1967
13. Blum M, Weiss B, Hernberg J: Evaluation of thyroid nodules by A-mode echography. Radiology 101:651, 1971
14. Hamburger JI, Miller JM, Kini S: Clinical-Pathological Evaluation of Thyroid Nodules. Handbook and Atlas. Private Publication, Southfield, 1979, pp 7–9
15. Mustard RA: Discussion of Walfish PG, Hazani E, Strawbridge HTG, Miskin M, Rosen IB: A prospective study of combined ultrasonography and needle aspiration biopsy in the assessment of the hypofunctioning thyroid nodule. Surgery 82:474, 1977
16. Blum M, Goldman AB, Herskovic A, Hernberg J: Clinical applications of thyroid echography. N Engl J Med 287:1164, 1972
17. Stoffer SS, Szpunar WE, Hawker CD: Differentiation of thyroid from parathyroid cysts. JAMA 243:1422, 1980
18. Miller JM, Horn RC, Block MA: The autonomous functioning thyroid nodule in the evaluation of nodular goiter. J Clin Endocrinol Metab 27:1264, 1967
19. Greenspan FS: Thyroid nodules and thyroid cancer. West J Med 121:359, 1974
20. Walfish PG, Hazani E, Strawbridge HTG, Miskin M, Rosen IB: A prospective study of combined ultrasonography and needle aspiration biopsy in the assessment of the hypofunctioning thyroid nodule. Surgery 82:474, 1977
21. Boehme CJ, Winship T, Lindsay S, Kypridakis E: An evaluation of needle biopsy of the thyroid gland. Surg Gynecol Obstet 119:831, 1964
22. Clark OH: Thyroid nodules and thyroid cancer: surgical aspects. West J Med 133:1, 1980
23. Clark OH, Greenspan FS, Coggs GC, Goldman L: Evaluation of solitary thyroid nodules by echography and thermography. Am J Surg 130:206, 1975
24. Miller JM, Zafar SU: The cystic thyroid nodule: recognition and management. Program of the 48th Meeting of the American Thyroid Association, Chicago, September 20–23, 1972, p 70
25. Miskin M, Rosen IB, Walfish RG: B-mode ultrasonography in assessment of thyroid gland lesions. Ann Intern Med 79:505, 1973
26. Crockford PM, Bain GO: Fine needle biopsy of the thyroid. Can Med Assoc J 110:1029, 1974
27. Clark OH, Demling R: Management of thyroid nodules in the elderly. Am J Surg 132:615, 1976
28. Hamburger JI: Thyroid nodules and ultrasound. Ann Intern Med 80:112, 1974
29. Witt TR, Meng RL, Economou SG, Southwick HW: The approach to the irradiated thyroid. Surg Clin North Am 59:45, 1979
30. Clark OH: Nodules in irradiated thyroids. N Engl J Med 302:1150, 1980

31. Crile G Jr, Esselstyn CB Jr, Hawk WA: Needle biopsy in the diagnosis of thyroid nodules appearing after radiation. N Engl J Med 301:997, 1979

32. Hubert JP, Kiernan PD, Beahrs OH, McConachey WM, Woolner LB: Occult papillary carcinoma of the thyroid. Arch Surg 115:394, 1980

33. Rodolfo RV, Waisman J, VanHerle AJ: Cystic papillary carcinoma of the thyroid gland. Diagnosis by needle aspirations with transmission electron microscopy. Acta Cytol 22:38, 1978

34. Clark OH: Parathyroid cysts. Am J Surg 135:395, 1978

35. Reiner M, Beck AR, Rybak B: Cervical thymic cysts in children. Am J Surg 139:704, 1980

36. Bruns P: Beobachtungen und Untersuchungen uber die schilddrusen be handlung des Kropfes. Beitr Klin Chirurg 16:521, 1896

37. Clark OH: TSH suppression in the management of thyroid nodules and thyroid cancer. World J Surg (in press)

38. Schneider AB, Stachura ME, Arnold J, et al.: Incidence prevalence and characteristics of radiation-induced thyroid tumors. Am J Med 64:243, 1978

39. Gobien RP: Aspiration biopsy of the solitary thyroid nodule. Radiol Clin North Am 17:543, 1979

Chapter 9

Do All Nodules Appearing in Patients Subsequent to Radiation Therapy to the Head and Neck Areas Require Excision?

Joel I. Hamburger, M.D.
J. Martin Miller, M.D.
Michael Garcia, M.D.

INTRODUCTION

Since the 1950 report of Duffy and Fitzgerald[1] there has been increasing awareness that radiation therapy to the upper body administered to infants, children, and even young adults may induce carcinoma of the thyroid 10 to 30 years later. Between 1950 and 1975 numerous publications provided support for this concept. It was generally appreciated that these malignancies were usually papillary carcinomas, easily cured surgically.

As long as reports were confined to the medical literature their implications were kept in proper perspective. Patients with thyroid nodules were asked if they had received prior radiation therapy, and if so this information was included as part of the total assessment of cancer probability.

In 1975 prior radiation therapy as a cause of thyroid cancer received extensive attention in the lay media, including newspapers and television. A "Marcus Welby, M.D." television drama depicted a young and beautiful female professional tennis player with a "time bomb" in her neck threatening her career and her life as well. Fortunately Dr. Welby saved her, just in the nick of time. As a consequence of this and other media events the lay public demanded action in the form of recall and public information programs. The medical profession by and large was bewildered. Endocrinologists had been aware of the problem for 25 years, but could see no reason for hysteria. After all, hardly anyone could recall a death from a radiation-related thyroid cancer. Many endocrinologists were more concerned that inappropriate surgical treatment for irradiated patients might lead to greater mortality and morbidity than the disease itself, if allowed to pursue its natural course. Nonendocrinologists were deluged with calls from anxious patients, some of whom had indeed received radiation therapy, but others only had ultraviolet treatments, diagnostic x-ray procedures, and who knows what else. The fires were kept fueled by a spate of public announcements by physicians, many of whom were not entirely disinterested in the issue. The flood of consultations was good for business, especially for nuclear medicine physicians whose imaging devices worked overtime. For academic physicians this was a marvelous opportunity for epidemiologic studies. Some physicians seemed passionately convinced that they were saving sizable numbers of lives.

Frankly we were not impressed; and nothing has happened since 1975 to change our opinion that the issue of radiation-related thyroid cancer has been a vastly overemphasized nonproblem.

In the first 1000 patients we screened we found 20 (2%) thyroid cancers. Details for the first 800 patients were published.[2] Most of the cancers were the same small papillary carcinomas which we were detecting in nonirradiated patients. In 19 years about 500 patients with papillary carcinoma have been seen at Northland Thyroid Laboratory, and 11% gave histories of prior radiation therapy. None have died from these cancers. Some patients with papillary carcinoma do die, but not many. Those who do are usually older patients who may well have biologically more aggressive lesions which, when first seen, are already large, invasive, and not readily curable tumors. For most patients with papillary or follicular carcinoma, surgery followed by radioiodine therapy, when indicated, and thyroid hormone cure the patient. This is true for younger patients even with extensive regional metastases. Surely there is no evidence that removal of these thyroid cancers when they are smaller than 1.5 cm (the size at which they become easily detectable by physical examination) reduces morbidity or mortality. For these reasons we have argued against the need for widespread screening programs of irradiated patients, and also against routine imaging of those who have a history of radiation therapy to detect "impalpable" nodules.

Similarly we have not advocated removal of all thyroid nodules in such patients. Most of these nodules are benign. We are unimpressed with the argument that the presence of a nodule, even though benign, may indicate an increased probability of an occult cancer elsewhere in the thyroid gland. We have already emphasized the unimportance of early diagnosis of occult thyroid cancer. Occult cancer may be found in 13% of thyroid glands carefully studied at autopsy.[3] Another report showed no deaths from thyroid cancer in 137 patients with occult papillary carcinomas after an average follow-up of 25.3 years.[4] Attempting to remove all occult thyroid cancers would present staggering logistic problems and doubtless cause more deaths than would be prevented. Nevertheless, a discussion by physicians with different points of view of the issues relating to thyroid nodules in irradiated patients should be useful. These issues include the following:

(1) Is a history of radiation therapy alone enough to indicate the necessity for surgical intervention whenever a thyroid nodule is discovered?

(2) If needle biopsy indicates that the nodule is benign, is operation still indicated?

(3) If the lesion is an autonomously functioning nodule (AFTN), or a cyst which disappears after needle aspiration, is operation still necessary?

To provide data which might be of assistance in a resolution of these issues we have reviewed our experience with thyroid nodules during the past 4 years in which we have been actively pursuing a program of routine needle biopsy to provide cytohistologic data to assist in the selection of nodules for operation.[5] Findings for patients with histories of radiation therapy will be compared with those for patients who were not irradiated.

EXPERIENCE OF NORTHLAND THYROID LABORATORY

Table 9-1 lists the number of nonirradiated and irradiated patients studied, those operated upon, and the percentage of malignancy. Although more irradiated patients had thyroidectomy, fewer nodules were malignant. More irradiated patients were operated upon precisely because of histories of radiation therapy. This was an important consideration in the decision to operate, as is illustrated by Case 1.

CASE 1: NEEDLE BIOPSY OF A "COLD" NODULE IN AN IRRADIATED PATIENT

A 42-year-old woman was referred for consultation for a hard 1.5-cm nodule in the left thyroid lobe. She had received radiation therapy to the tonsils and adenoids at age 10 years. The patient was euthyroid. Antithyroid antibodies were negative. Thyroid imaging showed a "cold" nodule. A fine needle biopsy specimen was benign. She was treated with levothyroxine for 6 months with no change in the nodule. A repeat needle biopsy specimen was benign. Because the nodule was hard and discrete and with the history of radiation therapy, the nodule was excised. It was a benign follicular adenoma. No malignancy was found although near-total thyroidectomy was performed.

Eleven irradiated patients with benign biopsies were operated upon. All 11 had benign disease. Of the 106 irradiated patients not operated upon, benign biopsy findings were obtained in 64.

Table 9-1. Number of nonirradiated and irradiated patients operated upon, and the number of malignancies detected.

	Nonirradiated	Irradiated
Number of nodules	1548	176
Number operated upon (%)	390 (25.2)	70 (39.8)
Number of malignancies (%)	146 (37.4)	19 (27.1)

Table 9-2. Age–sex distribution of irradiated and nonirradiated patients having surgery.

Age (years)	Nonirradiated patients		Irradiated patients	
	Males	Females	Males	Females
<20	2	21	1	3
20–29	8	61	7	9
30–39	14	69	7	16
40–49	15	63	6	5
50–59	21	63	6	7
60–69	8	27	0	2
70+	4	14	0	1
Total	72	318	27	43

Biopsies showed Hürthle cell tumors or cellular adenomas in 10 irradiated patients. Three patients refused operation. One nodule regressed on treatment with thyroid hormone. Another patient, in her 70s, had multiple myeloma, and hence was observed. Also observed were five patients with illnesses increasing the operative risk.

In spite of malignant biopsy findings operation was refused by one patient, and not advised for a second (because of inoperable pelvic malignancy).

The final 30 irradiated patients not operated upon had unsatisfactory biopsy specimens. One nodule disappeared on thyroid hormone. Three patients refused operation. Twenty-six patients were observed because the nodules were clinically not suspicious. There were ten additional patients with unsatisfactory biopsy specimens with clinically suspicious nodules which were excised. They are included in the 70 patients for whom surgical diagnoses are given.

Table 9-2 gives the age and sex distribution of the irradiated and nonirradiated patients who were operated upon.

Sex Distribution

The female to male ratio for the irradiated patients is only 1.6:1, compared to the more usual (for thyroid patients) ratio of 4.4:1 for nonirradiated patients. It is widely held that nodules in men are more often malignant than in women. This was so for the nonirradiated population for whom 31 (43.1%) of 72 males had malignant nodules, whereas 115 (36.2%) of 318 females had malignant nodules. Therefore, the inclusion of more males in the irradiated group having operation should have, if anything, increased the detection of malignancies. However, there were six (22.2%) malignancies in 27 irradiated men, whereas there were 13 (30.2%) malignancies in 43 irradiated women. Five of the ten operations performed in spite of benign biopsies were in men.

Age Distribution

Of irradiated patients 99 (56.3%) were less than 40 years old, and of those operated upon 43 (61.4%) were in this younger age group; compared to 175 (44.9%) of the nonirradiated group. Therefore part of the increased percentage of malignancy in the nonirradiated patients may be attributed to older age. This conclusion is strengthened by the finding that in irradiated patients 52.6% of the malignancies were in patients less than 40 years old, compared to 40.4% for the nonirradiated individuals.

Types of Malignancies Found

Table 9-3 gives the distribution of the types of malignancies in the two groups.

Table 9-3. Types of malignancies in nonirradiated and irradiated patients.

Type of malignancy	Nonirradiated	Irradiated
Papillary carcinoma	93	15
Follicular carcinoma	25	2
Hürthle cell tumor	2	0
Anaplastic carcinoma	5	0
Medullary carcinoma	5	1
Lymphoma	13	1
Metastatic carcinoma to the thyroid	3	0
Total	146	19

In the nonirradiated group there were 13 lymphomas, five anaplastic carcinomas, five medullary carcinomas, three metastatic carcinomas to the thyroid, and two Hürthle cell carcinomas. If only papillary and follicular carcinomas are considered, then the proportion of malignancies in the nonirradiated group becomes 118 (32.6%) of 362, and for the irradiated group 17 (25%) of 68.

Autonomously Functioning Nodules

Review of autonomously functioning thyroid nodule (AFTN) patients revealed that 20 (5.5%) of 361 gave a history of radiation therapy. Three patients with toxic AFTN were treated with ^{131}I. Two patients had thyroid cancers elsewhere in the gland, and were treated surgically. Two patients were operated upon only because of the history of radiation therapy. Both nodules were benign. The remaining 13 nodules have been observed, two for 13 years, one for 5 years, and six for 1 to 2 years. Case 2 is illustrative.

CASE 2: NONTOXIC AFTN IN AN IRRADIATED PATIENT

A 24-year-old euthyroid woman had a 1.5-cm nodule in the right thyroid lobe. There was a history of radiation therapy to the thymus at birth. Imaging studies confirmed an autonomously functioning nodule.

In the succeeding 13 years the nodule gradually doubled in size. The patient remained euthyroid, although no increase in the serum TSH(RIA) level was observed after intravenous TRH. Ultrasound evaluation showed partial cystic degeneration. The patient is a medical secretary at a local hospital. House officers, upon learning that she had received thymus radiation, repeatedly express shock that this nodule has not been removed.

Four patients have not returned for follow-up. Forty-nine additional AFTN in patients without histories of radiation therapy have been removed. All were benign. One patient did, however, have an 0.5-cm occult sclerosing papillary carcinoma within a 3.5-cm toxic AFTN.

Cystic Nodules

Seven of 153 patients with cystic nodules had received radiation therapy. Three patients had the cysts eliminated by aspiration. One patient had recurrent bloody fluid aspirated. The nodule was excised and was a benign Hürthle cell tumor. Two additional patients were advised to have operation because of poor responses to aspiration, but refused. One patient was lost to follow-up. Of six carcinomas in cystic lesions at Northland Thyroid Laboratory, none had a history of radiation therapy.

DISCUSSION

Does the Risk of Occult Cancer Justify Operation for All Nodules?

Should all nodules which are detected in patients who have received prior radiation therapy to the neck be removed surgically? Those who answer in the affirmative claim that the nodules are often malignant, and if not there may be occult malignancy elsewhere in the gland. Those who respond negatively observe that most nodules are benign, even in irradiated patients, and even in the reports of those enthusiastically in favor of operation.[6] Also, occult thyroid cancer, i.e., the lesion which is impalpable by an experienced clinician, has a negligible risk of future morbidity or mortality.[7] There is no evidence that delay in diagnosis of occult lesions until they become palpable adversely affects the prognosis. Indeed, even those who have followed sizable numbers of patients with larger cancers for which diagnosis was delayed have reported a mortality rate of less than 1%.[4,8]

Does a High Mortality Rate Justify Operation for All Nodules?

In spite of a massive effort by the Michael Reese group[6] in recalling irradiated patients, and the discovery of many cancers, these workers found only one patient who died of a radiation-related cancer, and that was in 1969, long before their studies began. Since those authors were so diligent in their search for a cancer death, it seems they should have mentioned the operative death which occurred in the Chicago area since the irradiation recall programs began. Although they and others operate on patients with impalpable "nodules" detected by thyroid imaging they do not say how many times they "went to the well" on this basis and "came up dry." If they have not, others have, as was reported at the Chicago conference.[9] They might also have surveyed the area-wide operative mortality for thyroidectomy and compared it to the mortality for potentially curable thyroid cancers. After all, the widely disseminated information indicating the high risk of cancer in nodules in irradiated patients has had an impact not only on practices at large teaching centers where the most experienced physicians and surgeons are found, but throughout all of the medical care facilities in this country and abroad. We, and others, have been concerned that this might lead to a "cure" far worse than the disease.

Our concern long antedates the recent radiation hysteria. For many years we have believed that the greater risk to the public health relative to the thyroid nodule was not thyroid cancer, but rather the many unnecessary operations performed only for the removal of benign nodules. This concern may be placed in proper perspective if it is appreciated that it is meant to be applied to operations for nodules which are not obviously malignant. If the obviously malignant lesions are deleted from consideration the percentage of malignancy in most surgical series would drop considerably from the usual 10–20% figures. The figure was 3% in one large community hospital in the Detroit area.

Usefulness of Needle Biopsy

In the past few years there has been a revival of interest in needle biopsy techniques which permit accurate diagnosis for most thyroid nodules. Needle biopsy is now available in most major medical centers. We reported previously that needle biopsy reduces the number of unnecessary thyroidectomies for benign disease by 75%.[10] The data in this report show that a history of radiation therapy does not alter the validity of needle biopsy findings. These data support published opinions that a nodule in an irradiated patient can be investigated just "as it would be in any patient,"[11,12] the opinions of others[13,14] to the contrary notwithstanding.

Nodules in Irradiated Patients May Be More Common, but Are Not More Often Malignant, than in Nonirradiated Patients

We wish to emphasize that we do not maintain, as some have suggested,[15] that there is no increase in thyroid nodules in irradiated patients. We believe that there is such an increase. However, we suggest that there has been an overemphasis on the probability of cancer in these nodules, ignoring the fact that benign nodules not only occur, but are much more common.[16–22] Our data indicate that even though thyroid nodules may be more common in irradiated patients, any given nodule has no greater probability of being malignant than a nodule in a nonirradiated person. Hence we agree with Utiger[12] that the mere detection of a nodule need not mean cancer, but only the need for the same investigation appropriate for a nodule in any other patient.

Management of Nodules in Irradiated Patients

Currently the key diagnostic study is needle biopsy. If the nodule is too small, or so situated as to make needle biopsy impractical, or if it is impossible to obtain an adequate specimen, one may proceed to judge the malignant probabilities using the conventional criteria which have served for many years.[2,23] This approach may be necessary where needle biopsy is unavailable, and the patient is unable to travel to a location where it can be done. If observation is elected thyroid hormone should be administered, unless contraindicated, and the patient examined at 6-month intervals for the first 2 years, then annually, assuming no growth or, with luck, some regression of the nodule. Enlargement in spite of treatment with thyroid hormone (again assuming the nodule is neither an AFTN, nor has enlarged because of central hemorrhagic degeneration) suggests the need to reconsider biopsy or operation.

This attitude is conditioned by our experience that thyroid cancer patients do not seem to be dying or otherwise suffering from delayed diagnosis, whether the lesions are radiation-related or not. On the contrary our concern continues to be for the many unnecessary thyroid operations. Four of approximately 1000 patients seen in the Northland Thyroid Laboratory who subsequently underwent thyroidectomy (three on our advice, one against it) failed to survive the operation. We approach every potential surgical candidate as if he may be number 5. We believe the reports indicating that death from thyroidectomy is an inescapable reality of life,[24] probably related more to the anesthesia than the surgeons. These deaths are unpredictable and unpreventable.

Management of AFTN and Thyroid Cysts in Irradiated Patients

In 1971 we suggested that radiation therapy might predispose to the development of AFTN, just as it seems to for other benign and malignant thyroid nodules.[25] Our subsequent experience would not cause us to modify that statement. In the absence of evidence for cancer elsewhere in the thyroid we see no reason to be more concerned for cancer in these AFTN than in any other AFTN.

With respect to thyroid cysts we would say the same thing. If the lesion is eliminated by simple aspiration, and does not return on follow-up examinations, the problem is solved. If there is a solid residual or the cyst recurs after several aspirations, we would give serious consideration to needle biopsy or removal (see Chapter 7).

COMMENTARY

Robert G. Carroll, M.D.

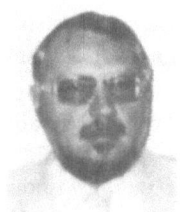

Screening Program for Irradiated Individuals

The American Medical Association and the American Hospital Association issued a joint statement on October 17, 1975, urging hospitals and physicians to work together in their communities to develop guidelines and procedures for public education and for screening of radiation-exposed individuals.[26] The joint AMA-AHA position paper sent to state medical societies carefully outlined the responsibilities of physicians and hospitals in educating the public. The AMA cover letter stated:

> Death from thyroid carcinoma is a rare occurrence. The "malignancy" of the thyroid nodules associated with radiation therapy discussed in the available studies was determined by pathologic examination, not by clinical course. Therefore, screening is a conservative measure, and the medical communities' response to possible findings also should be appropriately conservative. While surgery may be indicated in some cases, suppressive therapy or regular observation may serve other patients better. The predictable risks of mortality and morbidity from surgery should not be discounted as a community plans to respond to the possible threat of radiation-induced thyroid carcinoma.[26]

In keeping with the National AMA-AHA guidelines, the Allegheny County Medical Society in cooperation with the Hospital Council of Western Pennsylvania launched a major campaign to inform patients of the hazards of exposure to therapeutic irradiation received for benign conditions from approximately 1930 through the 1950s. The medical society endorsed participation in this project because of its public health benefit. "The profession of medicine as well as the hospitals in this community have a moral obligation to inform the public of the risk of this exposure with regard to the development of thyroid cancer. . . . The scientific data supporting this position are well founded and cannot be honestly disputed."[27] The bulletin of the county medical society carried the following recommended steps in patient management for those exposed to therapeutic radiation for benign conditions.[27]

(1) Perform a careful physical examination of the thyroid and salivary glands. Skin tumors and breast tumors must also be looked for.

(2) Patients with thyroid abnormalities on physical examination must have a thyroid imaging procedure with technetium and the gamma camera (thyroid scan).

(3) Individuals with a documented record of exposure to therapeutic amounts of radiation should have a gamma camera thyroid image.

(4) Individuals irradiated for acne with therapeutic x rays must be evaluated. The exact incidence of thyroid cancer in this group has not yet been documented; however, we believe it is significantly above that of the unexposed population.

(5) Yearly physical examination is mandatory for all individuals exposed to therapeutic radiation for all benign conditions.

(6) Thyroid gamma camera images should be performed at 5-year intervals in those with documented therapeutic radiation exposure.

Management of Irradiated Patients

These diagnostic guidelines were combined with many seminars on the appropriate management of nodular thyroid disease. There was no rush to surgery. It is a tribute to the effectiveness of this educational campaign that the overall pooled area hospital statistics revealed a 10.9% malignancy rate in thyroidectomy specimens obtained in the 17 months prior to the campaign and a 15.8% thyroid cancer rate in the specimens obtained in the 17 months after the campaign.[28] Management of patients with nodular thyroid disease who had a radiation history was substantially identical to management of patients with nodular thyroid disease without a history of radiation exposure, with the exception that multinodular thyroid disease has an appreciable incidence of thyroid cancer in irradiated patients and should be subjected to biopsy or surgical exploration in this group, whereas it might be simply watched in the nonexposed group.[29] The other difference in management deals with the obligation to carefully examine areas other than the thyroid which were within the field of radiation exposure. There is excellent evidence that therapeutic levels of ionizing radiation are carcinogenic to all tissues within the beam.[30] Thus, patients with head and neck exposure should have careful examination of the breast tissue and the salivary glands. A nodule in the thyroid of a patient should be evaluated by imaging using ^{123}I or ^{99m}Tc-pertechnetate. Nodules which do not take up radioiodine should then be evaluated by ultrasound to determine their cystic or solid nature. Solid lesions of the thyroid which do not take up radioiodine have approximately a one-third chance of being malignant.[29] If needle biopsy proves to be sensitive and specific in the separation of benign from malignant solid cold nodules, then it should be employed as a preoperative screening method. Those patients who have thyroid carcinoma diagnosed by biopsy or at operation should have a lobectomy on the affected side and a subtotal thyroidectomy on the contralateral side with great care taken to preserve parathyroid function. Postoperatively, the patient should be studied with ^{131}I while hypothyroid to determine if metastatic tissue is present in the neck or chest. Patients with metastatic lesions should be treated with ^{131}I according to the protocol of Beierwaltes.[31]

Benefit of Early Diagnosis of Papillary Thyroid Cancer

Mazzaferri et al. have convincingly demonstrated the efficacy of surgery, ^{131}I, and thyroid hormone in the management of papillary thyroid carcinoma.[8] The Allegheny County Medical Society approach was formulated after studying the work of a number of authors. Arnold et al.[32] studied 1452 patients who had x-ray therapy to the neck for benign conditions 18–35 years previously. Thyroid abnormalities were found in 21% of the examined patients. Those patients with abnormal palpation or images who had surgical exploration had a 29% carcinoma rate. Thyroid imaging detected 96% of the abnormalities, 40% of which would not have been unequivocally established by physical examination alone. Hempelmann et al.[33] surveyed 2872 young adults given x-ray treatments in infancy. The risk of cancer was proportional to the thyroid dose, with a linear risk coefficient of 2.5 thyroid cancers per year per million people exposed to 1 rad. Favus et al.[29] examined 1056 individuals who received irradiation with 200 kV x rays at a skin-source distance of 50 cm between 1939 and 1962. Clinical palpation and thyroid gamma camera pinhole images were obtained on all individuals. The ability of the examiners to detect thyroid abnormalities was significantly influenced by the scan. Palpable nodular thyroid disease was found in 16.5% of the examined population and nonpalpable lesions were detected by ^{99m}Tc thyroid imaging in an additional 10.7%, for a total prevalence of 27.2%. A careful weighing of all available literature regarding the relationship of head and neck irradiation to the subsequent development of thyroid neoplasms appeared in *Seminars in Nuclear Medicine* in October, 1976.[34]

A major issue is the mortality associated with thyroid cancer. Mazzaferri et al.[8] have clearly demonstrated that the proportion of individuals dying from this disease is significantly greater when the diagnosis is made after age 40 for males and after age 50 for females. Cady et al.[35] performed a 20-year gross mortality study for differentiated thyroid carcinoma. In men, diagnosis of differentiated carcinoma before the age of 40 is associated with a mortality rate of 5%; in the age group 40–50 years, a 16% mortality rate; and in the age group above 51, a 42% cancer mortality rate. If one looks only at papillary and mixed thyroid carcinomas, the 20-year gross mortality rate for those men and women diagnosed after age 50 is 29%.[35] The benefit of diagnosing asymptomatic disease is demonstrated by the extensive study of Mazzaferri et al.[8] which demonstrated a recurrence rate of 21% when the thyroid lesion was symptomatic (causing pain, hoarseness, or difficulty swallowing) or showed signs of rapid growth. Recurrences occurred in only 4.7% of asymptomatic patients. The recurrence rate for individuals with lesions of 2.5 cm or larger was 10.8%, in contrast with a recurrence rate of 5.8% for those individuals with primary lesions smaller than 2.5 cm. The recurrence rate of occult papillary carcinoma (i.e., a tumor smaller than 1.5 cm) was 4.7%.[8] The study of Young et al.[36] has proved a similar overview of the prognosis for pure follicular thyroid carcinoma. They found that patients who were likely to die of follicular carcinoma had distant metastatic disease at the time of initial presentation. Halan demonstrated a direct correlation between age at the time of diagnosis and mortality from thyroid cancer.[37]

Benefit of Recall Campaigns

What is the patient receiving in terms of benefit from the recall campaign? Most of the individuals who were found to have thyroid carcinoma were in their 30s.

All of the individuals who were diagnosed had entirely asymptomatic thyroid glands. There is excellent evidence in the literature that younger age and absence of symptoms at the time of diagnosis are associated with a lower mortality rate and a lower recurrence rate.[8,36,37] A follow-up study demonstrated that a minimum of 100 excess thyroid carcinomas were detected in asymptomatic individuals because of the Allegheny County Medical Society–Hospital Council of Western Pennsylvania–University Health Center of Pittsburgh Joint Recall Project.[28] The recall campaign has been responsible for the early discovery of thyroid cancers with favorable prognosis. Decreased mortality and morbidity results may be expected to follow this early diagnosis of disease.[8,36,37]

There is general agreement that the incidence of nodular thyroid disease is much higher in irradiated patients as compared with nonirradiated controls. There is also general agreement that the percentage of thyroid nodules which are found to be malignant is similar in both irradiated and nonirradiated groups. The focus of our efforts in screening radiation-exposed individuals is to locate those individuals who are at high risk for developing nodular thyroid disease. In the irradiated patient, multinodularity does not decrease suspicion of possible thyroid carcinoma. Patients with solitary thyroid nodules who have a history of irradiation should be handled in substantially the same way as patients with solitary thyroid nodules who do not have a history of radiation exposure. There is no evidence to suggest that thyroid cancer arising in irradiated thyroids behaves in a biologically different manner than thyroid cancer arising spontaneously.

COMMENTARY

Israel Doniach, M.D.

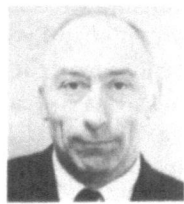

Nonsterilizing doses of ionizing radiation administered to the thyroid in infancy and childhood are carcinogenic. Prophylactic irradiation of the thymus of infants and radiation treatment of enlarged tonsils and adenoids, facial acne, and epilation of the scalp have all given rise, after a latent period of a varying number of years, to papillary carcinoma of the thyroid. Prospective and retrospective studies have shown the risk factor to lie between three and six cases per million people/year/rad administered to the thyroid gland. Thus, for example, out of 100 children receiving 500 rads to the thyroid, about five will develop thyroid carcinoma within 20 years. Against this background, it is evident that a lump in the thyroid gland in a patient with a previous history of radiation therapy to the upper body will arouse a strong suspicion of malignancy. Whether such a patient should be dealt with more radically than a nonirradiated person with a thyroid nodule has aroused considerable controversy. A further and understandable controversial problem is physician anxiety as to whether people who received thyroid irradiation in childhood should be sought out and examined regularly for the presence of a thyroid lump. This is a staggering problem in view of the enormous number of children in certain areas of the United States given external radiotherapy in the past for nonmalignant conditions of the head and neck.

Is Early Diagnosis of Radiation-Related Thyroid Cancer Essential?

In the preceding chapter, Hamburger et al. gave a succinct account of these problems and their experience with nodules in 1548 nonirradiated patients and 176 irradiated patients. After discussion of their own and others' experience, they conclude that the general problem has been vastly overemphasized and that a history of previous irradiation should make no difference to the investigation and management of a patient with a thyroid nodule. They describe the publicizing of the cancer risk in 1975 in the lay media, especially television, and the resultant mobilization of the lay public with demands for patient recall and public information programs as an induction of mass hysteria. I think that they are unjustifiably hard on the originators of the publicity who doubtless believe that catching the cancers early is in the best interests of the patients. Hamburger et al. point out that there is no evidence that the detection of thyroid cancers smaller than 1.5 cm in diameter by routine imaging, and their immediate surgical removal, leads to any improvement in morbidity or mortality. But it can be argued that future long-term follow-up of the new crop of patients so treated is required before this view is verified. However, since conventional treatment of a clinically palpable papillary carcinoma in young adults gives excellent results, it is difficult to see how earlier diagnosis could improve them. Moreover, the diagnosis of occult carcinomas might lead to unnecessary thyroidectomies for micropapillary tumors that are nonprogressive, nonaggressive, and possibly self-healing.

Are Nodules in Irradiated Patients More Often Malignant?

The alerting of the public and physicians of the cancer risk brought an influx of patients with palpable thyroid nodules to thyroid specialists. Previous irradiation produces benign as well as malignant nodules, but in far greater number are the spontaneous benign nodules that are commonplace in the population around Lake Michigan. In their own series of surgically removed nodules, Hamburger et al. found no material difference in incidence of malignancy in irradiated and nonirradiated patients. However, a greater proportion of the irradiated patients were less than 40 years old. In the irradiated patients 52.6% of the malignancies were in patients under age 40, compared to 40.4% for the nonirradiated patients. The findings do not indicate that irradiation of the thyroid is noncarcinogenic since we do not know the proportions of the total populations from which the two groups were drawn. But they do indicate the important practical point that there was no excess malignancy in the nodules selected for operative removal from irradiated patients. These negative findings might apply in general to districts where nodular goiter is common. But it is conceivable that where spontaneous nodular goiter is comparatively rare, there might be an increase in proportion of malignancy in the nodules of irradiated patients.

How Should Irradiated Patients Be Managed?

There is much controversy over the management of irradiated patients in whom thyroid nodules are detected. This is doubly difficult since there is lack of agreement as to the appropriate investigations and treatment of thyroid nodules in nonirradiated patients. Each center has its own conventional approach and treatment. These may vary considerably. But, the end results in general appear very good in the case of papillary carcinoma in patients less than age 40. Since there is as yet little or no indication that postirradiation thyroid cancers are any more aggressive than spontaneous ones, it is logical to apply the regimens already approved for the treatment of papillary cancers in nonirradiated patients. Hamburger et al. are acknowledged experts in interpretation of thyroid needle biopsy cytohistology, which they have applied effectively in the selection of patients for operation. Unfortunately, their method and the interpretation of the straight histology of thyroid needle biopsies, excellent when carried out by experts, are still far from being widely available. The same might be said of surgical thyroidectomy which in nonexpert hands still carries a definite morbidity, and even in expert hands a small mortality. The authors are rightly concerned with the occasional mortality from surgical thyroidectomy and use this among other arguments for the case against being extraradical in the approach to an irradiated patient with a thyroid nodule.

Granted acceptance of the arguments in support of a "normal" approach to an irradiated patient with a thyroid nodule, one is still left with the problem of recall of all irradiated persons. Hamburger et al. agree with others that irradiation leads to an increase in thyroid abnormalities. The necessity for recall cannot be dismissed out of hand. It is the extent of the exercise and the amount of anxiety produced in the families concerned that are so problematic, especially where spontaneous nodular goiters are common in the population. Hamburger et al. state their opinion "that the issue of radiation cancer has been a vastly overemphasized nonproblem." Since the authors accept that radiation is carcinogenic to the human thyroid it is not logical to dismiss radiation thyroid cancer as a nonproblem, although the "Marcus Welby, M.D." television drama does seem to be an example of overemphasis. Ideally, irradiated patients should be examined by a physician at regular intervals. If any abnormality is detected, the patient should seek advice from a thyroid specialist who, one hopes, will not recommend inappropriate surgical treatment.

COMMENTARY

Edwin L. Kaplan, M.D.

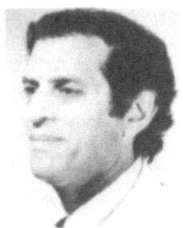

Hamburger et al. have clearly expressed their views concerning the importance, or should I say, the lack of importance, that they give a history of irradiation to the neck when evaluating a patient with a thyroid nodule. Their treatment program for thyroid nodules is based on the following assertions:

(1) Most radiation-induced cancers are papillary; they are usually small and occult, i.e., nonpalpable.

(2) Papillary cancers in the young do well no matter what treatment is elected.

(3) There is no need to search out these small lesions since no one dies of small papillary cancers.

(4) At postmortem examinations many incidental occult papillary thyroid cancers are found which did the patient no harm.

(5) Radiation results in more benign than malignant nodules.

(6) There is no increase in the incidence of thyroid cancer in nodules of irradiated patients.

(7) Needle biopsy of the thyroid is excellent in determining which thyroid lesions are benign and which are malignant, whether or not a history of radiation is documented.

The "greater risk to the public health relative to the thyroid nodule [is] not thyroid cancer," they say, "but rather the many unnecessary operations performed only for the removal of benign nodules." This is true, they feel, since in their experience four of perhaps every 1000 patients undergoing a thyroidectomy might be expected to die from this operation.

They conclude that radiation-induced thyroid cancer is a "nonproblem" which has been vastly overemphasized. This has occurred because of overdramatization of the relationship between radiation and thyroid cancer by the lay press which then led to public demand for massive screening programs. This hysteria was fanned by physicians who benefited either financially or, as they express it, "for academic physicians this was a marvelous opportunity for epidemiologic studies." Thus, they feel that a history of low-dose radiation should not change one's general way of treating a thyroid nodule.

The authors' views differ markedly from our opinions and from those of most investigators who have studied this problem. Our interest in radiation-induced thyroid cancer at the University of Chicago Medical Center began soon after the original description of this relationship by Duffy and Fitzgerald in 1950.[1] By 1955, Clark[38] reported that each of 15 children with thyroid cancer whom he operated upon had a previous history of low-dose radiation therapy to the head and neck. Since then, others from this institution have studied this problem and have made significant contributions toward an understanding of this disease state.[39–44] A recent culmination of these efforts has been the conference on radiation-associated thyroid carcinoma held at the University of Chicago in 1976.

The Basis for Our Attitude Toward Nodules in Irradiated Patients

Before answering whether all thyroid nodules appearing in patients subsequent to radiation therapy require excision we would like to develop the data which have led to our present mode of therapy. First of all, we have demonstrated that a history of low-dose radiation to the head and neck is very important. In 200 consecutive individuals who were examined at our institution in recent years because of a history of radiation to that area, 25% (51 persons) were found to have a palpable thyroid abnormality on physical examination.[42] Most of them had single or multiple nodules present. Other investigators have found remarkably similar results.[45] It is important to note that in our study anyone who was aware of a thyroid problem or was referred for a thyroid abnormality was excluded from consideration. Thus, these patients were unselected except for the history of irradiation. Operation was recommended for about 75% (35 of 51) of those with a palpable thyroid abnormality. Twenty-three of these 35 patients have thus far undergone operation. In nine of 23 (39%) of those operated upon, a carcinoma of the thyroid was found. Looked upon in a different way, at least 4.5% of all of the irradiated individuals whom we examined (and presumably others with the same exposure) harbored carcinoma. Other cancers will certainly be found when additional members of this group are operated upon. This is a very high prevalence of cancer of the thyroid.

To put these findings into proper perspective we have examined 74 members of our hospital community who were matched for age and sex with the irradiated group. None had a history of irradiation. Only five (7.5%) had a palpable thyroid abnormality and only one (1.4%) had a nodule. Thus, there is no question in our mind that low-dose irradiation to the thyroid gland results in a considerable increase of thyroid abnormalities.

We examined another 35 patients who were referred to us because a thyroid abnormality was suspected in a patient with a history of low-dose irradiation. Once more, operation was advised in 75% (24 of 35) of the patients. Nineteen of 24 of these individuals have been operated upon thus far, and seven of the 19 (40%) harbored cancer of the thyroid. Thus, in the total group of 35 patients, seven (20%) had cancer of the thyroid.

Is There a Greater Incidence of Thyroid Cancer in Patients Who Are Operated Upon for a Nodule and Who Have a History of Irradiation?

Hamburger et al. would have us believe that more cancers occur in the nonirradiated group; however, by their own data 9.4% (146 of 1548) of nonirradiated nodules are known to be cancerous while 10.8% (19 of 176) of the irradiated group are already known to have cancer because these were operated upon. It is interesting that 12 additional patients within their irradiated group had lesions which, on needle biopsy, were either known to be a cancer or were highly suggestive of a cancer but were not operated upon for one reason or another (Hürthle cell tumors or cellular adenomas, ten; malignancy, two). Thus, if these are included, as many as 19% of their irradiated group as a whole might have cancer and as many as 38% of the operated group might prove to have cancer. [A similar proportion of nonirradiated patients with these findings did not have operations for similar reasons.—Editor]

These findings then become very similar to those reported by others in the Midwest. At operation, a radiated thyroid gland with a single nodule or multiple nodules was found to contain cancer in 35–54% of cases.[44–47] At the University of Chicago Hospitals a nodule without a history of irradiation was found at operation to be malignant in only 12% of cases,[44] a figure which is similar to that of many other surgical series. Thus, in most surgical series the likelihood of finding a carcinoma is two to three times greater when a thyroidectomy is performed for a nodule with radiation than when no radiation exposure was present.

When it is further recognized that increases in the numbers of salivary gland tumors, basal and squamous cell skin cancers, meningiomas and malignant brain tumors,[48] parathyroid adenomas,[49] and even breast cancers[50] have been reported to occur after low-dose irradiation to these respective areas, we conclude that low-dose irradiation is a true health problem that hopefully has been largely eliminated. Unfortunately, since the latent period from exposure to disease has been shown to be up to 35 years or longer, such patients who have been irradiated will continue to be our concern for some time in the future.

Is Early Diagnosis of Thyroid Cancer Important?

The authors contend that there is no need to worry about finding thyroid cancers early since most are papillary and do the patient no harm. They draw these conclusions largely from the work of Nishiyama et al.,[3] who found occult papillary cancer as an incidental finding in the thyroid gland in 13% of autopsy examinations. However, the authors know, as well as we, that the tumors found by Nishiyama were all 8 mm or smaller in size and that in order to find them, each thyroid gland was entirely sectioned into 2- to 3-mm slices which were then subjected to multiple microscopic sections. This technique was not utilized by our pathologists or by any of the other authors whose data were cited. Furthermore, it is important that the majority of Nishiyama's patients whose thyroids were examined were elderly and many died of other cancers. A more realistic age-matched control group might well be the 137 autopsy studies of military personnel between the ages of 20 and 39 years which showed only one thyroid cancer to be present (0.7%) in this group.[51]

Will a Small Thyroid Cancer in a Young Person Remain Small and Nonaggressive throughout the Patient's Life?

Few physicians would be willing to assume that this is the case. Papillary cancer has a worse prognosis when diagnosed in individuals who are 40 to 45 years old or older. Undoubtedly, many of these cancers were present for years before.

Are Papillary Cancers Our Only Concern?

In the University of Chicago series, between 1950 and 1975, the majority of tumors were papillary; however, 14% were follicular.[52] Since then four of 16 (25%) of the more recent radiation-induced cancers were pure follicular. In another large series,[53] 29% of all radiation-induced cancers were follicular. These lesions do not have as good a prognosis as do papillary cancers. Furthermore, they are much more difficult to diagnose correctly by needle biopsy, as will be discussed below.

Are Radiation-Associated Thyroid Cancers as Aggressive as Other Thyroid Cancers?

Of additional interest is the fact that 90% of all radiation-associated cancers in our study were 0.5 cm in diameter or greater, 70% were 1 cm or greater, and 51% were 1.5 cm or greater.[52] Thus, these lesions were at least as large as others in our nonirradiated group of thyroid cancers. Virtually all of those 1 cm in diameter or greater were palpable when examined by a number of experienced physicians in our thyroid clinic. Furthermore, radiation-associated cancers are more likely to be multifocal, to present with clinically palpable lymph nodes, and to have either distant metastases or significant invasion of adjacent neck structures at the time of diagnosis than are nonirradiated cancers.[52,53] Thus, we hold that these lesions are at least as aggressive as those of similar morphology in nonirradiated patients.

Radiation-induced thyroid cancers do kill. Block[53] reported three deaths from these tumors in the Detroit area. One of our young male patients died from metastatic cancer of the thyroid, as well; several others are known to have widely metastatic disease at this time. Thus, once more we point out that radiation-induced cancers of the thyroid are important and deaths do occur from this disease.

How Are these Nodules best Detected?

Presently we feel that the most important tool for the evaluation of patients with or without a history of radiation exposure is a good physical examination. Virtually all operations have been performed because single or multiple nodules were felt by several of our experienced thyroid clinic physicians. Neither the measurement of thyroid antibodies, thyroglobulin (except in advanced cases), nor C.E.A. has been helpful in most instances. Isotopic imaging of the thyroid may be useful when a palpable abnormality is felt; but, contrary to others,[45] we have rarely if ever operated on anyone because of a scan defect in a patient without a palpable abnormality. We have used the ultrasound examination in evaluating many thyroid patients. However, in the radiated group essentially all of our nodules have been cold on scan and solid on ultrasound.

How Should Cystic and "Hot" Nodules Be Treated?

As Hamburger et al. point out, both cystic lesions and "hot" nodules are rare in the irradiated patient. Our experience with cysts in nonirradiated patients is that the nodule usually returns despite repeated aspirations. Many young individuals elect to have these cysts removed despite assurances of their benign nature. Only one of 205 isotopic scans in our irradiated patients was interpreted as being "hot." In this individual, a physician, a needle biopsy was attempted but was not conclusive. He elected to have the lesion removed and it proved to be benign. However, a small papillary carcinoma and a second benign lesion were found in other parts of his gland. We agree with Hamburger et al. on the management of these two small subgroups of patients. However, again we point out that the main problem is management of the patient with a cold, noncystic nodule.

What About the Use of Needle Biopsy of the Thyroid?

We have utilized both core needle biopsy and more recently needle aspiration biopsy with cytologic examination in selected individuals. We have been impressed by both the false negative and false positive results which we have occasionally obtained using either of these techniques. Our endocrine pathologist has been unhappy with these procedures since both sampling errors and errors of interpretation may occur. Not infrequently, especially in follicular lesions, penetration of cells beyond the capsule of the nodule is very important in the final evaluation of malignancy. This is not assessed in either of these techniques. The

Karolinska group[54] and others[55] suggest that all cellular follicular specimens should be operated upon since follicular carcinoma and adenoma cannot be differentiated by these techniques.

We have not used needle biopsies in evaluating patients with a history of radiation except in the one instance cited above. The glands of irradiated patients are more likely to be multinodular and the lesions may be small, making sampling errors more likely and the needle biopsy more hazardous. Remember that up to 25% of our most recent patients exhibited follicular cancer, and these are the most difficult to diagnose by either core biopsy or needle aspiration cytology. Finally, the fact that 40% of patients undergoing thyroidectomy will be found to have cancer has been persuasive. We know of no long-term trial which suggests that these lesions should not be treated surgically as they are found. We agree that unnecessary operations should be prevented but we do not feel that patients with nodules and a history of radiation exposure fall into this category.

What Are the Risks of Thyroidectomy?

Our approach has been influenced by the success of operation upon the thyroid at our institution and at other comparable hospitals. If patients are selected properly, thyroidectomy for a nodule should assume little more risk than the hazard of general anesthesia itself which is approximately one death per 10,000 cases. Furthermore, the morbidity should be low if an experienced neck surgeon performs the operation. In a personal series of over 100 radiation-induced lesions, neither a permanent recurrent nerve injury nor an instance of permanent hypoparathyroidism has occurred.

Weighing both sides of the issue, we and the majority of our colleagues feel that our approach of operating upon the vast majority of palpable cold nodules in individuals with a history of definite radiation exposure is appropriate. As new long-term data appear concerning the reliability and accuracy of other diagnostic techniques, we may modify this position in the future. However, at present, we feel that our approach is quite satisfactory.

Finally, I remember vividly the words of a well-known endocrinologist who recently stated that the only time he would ever operate upon a thyroid nodule was if distant spread or a serious complication such as hoarseness occurred. Thus, a discussion of the management of thyroid nodules is still very timely and certainly worthy of reappraisal.

COMMENTARY

Robert D. Utiger, M.D.

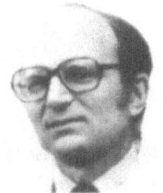

Questions concerning the significance of solitary thyroid nodules and the proper evaluation and management of patients found to have such lesions have bedeviled clinicians for years. A nodule may be a thyroid carcinoma, an adenoma, a cyst, a region of thyroiditis, an adenomatous nodule which is part of an unrecognized multinodular goiter, or rarely of nonthyroid origin, e.g., a lipoma or parathyroid adenoma. The key question is how to identify the thyroid carcinoma, since the other lesions pose little or no risk to the patient. The question has gained added importance in recent years because of the recognition that radiation of the head and neck for various benign diseases, at least when given in infancy and early childhood, is a risk factor for the development of thyroid disease in general and thyroid carcinoma in particular. The evidence that such radiation therapy is a risk factor is substantial, although most studies are not well controlled, and will not be reviewed here. The question to be addressed in this commentary is not that of frequency, but rather whether the thyroid diseases found in patients who had head and neck irradiation in infancy differ in type and/or natural history from those in patients without such exposure. This is a more general statement of the title of the immediately preceding chapter by Hamburger et al. The questions are really the following three:

(1) Is a thyroid nodule more often a carcinoma in patients who had radiation therapy?

(2) Is the type or natural history of thyroid carcinoma different in these patients?

(3) Are different methods of diagnosis and treatment required in patients with radiation-associated thyroid disease?

Is a Thyroid Nodule in a Patient Who Was Exposed to Radiation More Often a Thyroid Carcinoma?

The answer appears to be no. Thyroid carcinomas account for from 10 to 40% of the lesions found at surgery, whether or not there was a history of radiation therapy.[28,56–59] Ideally this question should be answered by studies in which patients with and without a confirmed radiation history are evaluated by the same investigators and surgery is based on the same criteria. This was done in the study of Royce et al. although that study is marred by small sample size and the facts that the subjects were largely adolescents when irradiated and the study perhaps was done too soon after irradiation.[15]

The results presented by Hamburger et al. support the same conclusion, although the history of radiation in that subgroup was not documented. Other studies, done in differing populations by different investigators, also support the conclusion that thyroid carcinoma is no more often the cause of a thyroid nodule in irradiated than in nonirradiated patients. However, some reports do not provide clear information concerning whether the carcinoma was the lesion which led to the decision to operate or whether it was a clinically unrecognized lesion found elsewhere in the thyroid. Therefore, the clinically detected lesion may be a carcinoma less often, especially in irradiated patients, since that history alone has been used as an indication for surgery. For example, in the studies of irradiated patients of Schneider et al.,[6] 26% of the patients who were operated on had carcinomas 5 mm or less in diameter and 40% were from 6 to 15 mm in diameter. Surely all of the former and many of the latter would have been clinically undetectable.

The clinically unrecognized ("occult") carcinoma should not enter into the overall question for several reasons. First, such lesions unquestionably occur in patients with otherwise entirely normal thyroid glands, although the frequency of their identification varies greatly.[60] Second, since patients who have such lesions have no reduction in survival,[61] there is no reason to believe that those whose lesions remain unrecognized in situ are at risk for the development of metastatic thyroid carcinoma.

Is the Type or Natural History of Thyroid Carcinoma Different in Those Patients Who Had Head and Neck Irradiation?

In such patients, the tumors are nearly always well-differentiated papillary or follicular carcinomas,[6,28,57] the most "benign" of the histologic types of thyroid carcinoma. These types of tumor are also most common in the nonirradiated patient; in the series of Hamburger et al. 89% of the tumors in the irradiated patients and 81% of those in the nonirradiated patients were of these types. This is probably a reflection of the younger age of the irradiated patients, since papillary and follicular carcinomas have long been known to account for nearly all thyroid carcinomas in younger patients. Regarding natural history, Roudebush et al.[62] compared the clinical course in 91 patients with radiation-associated thyroid carcinoma and 72 nonirradiated patients operated on at the same institution. All irradiated patients had papillary or follicular carcinoma; the control group was selected to have the same. Males constituted 35% of the irradiated group but only 20% of the controls; similar figures were recorded by Hamburger et al. The proportion of patients having a solitary nodule and the proportion having a nodule that was hypofunctioning on thyroid isotope scan was the same (70%) in the two groups. The overall size distribution (approximately 50% less than 1.5 cm) was also the same, although the proportion with multifocal lesions was higher in the irradiated patients. Initially, 10% of the irradiated patients and 4.2% of those not exposed had evidence of invasion of neck structures or distant disease. During follow-up, which averaged about 10 years, recurrent disease developed in 6.5% of the irradiated patients and 1.4% of the controls, even though more irradiated patients underwent total thyroidectomy and received postoperative ^{131}I therapy. These data do suggest that thyroid carcinoma in irradiated patients is somewhat more aggressive. There is no information to suggest that the histologic or functional spectrum of benign adenomas or other thyroid diseases differ in irradiated and nonirradiated patients.

Does the Patient with a History of Head or Neck Irradiation Require Special Evaluation?

If there are no palpable abnormalities, of what should evaluation consist? Information concerning the rate of enlargement, the presence of symptoms, and the palpatory characteristics of nodule(s) present allows experienced clinicians to make reasonably accurate predictions of the nature of the lesion.[56,59,63] A commonly used protocol for the evaluation of patients with a solitary nodule calls for a thyroid isotope scan, followed by ultrasonography if the lesion is hypo- or nonfunctional. The major purpose of the isotope scan is to identify those patients who have an autonomously functioning thyroid adenoma or a clinically unrecognized multinodular goiter, in whom the likelihood of thyroid carcinoma is minimal. Although virtually all thyroid carcinomas concentrate radioisotope poorly if at all, the same is true of most thyroid adenomas. Hence, such scan results alone have little diagnostic value.[64,65] Since ultrasonography allows reliable detection of cystic lesions, nearly all benign, which can often be treated effectively by aspiration (see Chapter 8), this procedure should always be done before surgery is contemplated. Other options include observation, with or without thyroid therapy, and needle or aspiration biopsy. The use of fine needle aspiration biopsy has become widespread, and appropriately so, in view of its simplicity, safety, and reliability.[58,66,67] The evidence[4] indicates this is so in those patients with a history of irradiation as well as in those patients without such a history. Measurements of serum thyroid hormone, TSH, and thyroglobulin concentrations are not helpful in identifying patients who are likely to have thyroid carcinoma whether or not they have a history of head and neck irradiation.[57,59,68] Thus, while the diagnostic efficacy of any of these procedures has not been rigorously tested simultaneously in patients both with and without a history of irradiation, there is no evidence that they are not equally applicable, or inapplicable, to both groups.

In sum, there is little or no evidence (1) that thyroid carcinoma is more often the cause of a thyroid nodule in patients with a history of head and neck irradiation; (2) that the type or natural history of thyroid carcinoma is different in such patients; or (3) that current methods of evaluation are inadequate or unreliable in such patients. It follows that the mere fact that a patient has such a history is not reason to undertake more extensive evaluation or treatment than would otherwise be indicated.

SUMMARY—CHAPTER 9

As expected the issues raised in this chapter provoked responses which highlight differences of opinion. Nevertheless, there is a remarkable degree of agreement on the major considerations upon which clinical judgments are based.

Areas of Agreement

(1) Does a history of radiation therapy to the upper body increase the chances of subsequent development of thyroid nodules or cancer? All participants agree that it does. The prevalence of cancer in these irradiated patients, whether the "at least 4.5%" indicated by Kaplan, the 2% reported by Hamburger,[2] or the 1% in a very recent publication,[69] is substantially higher than would be expected in controls.

(2) How should nodules be detected in irradiated patients? Again, all parties agree that physical examination should be the primary diagnostic method, with imaging reserved for those with palpable abnormalities.

(3) Should all irradiated patients with thyroid nodules be advised to have thyroidectomy? Here too there is agreement that operation is not always necessary. Carroll, Doniach, and Utiger state that one should deal with the irradiated-nodule patients the same as any other nodule patient. Kaplan advises operation for "the vast majority," but still not all such patients.

Areas of Disagreement

(1) Is radiation-related thyroid cancer a major public health problem? Hamburger et al. are not impressed with the urgency for mass screening programs to identify thyroid cancers as early as possible. Although these programs have led to the identification of many thyroid cancers, undoubtedly many others have not been discovered since screening programs only reach a minority of affected people. Nevertheless, there are no data suggesting an increased morbidity or mortality from these tumors. Approximately 1100 people die of thyroid cancer every year. Detroit area figures suggest that no more than 15% (165) of these will be radiation related. If even 25% of these deaths were preventable by early diagnosis (an optimistic figure as judged by my experience), the cost of the screening program necessary to perhaps save these 41 people would be prohibitive. Carroll and Doniach point out that early diagnosis is in the best interests of these people. Kaplan emphasizes that, "Radiation-induced thyroid cancers do kill," as illustrated by one of his patients and three reported by Block.[53] However, two of Block's patients had anaplastic cancer, and the third had a long-neglected papillary carcinoma

which ultimately killed her in her 70s. The question is not whether these thyroid cancers can kill, but how often. As a rule lethal thyroid cancer is very infrequent in irradiated patients (excluding anaplastic lesions which are generally incurable and mercifully very rare). Hence, concern for untoward consequences of unnecessary thyroid surgery seems reasonable. Kaplan says that thyroidectomy for a nodule *should* carry a mortality rate of only about one in 10,000 (0.01%). However, the survey of Foster[24] showed that actual results have not been that good, the mortality rate ranging from 0.02 to 2.8%, depending upon the indication and age of the patients, the highest figure for malignant lesions in patients 50 years or older. Academic physicians do not always consider that their statements influence practice habits in community hospitals where optimal results are seldom achieved.

(2) Are nodules in irradiated patients more often malignant than those in nonirradiated patients? Contrary to Kaplan's interpretation, Hamburger et al. do not "believe that more cancers occur in the nonirradiated group." A greater proportion of excised nodules in nonirradiated patients were malignant, but considering differences in age and type of malignancy in the two groups the difference in percentage malignancy was not material. Kaplan ignored these considerations when he related the number of malignancies to the total number of nodules to show that there was a slightly greater proportion of malignant nodules in irradiated (10.8%) than nonirradiated (9.4%) patients. This calculation gives inappropriate weight to many nodules in older patients which were benign by both clinical and biopsy evaluation. Carroll and Utiger agree that the likelihood of malignancy is similar in nodules whether in irradiated or nonirradiated patients; but Doniach allowed for the possibility that the findings might be different in localities where spontaneously developing nodules are less common. Nevertheless, Kaplan showed that only 12% of the nodules excised in his institution from nonirradiated patients were malignant, whereas the figure was nearly 40% for irradiated patients, a sizable differential. However, a rate of malignancy as low as 12% can only be achieved if nodule patients are operated upon almost without selection. Therefore Hamburger et al. would better have said that there is no important difference in percentage malignancy for nodules excised for the two groups, providing the operations were performed for nodules for which there were clinical or biopsy findings consistent with malignancy. When nearly all nodules are removed the vast numbers of benign degenerated nodules in older people, usually not irradiated, will introduce a bias.

(3) How dangerous are small thyroid cancers? Mazzaferri et al.[8,36] and others[70–72] showed that small papillary and follicular cancers, not already associated with distant metastases, are almost never lethal. Carroll uses these data to argue for early diagnosis and treatment. Older patients do have larger and more malignant forms of papillary and follicular carcinoma, suggesting that Kaplan is correct to argue that there is no guarantee that small lesions left in situ will remain small. Again, the issue is not whether small curable nodules ever become large and incurable, but rather how frequently and how rapidly this happens. Review of the histories of lethal differentiated carcinomas indicates that almost always death was preceded by many years of neglect, often compounded by surgical procedures

as inadequate as they were delayed. In spite of delayed diagnosis and inadequate treatment, so few differentiated thyroid cancers are ever lethal that one might infer that the lethal lesions are inherently different, and may have a poor prognosis regardless of treatment. In any event, observation does not imply the gross neglect that permits a small malignant tumor to grow to the point of incurability.

(4) Are too many irradiated patients having unnecessary thyroidectomies? Carroll does not object to a 15.8% malignancy rate in surgical specimens in his locality; i.e., 84.2% were operated upon for benign disease. Hamburger et al. advised operation for 11 patients in spite of benign needle biopsy data, primarily because of radiation histories. In Kaplan's surgical series 60+% of the patients did not have cancer. To consider this "quite satisfactory" without trying to do better suggests a level of complacency which many would find unacceptable.

(5) Can needle biopsy reduce the number of unnecessary operations in irradiated patients? Utiger thinks so. Doniach regrets that the procedures are not yet available everywhere. Carroll is still withholding judgment, pending greater experience. However, Kaplan has rejected needle biopsy for reasons deserving comment:

(a) He has had false negative results. It is improbable that false negative biopsy diagnoses can be eliminated completely, but with experience this problem can be reduced to a very low level. Not performing needle biopsy and not comparing the findings with those from surgical specimens ensures that the requisite experience will not be obtained. A false negative diagnosis is not equivalent to death. Further developments may suggest cancer while the lesion is still curable. To eliminate all false negative diagnoses means that all nodules must be removed. This has been considered unacceptable for nonirradiated patients. Even Kaplan does not recommend operation for all, although 40% of his patients had cancer. Should Carroll, who had only 15.8% malignancy, advise operation for all of his patients?

(b) Kaplan's concern for unreliable needle biopsy diagnoses in follicular tumors is based upon a conceptual misunderstanding. Many follicular cancers are easily diagnosed by needle biopsy. Those that are difficult to distinguish from benign follicular neoplasms do not present findings suggesting benign nodular goiter, but those of a cellular neoplasm. Therefore it must be appreciated that such a needle biopsy diagnosis is consistent with malignancy, and one would act accordingly. Also, only 15% of our first 1000 biopsy patients had these inconclusive findings. For the rest, from whom adequate biopsy specimens were obtained, highly accurate diagnoses of benign or malignant lesions could be made.[73]

(c) Kaplan's concern for false positive needle biopsy diagnoses seems inappropriate since he made 60% false positive diagnoses by operating upon the vast majority of nodules. It is unlikely that he could have done worse had needle biopsy data been obtained.

(d) Finally, Kaplan noted that some nodules in irradiated patients may be too small for needle biopsy. Since biopsies of some form can be done on nodules as small as 1 cm, smaller if favorably placed, this objection is applicable to very few palpable lesions. For these patients, those who fear that small malignant nodules may progress to incurability so rapidly that only immediate operation will save the patient obviously will advise surgery. Those more concerned about unnecessary surgery will advise observation.

Needle biopsy diagnoses are not perfect, but they are more reliable than any other method for preoperative diagnosis of thyroid nodules. To obtain the best possible results from needle biopsy requires considerable effort and experience. Those who will not try, cannot succeed.

J. Martin Miller, M.D.

REFERENCES

1. Duffy BJ Jr, Fitzgerald PJ: Cancer of the thyroid in children: a report of 28 cases. J Clin Endocrinol 10:1296, 1950
2. Hamburger JI, Stoffer SS: Late thyroid sequelae of radiation therapy to the upper body. In DeGroot LJ (ed): Radiation-Associated Thyroid Carcinoma. New York, Grune & Stratton, 1977, pp 17–31
3. Nishiyama RH, Ludwig GK, Thompson NW: The prevalence of small papillary thyroid carcinomas in 100 consecutive necropsies in an American population. In DeGroot LJ (ed): Radiation-Associated Thyroid Carcinoma. New York, Grune & Stratton, 1977, pp 123–135
4. Hubert JP Jr, Kiernan PD, Beahrs OH, McConahey WM, Woolner LB: Occult papillary carcinoma of the thyroid. Arch Surg 115:394, 1980
5. Hamburger JI, Miller JM, Kini SR: Clinical-Pathological Evaluation of Thyroid Nodules. Handbook and Atlas. Private publication, Southfield, 1979, pp 10–19
6. Schneider AB, Favus MJ, Stachura ME, Arnold J, Arnold MJ, Frohman LA: Incidence, prevalence, and characteristics of radiation-induced thyroid tumors. Am J Med 64:243, 1978
7. Sampson RJ, Buncher KCR, et al. Papillary carcinoma of the thyroid gland; sizes of 525 tumors found at an autopsy in Hiroshima and in Nagasaki. Cancer 25:1391, 1970
8. Mazzaferri EL, Young RL, Oertel JE, Kemmerer WT, Page CP: Papillary thyroid carcinoma: The impact of therapy in 576 patients. Medicine 56:171, 1977
9. Dobyns BM: Discussion of "Diagnostic Procedures for Possible Cancer." In DeGroot LJ (ed): Radiation-Associated Thyroid Carcinoma. New York, Grune & Stratton, 1977, p 351
10. Hamburger JI, Miller JM, Kini SR: Clinical-Pathological Evaluation of Thyroid Nodules. Handbook and Atlas. Private publication, Southfield, 1979, pp 74–86
11. Crile G Jr, Esselstyn CV Jr, Hawk WA: Needle biopsy in the diagnosis of thyroid nodules appearing after radiation. N Engl J Med 301:997, 1979
12. Utiger RD: Is external irradiation a risk factor for thyroid disease and thyroid carcinoma? JAMA 242:2702, 1979
13. Schneider AB, Favus MJ, Frohman LA: Nodules in irradiated thyroids. N Engl J Med 302:1148, 1980
14. Nodules in irradiated patients. Letters to the editor. N Engl J Med 302:1149, 1980
15. Royce PC, MacKay BR, DiSabella PM: Value of postirradiation screening for thyroid nodules. A controlled study of recalled patients. JAMA 242:2675, 1979

16. Sheline GE, Lindsay S, McCormack KR, Galante M: Thyroid nodules occurring late after treatment of thyrotoxicosis with radioiodine. J Clin Endocrinol 22:8, 1962

17. Doniach I, Eadie DGA, Hope-Stone HF: The development of multiple thyroid adenomata in primary hyperthyroidism in previously irradiated thyroid glands. Br J Surg 53:681, 1966

18. Robbins J, Rall JE, Conrad RA: Late effects of radioactive iodine in fallout. Ann Intern Med 66:1214, 1967

19. Pincus RA, Reichlin S, Hempelmann LH: Thyroid abnormalities after radiation exposure in infancy. Ann Intern Med 66:1154, 1967

20. Pifer JW, Hempelmann LH, Dodge HJ, Hodes FJ II: Neoplasms in the Ann Arbor series of thymus-irradiated children; a second survey. Ann J Roentgenol 103:13, 1968

21. Conard RA, Dobyns BM, Sutow WW: Thyroid neoplasia as late effect of exposure to radioactive iodine in fallout. JAMA 214:316, 1970

22. Janower JL, Miettinen OS: Neoplasms after childhood irradiation of the thymus gland. JAMA 215:753, 1971

23. Hamburger JI: Clinical Exercises in Internal Medicine, Vol. I. Thyroid Disease. Philadelphia, Saunders, 1978, pp 205–212

24. Foster RS Jr: Morbidity and mortality after thyroidectomy. Surg Gynecol Obstet 146:423, 1978

25. Meier DA, Hamburger JI: An autonomously functioning thyroid nodule, cancer, and prior radiation. Arch Surg 103:759, 1971

26. Sammons JR, McMahon JA: Radiation Treatment and Thyroid Cancer: Letter to State Medical Societies. A Joint Recommendation of the American Medical Association and the American Hospital Association, October 17, 1975

27. Ellis LD: Moral Obligation. Editorial. Allegheny County Med Soc 65:267, 1976

28. Schramm VL Jr, Carroll RG: Radiation-associated disease: disease incidence and cost effectiveness of followup. Laryngoscope 89:529, 1979

29. Favus JJ, Schneider AB, Stachura ME, Arnold JE, Ryo UY, Penski S, Coleman M, Arnold MJ, Frohman LA: Thyroid malignancy occurring as a consequence of head and neck irradiation: evaluation of 1056 patients. N Engl J Med 294:1019, 1976

30. Miller RW: Radiation-induced cancer. J Natl Cancer Inst 49:221, 1972

31. Beierwaltes WH: The treatment of thyroid cancer with radioactive iodine. Semin Nucl Med 8:79, 1978

32. Arnold J, Penski S, Ryo UY, Frohman L, Schneider A, Favus M, Stachura M, Arnold N, Colman M: Technetium[99m] pertechnetate thyroidscintigraphy in patients predisposed to thyroid neoplasm by prior radiotherapy to the head and neck. Radiology 115:653, 1975

33. Hempelmann LH, Hall WJ, Phillips W: Neoplasms in persons treated with x-rays in infancy: 4th survey in 20 years. J Natl Cancer Inst 55:519, 1975

34. Carroll RG: The relationship of head and neck irradiation to the subsequent development of thyroid neoplasms. Semin Nucl Med 6:411, 1976

35. Cady B, Sedgwick CE, Meissner WA, Bookwalter JR, Romagosta V, Werber J: Changing clinical, pathologic, therapeutic, and survival patterns in differentiated thyroid carcinoma. Ann Surg 184:541, 1976

36. Young RL, Mazzaferri EL, Rahe AJ, Dorfman SG: Pure follicular thyroid carcinoma: impact of therapy on 214 patients. J Nucl Med 21:733, 1980

37. Halan KE: Influence of age and sex on incidence and prognosis of thyroid carcinoma: 344 cases followed for 10 years. Cancer 19:1534, 1966

38. Clark DE: Association of irradiation with cancer of the thyroid in children. JAMA 159:1007, 1955
39. Harper PV, Paloyan D: Thyroid carcinoma associated with radiation therapy. Surg Clin North Am 49:47, 1969
40. Wilson SM, Platz C, Block GE: Thyroid carcinoma following irradiation. Arch Surg 100:330, 1970
41. DeGroot L, Paloyan E: Thyroid carcinoma and radiation, a Chicago endemic. JAMA 225:487, 1973
42. Refetoff S, Harrison J, Karanfilski BT, et al.: Continuing occurrence of thyroid carcinoma after irradiation to the neck in infancy and childhood. N Engl J Med 292:171, 1975
43. Kaplan EL, Taylor J: Recent developments in radiation-induced carcinoma of the thyroid. Surg Clin North Am 56:199, 1976
44. Kaplan EL: An operative approach to the irradiated thyroid gland with possible carcinoma: Criteria, technique, and results. In DeGroot LJ, Frohman LA, Kaplan EL, Refetoff S (eds): Radiation Associated Carcinoma of the Thyroid. New York, Grune & Stratton, 1977, pp 371–382
45. Frohman LA, Schneider AB, Favus MJ, Stachura ME, Arnold J, Arnold M: Thyroid carcinoma after head and neck irradiation: Evaluation of 1476 patients. In DeGroot LJ, Frohman LA, Kaplan EL, Refetoff S (eds): Radiation Associated Carcinoma of the Thyroid. New York, Grune & Stratton, 1977, pp 5–14
46. Paloyan E: Operation for the irradiated gland for possible thyroid carcinoma. Criteria, technique, and results. In DeGroot LJ, Frohman LA, Kaplan EL, Refetoff S (eds): Radiation Associated Carcinoma of the Thyroid. New York, Grune & Stratton, 1977, pp 383–394
47. Southwick HW, Economu SG, Sadove AM, Gould VE: Surgery of the irradiated gland for possible thyroid carcinoma: Criteria, technique, and results. In DeGroot LJ, Frohman LA, Kaplan EL, Refetoff S (eds): Radiation Associated Carcinoma of the Thyroid. New York, Grune & Stratton, 1977, pp 395–404
48. Modan B, Ron E, Werner A: Thyroid neoplasms in a population irradiated for scalp tinea in childhood. In DeGroot LJ, Frohman LA, Kaplan EL, Refetoff S (eds): Radiation Associated Carcinoma of the Thyroid. New York, Grune & Stratton, 1977, pp 449–457
49. Tisell LE, Carlson S, Lindberg S, et al.: Autonomous hyperparathyroidism, a possible late complication of neck radiotherapy. Acta Chir Scand 142:367, 1976
50. Baral E, Larsson L, Mattsson B: Breast cancer following irradiation of the breast. Cancer 40:2905, 1977
51. Oertel JE, Klinck GH: Structural changes in the thyroid gland of healthy young men. Med Ann DC 34:75, 1965
52. Roudebush CP, DeGroot LJ: The natural history of radiation-associated thyroid cancer. In DeGroot LJ, Frohman LA, Kaplan EL, Refetoff S (eds): Radiation Associated Carcinoma of the Thyroid. New York, Grune & Stratton, 1977, pp 97–115
53. Block MA: Surgery of the irradiated thyroid gland for possible carcinoma: Criteria, technique, results. In DeGroot LJ, Frohman LA, Kaplan EL, Refetoff S (eds): Radiation Associated Carcinoma of the Thyroid. New York, Grune & Stratton, 1977, pp 353–370
54. Lowhagen T, Granberg P-O, Lundell G, Skinnari P, Sundblad R, Willems JS: Aspiration biopsy cytology (ABC) in nodules of the thyroid gland suspected to be malignant. Surg Clin North Am 59:3, 1979

55. Vickery AL Jr: Needle biopsy and the thyroid nodule. In DeGroot LJ, Frohman LA, Kaplan EL, Refetoff S (eds): Radiation Associated Carcinoma of the Thyroid. New York, Grune & Stratton, 1977, pp 339–345

56. Thomas CJ Jr, Buckwalter JA, Staab EV, Kerr CY: Evaluation of dominant thyroid masses. Ann Surg 183:463, 1976

57. Cerletty JM, Guansing AR, Engbring NH, Hagen TC, Kim HJ, Shetty KR, Rosenfeld PS, Wilson S: Radiation-related thyroid carcinoma. Arch Surg 113:1072, 1978

58. Crile G Jr, Esselstyn CB Jr, Hawk WA: Needle biopsy in the diagnosis of thyroid nodules appearing after radiation. N Engl J Med 301:997, 1979

59. Blum M, Rothschild M: Improved nonoperative diagnosis of the solitary "cold" thyroid nodule. JAMA 243:242, 1980

60. Sampson RJ: Prevalence and significance of occult thyroid cancer. In DeGroot LJ, et al. (eds): Radiation Associated Thyroid Carcinoma. New York, Grune & Stratton, 1977, pp 137–153

61. Hubert JP Jr, Kiernan PD, Beahrs OH, McConahey WM, Woolner LB: Occult papillary carcinoma of the thyroid. Arch Surg 115:394, 1980

62. Roudebush CP, Asteris GT, DeGroot LJ: Natural history of radiation-associated thyroid cancer. Arch Intern Med 138:1631, 1978

63. Hamburger JI: Clinical Exercises in Internal Medicine, Vol. I. Thyroid Disease. Philadelphia, Saunders, 1978, pp 199–226

64. Kendall LW, Condon RE: Prediction of malignancy in solitary thyroid nodules. Lancet 1:1071, 1969

65. Nelson RL, Wahner HW, Gorman CA: Rectilinear thyroid scanning as a predictor of malignancy. Ann Intern Med 88:41, 1978

66. Gershengorn MC, McClung MR, Chu EW, Hanson TAS, Weintraub BD, Robbins J: Fine needle aspiration cytology in the preoperative diagnosis of thyroid nodules. Ann Intern Med 87:265, 1977

67. Walfish PG, Hazani E, Strawbridge HTG, Miskin M, Rosen IB: Combined ultrasound and needle aspiration cytology in the assessment and management of hypofunctioning thyroid nodule. Ann Intern Med 87:270, 1977

68. Schneider AB, Favus MJ, Stachura ME, Arnold J, Ryo U, Pinsky S, Colman M, Frohman L: Plasma thyroglobulin in detecting thyroid carcinoma after childhood head and neck irradiation. Ann Intern Med 86:29, 1977

69. Maxon HR, Saenger EL, Thomas SR, Buncher CR, Kereiakes JG, Shafer ML, McLaughlin CA: Clinically important radiation-associated thyroid disease. JAMA 244:1802, 1980

70. Martin JW, Dozier WE: Carcinoma of the thyroid gland. A 15-year survey in private hospitals in Sacramento. California Med 108:166, 1968

71. Block MA: Management of carcinoma of the thyroid. Ann Surg 185:133, 1977

72. Woolner LB, Beahrs OH, Black BM, et al.: Thyroid carcinoma: general considerations and followup data on 1181 cases. In: Imperial Research Fund Symposium (2nd): Thyroid Neoplasia. London, Academic Press, 1968, pp 51–77

73. Hamburger JI, Miller JM, Kini SR: Clinical-Pathological Evaluation of Thyroid Nodules. Handbook and Atlas. Private publication, Southfield, 1979, p 76

Chapter 10

Is Lymphoma of the Thyroid a Disease Which Is Increasing in Frequency?

J. Martin Miller, M.D.
Sudha R. Kini, M.D.
John Rebuck, M.D.
Joel I. Hamburger, M.D.

INTRODUCTION

It has been said that primary lymphoma of the thyroid gland is rare.[1-9] The number of cases reported in the world literature has been cited at approximately 250.[9] Although this is probably an underestimate, it is a general indication of the frequency of this disease. Most of the tumors are histiocytic or lymphocytic lymphomas. Primary involvement of the thyroid gland by Hodgkin's disease is truly exceedingly rare.[10] The diagnoses have almost always been made retrospectively after operations for different presumptive diagnoses.

Since 1976 we have been employing needle biopsy for the diagnosis of thyroid nodules which were hypofunctional by radionuclide imaging. To our surprise lymphomas of the thyroid were identified much more often than previously.

The literature has emphasized the strong association of lymphoma of the thyroid with Hashimoto's thyroiditis.[1-4,7-9] Hashimoto's thyroiditis is probably the most common thyroid disease of all. Infiltration of lymphocytes, at times forming germinal centers, is characteristic of Hashimoto's thyroiditis. Hence, a needle biopsy specimen from a thyroid nodule which contains many cells which resemble lymphocytes might suggest to the pathologist a diagnosis of Hashimoto's thyroiditis—a very common disease, rather than lymphoma of the thyroid—a very uncommon disease. Since the two diseases commonly coexist, if the biopsy specimen samples an area of Hashimoto's thyroiditis, perhaps along with the lymphoma,[11] an incomplete diagnosis of just Hashimoto's thyroiditis may be made. This error is especially likely if the pathologist is told that the patient has clinical findings characteristic of Hashimoto's thyroiditis. These are some of the reasons why incorrect or incomplete needle biopsy diagnoses of Hashimoto's thyroiditis have been made on needle biopsy specimens.[12]

On the basis of our experience and our review of the literature we believe that the following issues deserve further discussion:

(1) Is lymphoma of the thyroid increasing in frequency?

(2) Does the strong association of Hashimoto's thyroiditis and lymphoma of the thyroid indicate that the latter is derived from the former? If so, why is lymphoma of the thyroid so uncommon, when Hashimoto's thyroiditis is so common?

(3) What are the clinical features which suggest lymphoma of the thyroid, especially early, when the disease is highly curable?

(4) What are the pitfalls in the needle biopsy diagnosis of lymphoma of the thyroid?

(5) Is it important to make the diagnosis of lymphoma of the thyroid preoperatively by needle biopsy?

We shall review our experience with lymphoma of the thyroid, diagnosed by needle biopsy, to serve as a basis for a preliminary discussion of these issues. Methods for fine needle aspiration biopsy (FNAB), which produces a specimen for cytologic evaluation, and large needle biopsy (LNB) techniques, which produce specimens for histologic evaluation, have been published elsewhere.[13] The lymphoma diagnoses in this chapter are designated according to the new working formulation of the National Cancer Institute; the designation in parentheses corresponds to Rappaport's current classification.

EXPERIENCE OF NORTHLAND THYROID LABORATORY (NTL)

Changing Frequency of Lymphoma

Between 1964 and 1976 only four patients with lymphoma of the thyroid were diagnosed at NTL, or 0.27 cases per year. Between 1976 and 1980, 14 cases were identified, or 3.5 cases per year. This represents a 13-fold increment in the frequency of the diagnosis of this disease. Part of this increase can be attributed to the growth in patient volume. In the 4-year period between 1976 and 1980 approximately as many new patient referrals were seen at NTL as had been seen in the 15 years previously. Therefore the increment in diagnosis of lymphoma of the thyroid at NTL, per equivalent patient volume, is approximately 3.5-fold.

Table 10-1 provides data from selected reports on this subject which may provide limited support for the impression that lymphoma of the thyroid may be increasing in frequency. The lower frequencies of Shimkin and Sagerman[6] and Cox[4] were in series accumulated prior to 1970. Burke et al.[8] have one of the largest series of these cases. The frequency of diagnosis is somewhat higher. Unfortu-

Table 10-1. Frequency of diagnosis of lymphoma of the thyroid at selected centers.

Author	Number of cases	Time period	Number of cases per year
Shimkin[6]	11	1934–1967	0.33
Cox[4]	6	1952–1962	0.6
Burke[8]	35	1951–1975	1.46
Woolner[2] (a)	21	1930–1955	0.84
Woolner[2] (b)	25	1955–1964	2.78
Crile[3] (a)	13	1927–1952	0.52
Crile[3] (b)	17	1952–1962	1.7
Sirota[9] (a)	4	1966–1974	0.5
Sirota[9] (b)	12	1975–1977	6
Hamburger (a)	4	1961–1976	0.27
Hamburger (b)	15	1976–1980	3.5

(a): First report; (b): Subsequent report.

nately they did not provide data on the number of cases which might have been detected more recently, compared to those from earlier years. However, this kind of information is available in reports from three centers.[2,3,9] At the Mayo Clinic[2] a 3.3-fold increment in the frequency of the diagnosis of lymphoma of the thyroid was achieved in the decade between 1955 and 1964, compared to the preceding 25-year period. At the Cleveland Clinic[3] a similar 3.27-fold increment in the frequency of the diagnosis was observed in the 10-year period between 1952 and 1962, compared to the preceding 25-year period. At the Mount Sinai Medical Center[9] an even more striking 12-fold increment in the diagnosis was observed in the 2-year period between 1975 and 1977, compared with the preceding 8-year period. These data resemble ours quite closely.

The NTL Series of Thyroid Lymphomas

Table 10-2 presents the principal data relevant to the 14 patients. There were nine women and five men, ranging in age from 27 to 80 years old (average 55.6). Case 1 is the youngest patient, and his youth was probably a factor which contributed to delay in diagnosis.

CASE 1: LYMPHOMA OF THE THYROID IN A YOUNG MAN FOR WHOM AN
EARLIER CLINICAL DIAGNOSIS WAS HASHIMOTO'S THYROIDITIS
A 27-year-old medical student requested a thyroid image after having detected a nodule on the right side of his neck. The mass was hypofunctional. A diagnosis of Hashimoto's thyroiditis was made and treatment with thyroid hormone advised. After 7 months' treatment the mass had enlarged to 5 cm, was very hard, and the patient requested a second opinion. Antithyroid antibodies were strongly positive. FNAB (Fig. 10-1) and LNB (Fig. 10-2) established a diagnosis of lymphoma. The surgical diagnosis was non-Hodgkin's lymphoma, diffuse

Table 10-2. Clinical data in 14 patients with primary lymphoma of the thyroid.

No.	Date of first contact	Age/ sex	Size of lesion (cm)	Recent growth	Local symptoms	Thyroid function	Titer Antithyro-globulin antibody	Titer Antimicro-somal antibody	FNAB	LNB	Surgical diagnosis	Associated HT	Treatment	Current status	Associated disease or condition
1	3/3/77	46/F	4	No	No	Normal	—	1/6400	HT	Lymphoma, ? carcino-ma	N-H L, LC immunoblastic (LC diffuse "histiocytic" and plasmacytoid features)	Yes	S	Alive	
2	9/2/77	70/F	6	Yes	No	Normal	—	1/1600	HT	Lymphoma and HT	N-H L, small lymphocytic (lymphocytic well-differentiated diffuse)	Yes	S, R	Alive	
3	10/6/77	62/M	2.5	No	No	Normal	—	—	Lymphoma	Lymphoma	N-H L, diffuse LC (LC diffuse "histiocytic")	No	S, R	Alive	
4	11/14/77	80/F	8	Yes	No	Hypothyroid	1/25,600	1/25,600	HT	Not done	N-H L, diffuse LC (LC diffuse "histiocytic")	Ab[c] only	R	Dead	On Cytoxan for 10 years prior to diagnosis of lymphoma for "lung tumor"; doubtful diagnosis

5	4/3/79	55/M	Diffuse goiter, cold area right	No	No	Augmented TRH response	—	—	HT[b]	Lymphoma	N-H L, small lymphocytic (lymphocytic well-differentiated diffuse)	No	S, R	Alive
6	5/3/79	27/M	5	Yes	No	On thyroid when first seen	26%[a]	1/25,600	HT, ? Lymphoma	Lymphoma	N-H L, diffuse LC (LC diffuse "histiocytic")	Yes	S, R	Alive
7	9/25/79	51/F	2.5	Yes	No	Normal	—	—	Benign	Lymphoma	N-H L, LC immunoblastic (LC diffuse "histiocytic" with plasmacytoid features)	No	C	Dead — Sjögren's syndrome
8	11/9/79	58/M	Bilateral masses, each 4	No	Hoarseness	Normal	—	1/25,600	Anaplastic carcinoma	Anaplastic carcinoma, HT	N-H L, diffuse LC (LC diffuse "histiocytic")	Yes	S, R	Alive
9	2/4/79	53/F	3	Yes	No	TSH elevated	—	1/100,000	Lymphoma	Lymphoma	N-H L, LC immunoblastic (LC diffuse "histiocytic" with plasmacytoid features)	Yes	S, R, C	Alive
10	3/12/80	66/F	5	No	No	Hypothyroid	11%	1/6400	Lymphoma, HT	Lymphoma	N-H L, diffuse LC (LC diffuse "histiocytic")	Yes	S	?
11	3/18/80	53/M	8	Yes	No	Normal	21%	1/25,600	HT	Lymphoma	N-H L, diffuse LC (LC diffuse "histiocytic")	Ab[c] only	S, C	Alive

Table 10-2. (continued)

No.	Date of first contact	Age/sex	Size of lesion (cm)	Recent growth	Local symptoms	Thyroid function	Titer		FNAB	LNB	Surgical diagnosis	Associated HT	Treatment	Current status	Associated disease or condition
							Antithyroglobulin antibody	Antimicrosomal antibody							
2	4/16/80	71/F	4	Yes	No	Hypothyroid	10%	1/1600	Lymphoma, HT	Histiocytic lymphoma	N-H L, follicular and diffuse LC (LC nodular and diffuse "histiocytic")	Yes	S	Alive	
3	4/24/80	38/F	5	?	Dysphagia, pressure	Normal	11%	1/25,600	Unsatisfactory	Poorly differentiated follicular arcinoma	N-H L, diffuse LC (LC diffuse "histiocytic")	Yes	S	Alive	
4	5/19/80	72/F	Diffuse goiter, cold area left	Yes	Hoarseness	Normal	—	—	HT, rule out lymphoma	Lymphoma	N-H L, diffuse LC (LC diffuse "histiocytic")	Yes	S, R	Alive	

C, chemotherapy; FNAB, fine needle aspiration biopsy; HT, Hashimoto's thyroiditis; LC, large cell; LNB, large needle biopsy; N-H L, non-Hodgkin's lymphoma; R, radiotherapy; S, surgery.
[a]Antithyroglobulin titers expressed in percent are performed by RIA. Normal is up to 10%; borderline, 10–12%; elevated >12%.
[b]Done at another institution.
[c]Ab, antibodies; thyroid tissue entirely replaced by lymphoma.

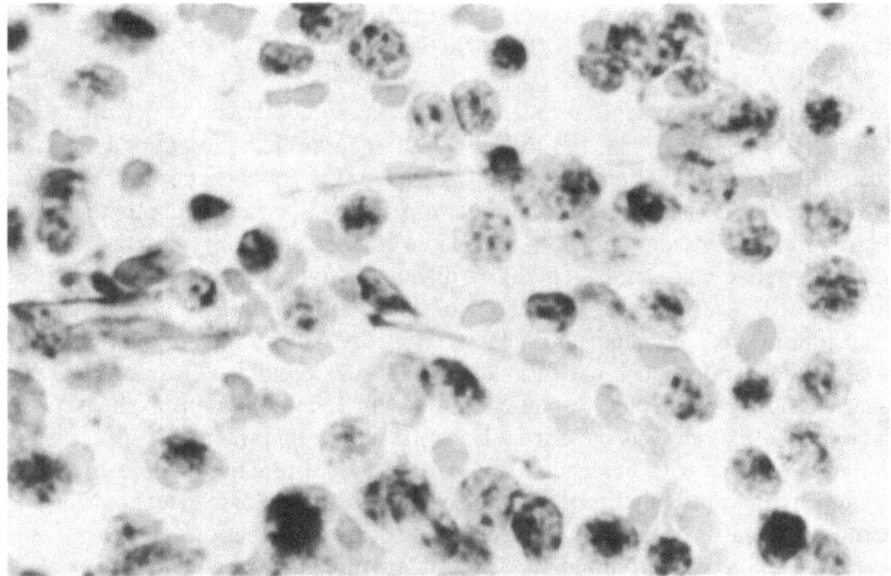

Figure 10-1. FNAB; lymphoma cells. Papanicolaou stain. × 630

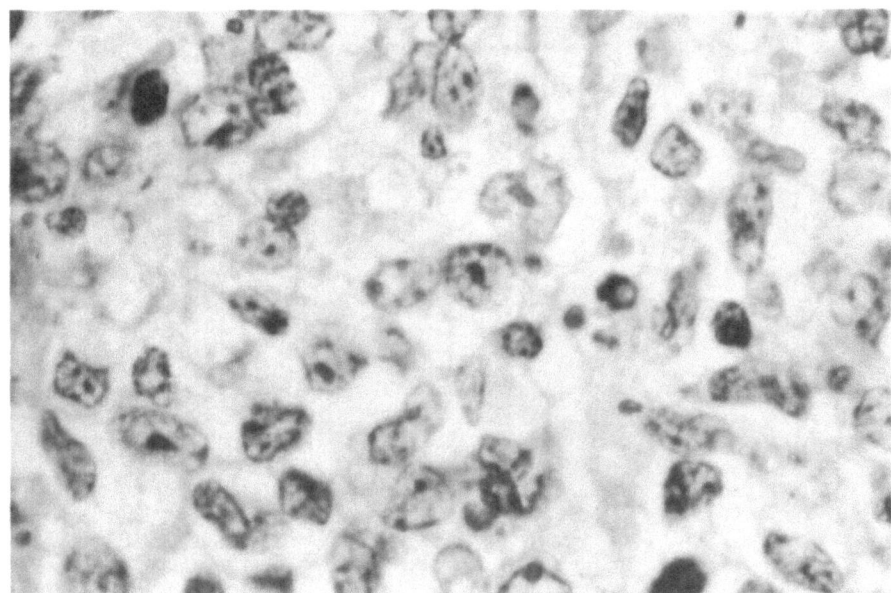

Figure 10-2. LNB; malignant lymphoma. Hemetoxylin and eosin (H & E). × 1000

large cell (malignant lymphoma large cell diffuse "histiocytic") (Fig. 10-3), arising in a background consistent with Hashimoto's thyroiditis (Fig. 10-4).

Eight of the 14 patients presented within the 9-month period preceding this writing, and ten presented within the prior 22 months. The presenting lesion was a single mass in 11 patients, bilateral masses in one patient, and diffuse goiters with large "cold" areas on imaging in two patients. For eight patients there was a history of recent enlargement of the nodule or goiter; however, only two patients had obstructive complaints. The early diagnosis which needle biopsy permitted limited the potential for further growth of these lesions and therefore reduced the opportunities for obstructive problems. Hypothyroidism was present in three patients. One additional patient had an elevated basal level of serum TSH, another had an augmented response in the serum TSH level to intravenous TRH, and one final patient was on thyroid hormone medication when first seen. Five of these six patients with evidence for impaired thyroid function had positive tests for antithyroid antibody titers and four of them had histologic evidence of Hashimoto's thyroiditis on either LNB, surgical specimens, or both.

FNAB diagnoses of lymphoma or possible lymphoma were made for six of 13 patients for whom specimens were interpreted by one of us (SRK). A diagnosis of anaplastic carcinoma was made for one additional patient. For four patients a diagnosis of Hashimoto's thyroiditis was made. Three of these were errors made early in our experience. Blind reevaluation 2 years later indicated that diagnoses

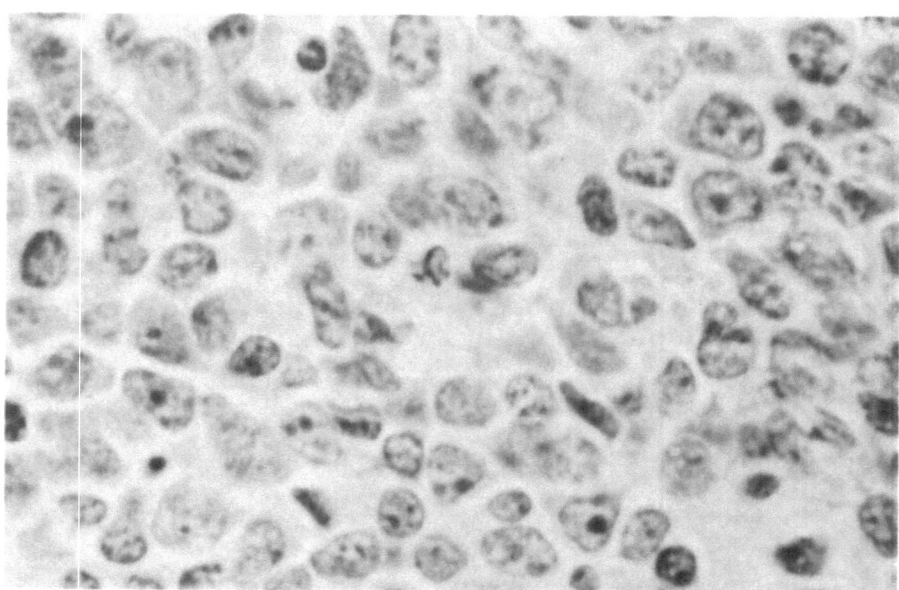

Figure 10-3. Microscopic section, surgical specimen; non-Hodgkin's lymphoma, diffuse large cell. H & E. × 1000

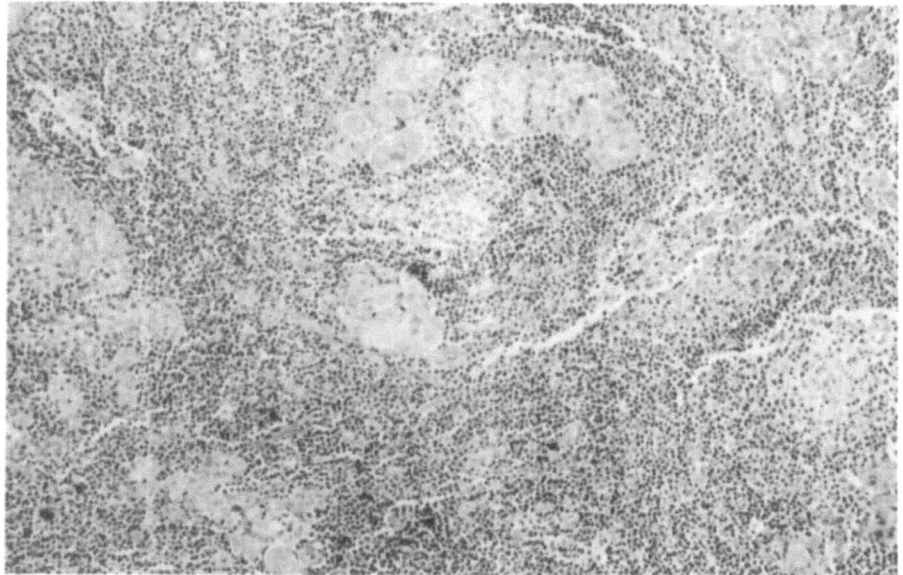

Figure 10-4. Microscopic section, surgical specimen; Hashimoto's thyroiditis. H & E. × 100

of lymphoma should have been made. The fourth specimen was diagnosed as Hashimoto's thyroiditis, even though it was known that a LNB specimen showed lymphoma. One specimen was called "benign." On retrospective review this specimen was called unsatisfactory. The final specimen was unsatisfactory for interpretation. One additional FNAB specimen was interpreted as Hashimoto's thyroiditis at another institution. The accuracy of LNB was considerably greater. Diagnoses of lymphoma were made or suggested for 11 of 13 patients. The other two cases were diagnosed as anaplastic carcinoma and poorly differentiated follicular carcinoma. Therefore, all of the LNB specimens were identified as representative of malignant disease. Cases 2–5 illustrate diagnostic errors by FNAB.

CASE 2: LYMPHOMA OF THE THYROID INCORRECTLY IDENTIFIED AS HASHIMOTO'S THYROIDITIS ON FNAB, CORRECTLY IDENTIFIED ON LNB

A 46-year-old woman had a 4-cm mass on the right side of the neck discovered on a routine examination. Thyroid imaging revealed a hypofunctional mass in the upper pole of the right lobe. The antimicrosomal antibody titer was positive at 1/1600. FNAB (Fig. 10-5) was interpreted as Hashimoto's thyroiditis; however, a LNB (Fig. 10-6) was diagnosed as lymphoma. The surgical diagnosis confirmed non-Hodgkin's lymphoma, large cell, immunoblastic (large cell "histiocytic"), (Fig. 10-7) in a background of Hashimoto's thyroiditis (Fig. 10-8). This was the first FNAB specimen from lymphoma of the thyroid seen by our cytopathologist. The same specimen was resubmitted for analysis (without the cytopathologist being aware that she had seen the specimen earlier) 2 years later and a diagnosis of lymphoma of the thyroid was made.

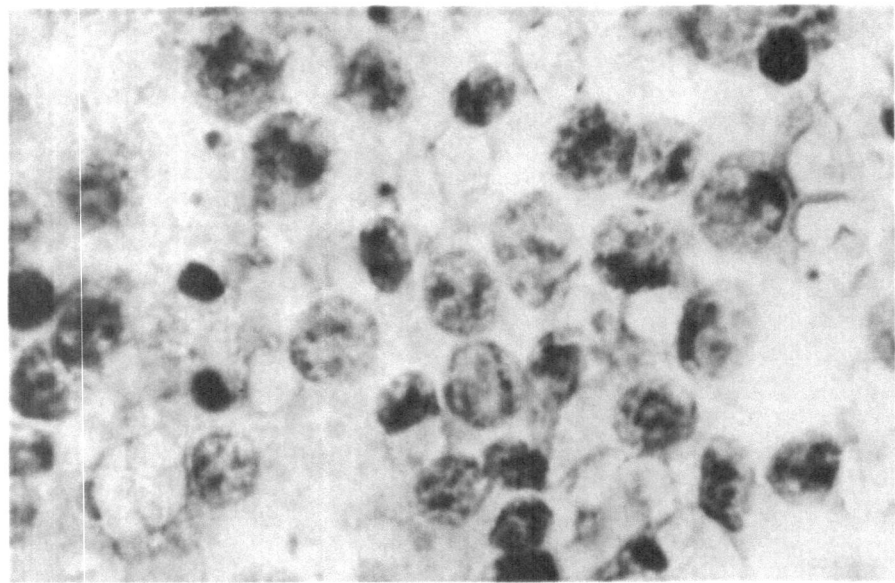

Figure 10-5. FNAB; malignant lymphoma. Papanicolaou stain. × 630 (This aspirate was initially interpreted incorrectly as Hashimoto's thyroiditis.)

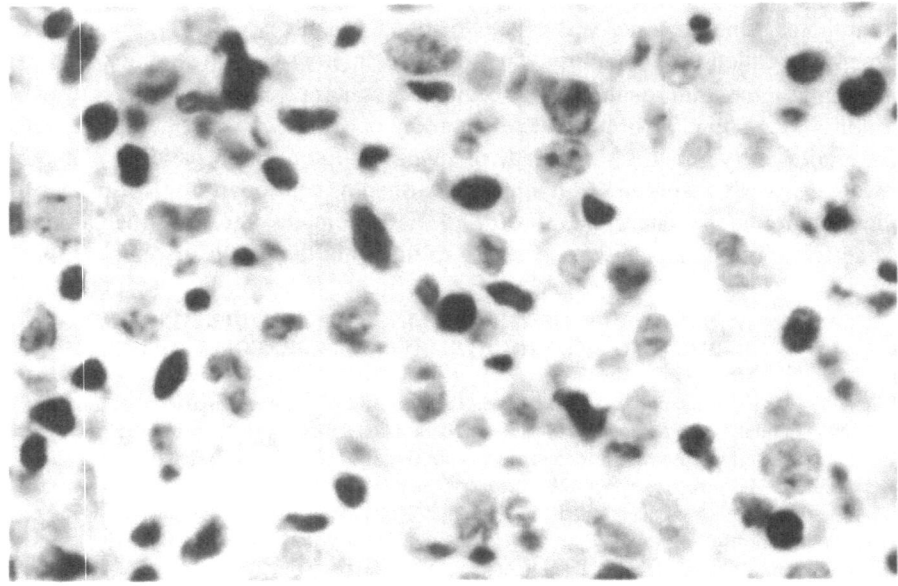

Figure 10-6. LNB; malignant lymphoma. H & E. × 1000

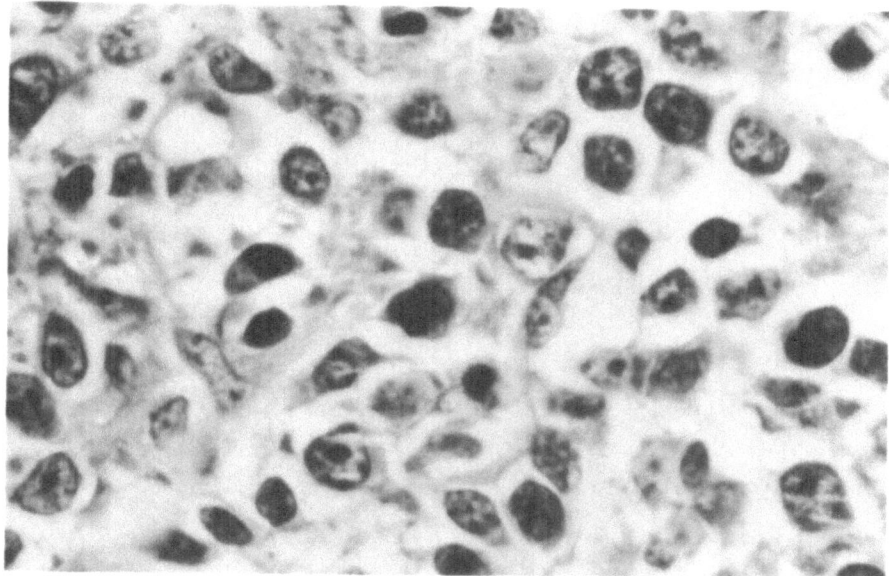

Figure 10-7. Microscopic section, surgical specimen; non-Hodgkin's lymphoma, large cell immunoblastic. H & E. × 1000

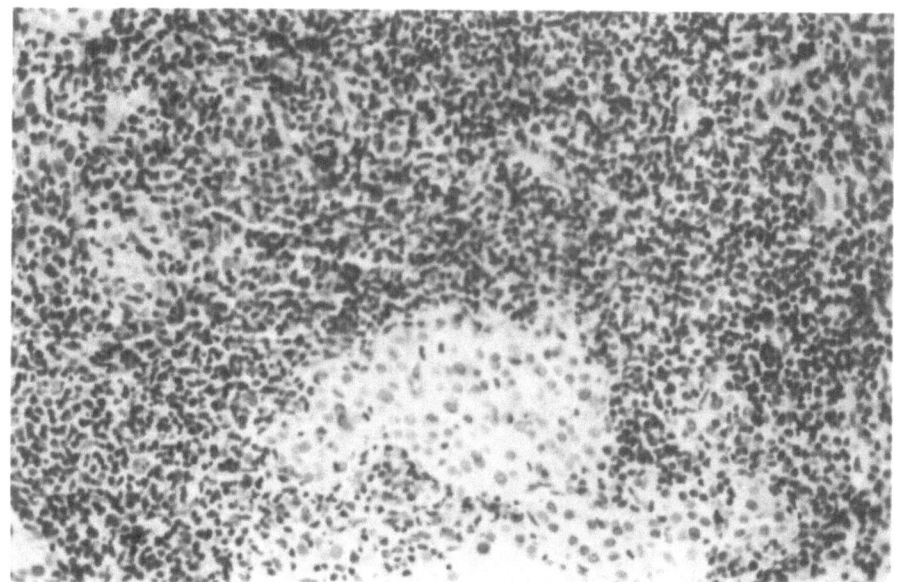

Figure 10-8. Microscopic section, surgical specimen; Hashimoto's thyroiditis. H & E. × 160

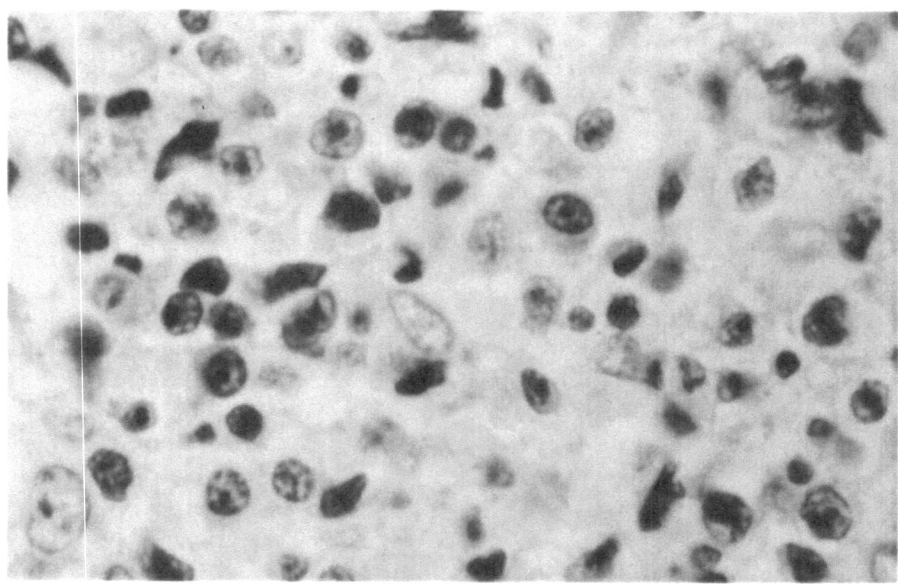

Figure 10-9. LNB; malignant lymphoma. H & E. × 1000

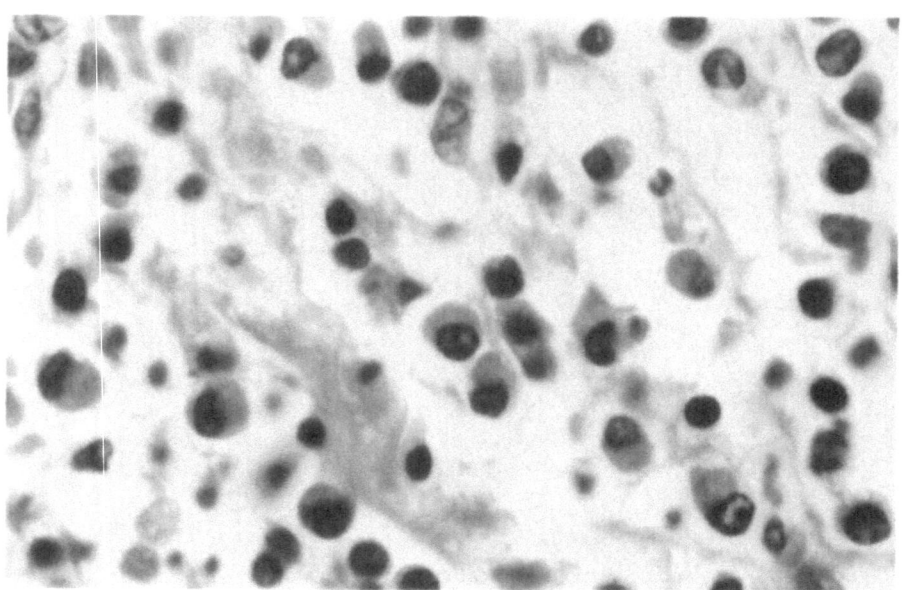

Figure 10-10. Microscopic section, autopsy specimen; non-Hodgkin's lymphoma, large cell immunoblastic. H & E. × 1000

CASE 3: LYMPHOMA ASSOCIATED WITH SJÖGREN'S SYNDROME

A 51-year-old woman with Sjögren's syndrome for 8 years had a small nodule in the lower pole of the left thyroid lobe. It enlarged to 2.5 cm in a 3-month period. Antithyroid antibodies were not detected. The mass was "cold" on thyroid imaging. A FNAB was interpreted as benign, but a LNB (Fig. 10-9) was diagnosed as non-Hodgkin's lymphoma, large cell immunoblastic (malignant lymphoma, large cell "histiocytic"). The patient went rapidly downhill to death in spite of chemotherapy. The autopsy confirmed the above diagnosis, with involvement of generalized lymph nodes, liver, and thyroid (Fig. 10-10).

CASE 4: A PATIENT WITH LYMPHOMA OF THE THYROID INCORRECTLY DIAGNOSED AS HAVING HASHIMOTO'S THYROIDITIS BY FNAB

An 80-year-old woman had an enlarging firm 8-cm mass in the left lobe of the thyroid, detected 6 months earlier. She had been treated with Cytoxan for the previous 10 years because of a diagnosis of a "lung tumor." She had received radiation therapy to the chest after operation for the "tumor" 10 years earlier. The records of that illness indicated that only fibrotic tissue without evidence of malignancy was removed. At this time the patient was clinically and biochemically hypothyroid. Antithyroid antibodies were present in high titer. Imaging revealed no functioning thyroid tissue. A clinical diagnosis of anaplastic carcinoma was made. The FNAB (Figs. 10-11 and 10-12) diagnosis was Hashimoto's thyroiditis. Treatment with thyroid hormone was instituted. She was asked to return for further evaluation. However, the mass enlarged rapidly and she was hospitalized for open biopsy at the insistence of her attending physician. A diagnosis of non-Hodgkin's lymphoma diffuse, large cell (large cell diffuse "histiocytic") was made (Fig. 10-13). Her course was rapidly downhill to death in 6 months, in spite of a temporary response to radiotherapy. Once again blind reevaluation of the FNAB specimen by the cytopathologist, after further experience, permitted a correct diagnosis.

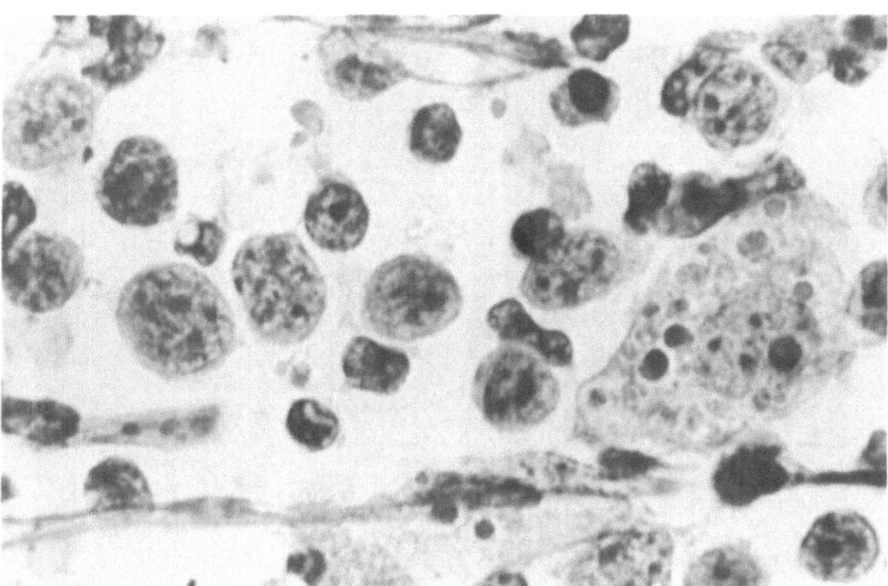

Figure 10-11. FNAB; follicle center cells. Note the entire range of transforming lymphocytes and the phagocytic histiocyte. Papanicolaou stain. × 1600

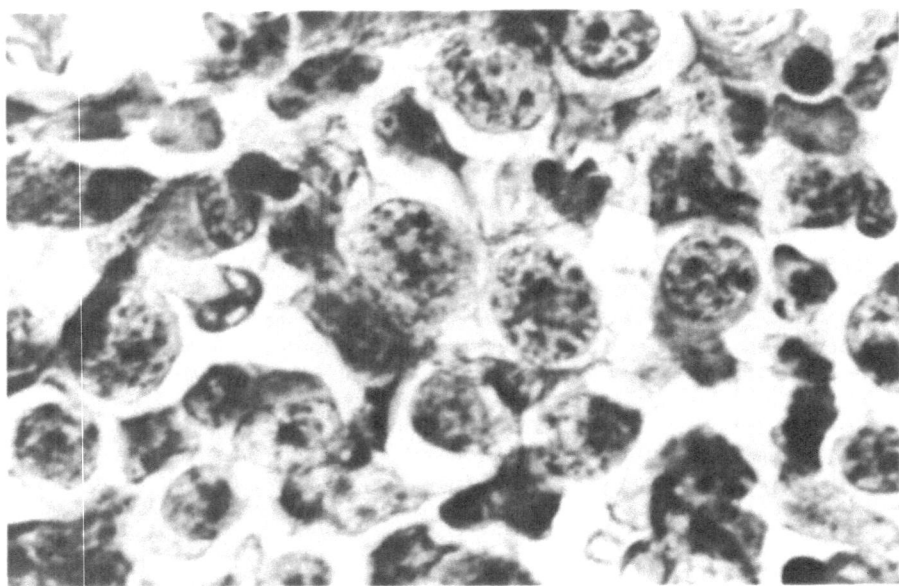

Figure 10-12. FNAB; The large aggregates of transformed lymphocytes illustrated were not appreciated at the time of the original review as suggestive of lymphoma because of the presence of follicle center cells in other areas of the smear (see Fig. 10-11). Papanicolaou stain. × 1600

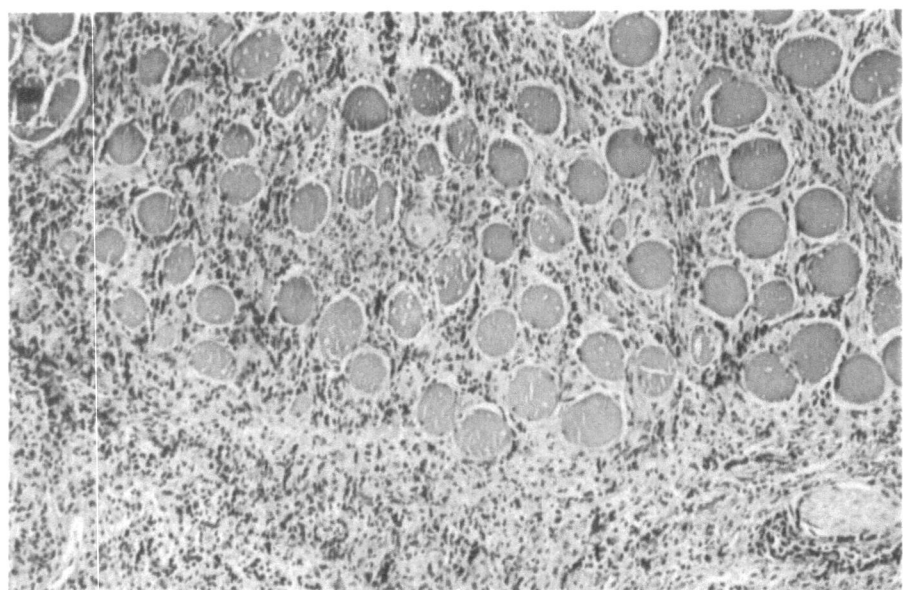

Figure 10-13. Microscopic section, surgical biopsy specimen. Non-Hodgkin's lymphoma, diffuse large cell, widely infiltrating the surrounding skeletal muscle. H & E. × 160

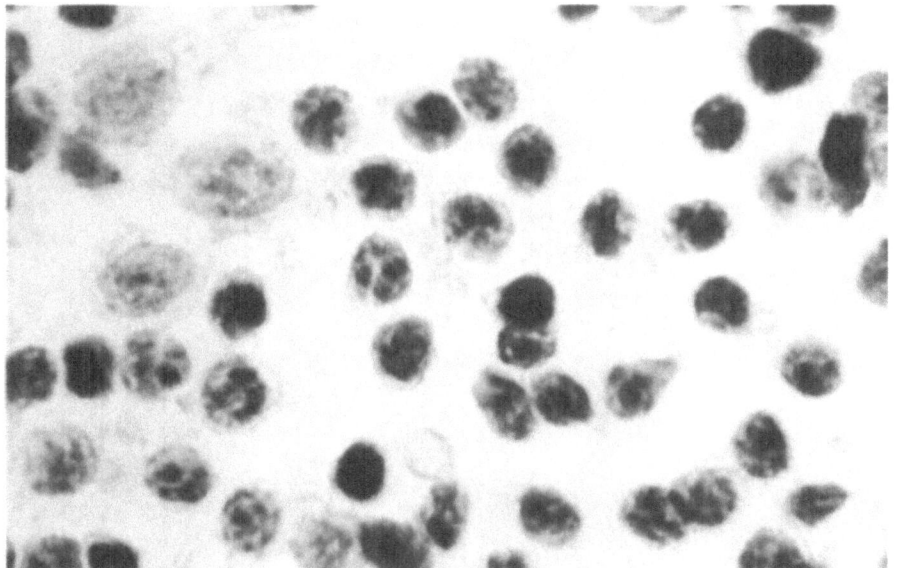

Figure 10-14. FNAB. This dense population of well-differentiated lymphocytes were responsible for the diagnosis of Hashimoto's thyroiditis originally made from this aspirate. Papanicolaou stain. × 630

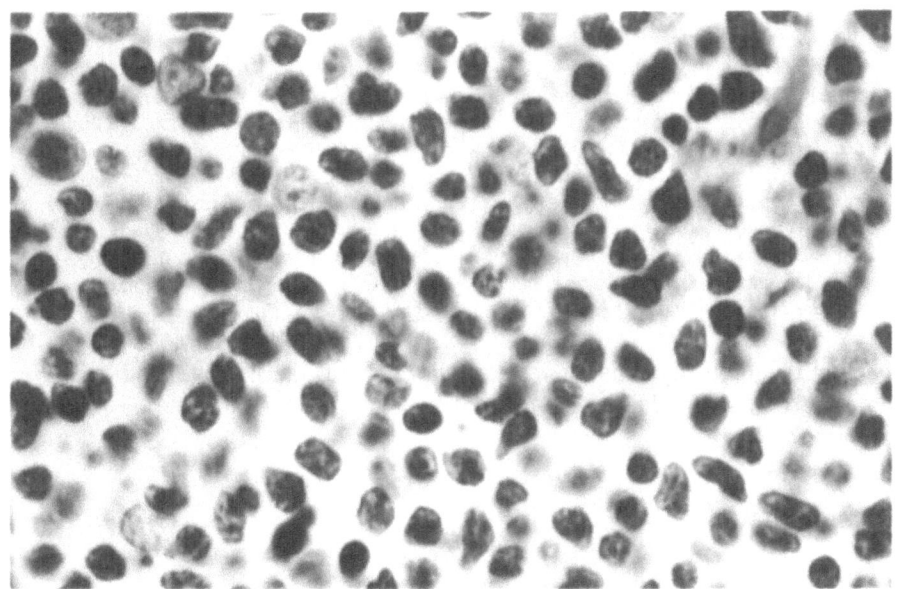

Figure 10-15. LNB; malignant lymphoma. H & E. × 1000

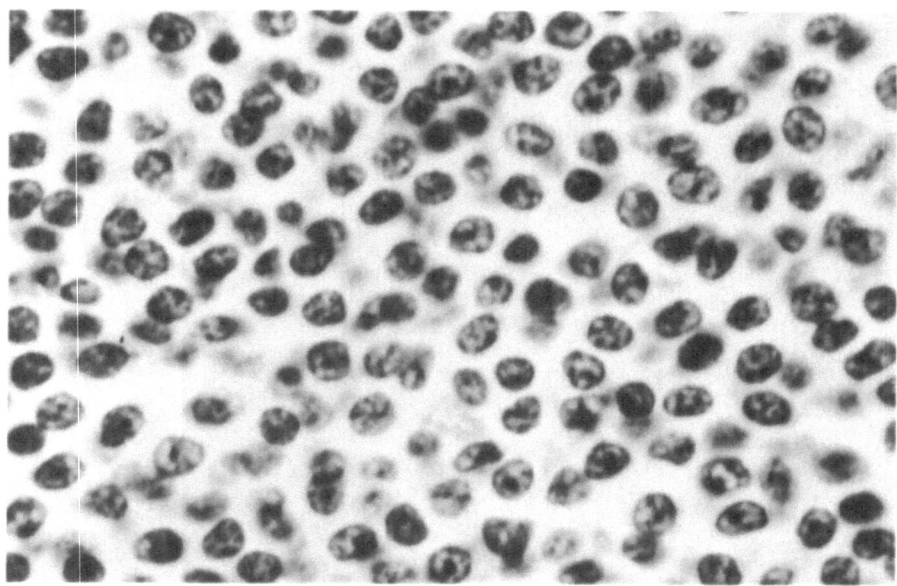

Figure 10-16. Microscopic section, surgical specimen. Non-Hodgkins's lymphoma, small cell lymphocytic. No evidence of Hashimoto's thyroiditis was appreciated. H & E. × 1000

CASE 5: LYMPHOMA OF THE THYROID, INCORRECTLY DIAGNOSED BY FNAB AT ANOTHER INSTITUTION, CORRECTLY DIAGNOSED BY LNB

A 55-year-old man was told he had a 3-cm mass in the right lobe of the thyroid, detected on physical examination. The mass was hypofunctional on imaging. A surgeon performed a FNAB (Fig. 10-14) and diagnosed Hashimoto's thyroiditis. However, the surgeon, suspicious of malignancy, advised thyroidectomy. The patient requested a second opinion. No discrete nodular mass was found. The thyroid gland was diffusely enlarged and firm, but review of the thyroid image revealed reduced function in the right lobe. Thyroid function studies were normal except for an augmented response of the serum TSH(RIA) level to intravenous TRH. Antithyroid antibodies were not detected. LNB was advised. A diagnosis of non-Hodgkin's lymphoma, small lymphocytic (lymphocytic well-differentiated diffuse) was made (Fig. 10-15). He is alive without evidence of disease after surgery and radiotherapy. The microscopic sections of the surgical specimen confirmed the above diagnosis (Fig. 10-16).

Only two of 13 patients for whom follow-up is available have died. However, eight of the patients have been diagnosed within the 9-month period preceding this writing.

DISCUSSION

Frequency of Lymphoma of the Thyroid

There is general agreement that primary lymphomas of the thyroid gland are rare;[1-9] however, our experience suggests that these lesions may be more common than generally appreciated. Also, the frequency of lymphoma of the thyroid may be increasing. We had initially assumed that the greater precision of diagnosis which is possible with needle biopsy might have accounted for the surge in our cases. However, as the number continued to rise we were forced to reconsider. In almost every patient there was either a large obviously malignant growth, or an enlarging mass which probably would not have gone undiagnosed for long even if needle biopsy were not available. Therefore, we believe that there is an increase in the frequency of this disease. This conclusion can be inferred from other reports on this entity.[2,3,9]

Association of Lymphoma of the Thyroid with Prior Radiation Therapy

The association of prior radiation therapy to the head or neck and the development of lymphoma of the thyroid has been reported for two patients,[9,14] as has Hashimoto's thyroiditis.[9] One of our patients received prior radiation therapy. Nevertheless, the small number of patients with such a history (all of our patients were specifically queried on this point) indicates that prior radiation therapy could only be a minor contributing factor.

Association of Hashimoto's Thyroiditis and Lymphoma of the Thyroid

Perhaps more important is the association of Hashimoto's thyroiditis with lymphoma of the thyroid. This relationship was documented for nine of our 14 patients. An additional two patients had antithyroid antibodies consistent with Hashimoto's thyroiditis. Table 10-3 shows the frequency with which lymphoma

Table 10-3. Association of Hashimoto's thyroiditis and lymphoma of the thyroid.

Author	Date of publication	No. of cases	No. with Hashimoto's thyroiditis
Lindsay[1]	1955	8	7
Woolner[2]	1966	46	10
Crile[3]	1963	17	10
Cox[4]	1964	9	3
Shimkin[6]	1969	11	1
Taylor[7]	1976	8	4
Burke[8]	1977	35	27[a]
Sirota[9]	1974	12	4

[a]In the 8 cases without evidence of Hashimoto's thyroiditis the tumor had replaced the thyroid parenchyma completely.

of the thyroid was accompanied by Hashimoto's thyroiditis in other reports. This association is too strong to be dismissed as inconsequential, as Mikal[5] has advised. Perhaps Mikal has missed the point. He emphasized that very few patients with Hashimoto's thyroiditis have lymphoma, which is correct. However, most patients with lymphoma of the thyroid also have Hashimoto's thyroiditis. Indeed, there seems to be an increasing acceptance of the proposal of Lindsay and Dailey[1] that lymphomas of the thyroid are an outgrowth of Hashimoto's thyroiditis.[8,9,15,16]

Some of the differences in the observed frequency of the association of Hashimoto's thyroiditis may relate to different criteria for the diagnosis of Hashimoto's thyroiditis.[4] In advanced cases the lymphoma may produce such extensive destruction of the thyroid parenchyma that it may not be possible to demonstrate the features of Hashimoto's thyroiditis.[4,17] This was the case for two patients in our series. Both had antithyroid antibodies in high titer. Although Cox[4] proposed that the presence of antithyroid antibodies in high titer indicates a concomitant or preexisting thyroiditis, others[6,18] have shown that this is not reliable because antithyroid antibodies may be found in lymphoma patients without histologic evidence of Hashimoto's thyroiditis in the associated thyroid parenchyma. For this reason it has been suggested that rather than arising from Hashimoto's thyroiditis, the lymphoma actually might induce the Hashimoto's thyroiditis.[17] However, Burke et al.[8] provide electron microscopic data supporting the concept that lymphoma of the thyroid develops from preexisting Hashimoto's thyroiditis, secondary to the "chronic antigenic stimulation or from a defect in immunologic surveillance resulting from the altered immune state." These authors also note the association of lymphoma of the thyroid with Sjögren's syndrome and other immunologic abnormalities, including prolonged immunosuppression by drugs. One of our patients had Sjögren's syndrome, and another had been taking Cytoxan (Table 10-2; Cases 4 and 7).

If lymphoma of the thyroid may be an outgrowth of preexisting Hashimoto's thyroiditis, then one might attribute the rise in the incidence of lymphoma of the thyroid to the increased frequency of Hashimoto's thyroiditis in recent years.[19]

Immunologic Considerations Relating Malignant Lymphoma to Hashimoto's Thyroiditis

Recent rapid advances in immunologic interpretations of malignant lymphomas have made more plausible the interrelation of Hashimoto's thyroiditis and the lymphomatous process. Reactive hyperplasia of the lymphoid follicles of lymph nodes, the sites of B-lymphocyte induction to large transformed lymphocytes, is rarely a prelude to lymphomatous transformation. Reactive hyperplasia of the multiplicative arm of the B-lymphocyte system, normally located in the medullary cords of lymph nodes, is a diffuse process marked by proliferation of the large transformed lymphocytes through mitotic divisions leading to increasing numbers of daughter cells showing step-wise differentiation to lymphoblasts, poorly differentiated lymphocytes, and finally lymphocytes with a parallel pyramidal proliferation of plasmablasts, proplasmacytes, and plasma cells. When the multiplicative arm of the B-lymphocytes, or follicular center cell system (FCC) as it is called, undergoes massive hyperplasia so as to replace normal thymic-dependent, follicular, and sinus sites, it is called angioimmunoblastic lymphadenopathy or simply immunoblastic lymphadenopathy. It is this latter atypical, diffuse hyperplasia of the multiplicative arm of the B- or FCC lymphocytic series that has a propensity for lymphomatous conversion by way of cloning out of the large transformed lymphocyte multiplier.

A similar process for Hashimoto's thyroiditis is proposed in which follicular hyperplasia of a transformational nature gives way to a diffuse proliferative hyperplasia of the multiplicative arm of the FCC with its inherent danger of cloning out the large transformed (large noncleaved) lymphocyte. This concept would explain both the lower frequency of follicular lymphomas of the thyroid (since follicular lymphomas exhibit a block in B-lymphocyte transformation) and the higher incidence of diffuse large cell lymphomas which are a cloning out of the multiplicative cells resulting from their transformation in the follicle.

Why Is Hashimoto's Thyroiditis so Common and Lymphoma of the Thyroid so Uncommon?

If lymphoma of the thyroid arises in many instances from preexisting Hashimoto's thyroiditis, why is it that Hashimoto's thyroiditis is so very common, while lymphoma of the thyroid, even if recognized more often of late, is still a distinctly uncommon disease? Since lymphoma of the thyroid is, by and large, a disease of the elderly, it might be assumed that Hashimoto's thyroiditis must be present for many years before it evolves into lymphoma. Probably other etiologic factors may be operative as well. One has already been noted, i.e., prior radiation therapy to the head or neck area. Prolonged TSH stimulation (accepted as a factor in the genesis of thyroid carcinoma) may play a role.[5] In time it is likely that other hereditary, pathophysiologic, or environmental factors will be elucidated.

Lymphoma of the Thyroid Is Easily Overlooked

With few exceptions lymphoma of the thyroid has been unsuspected until after excision of the tumor permitted a retrospective diagnosis.[1,2,4−9] It is easy to overlook the possibility of lymphoma of the thyroid, especially early. Many patients are elderly, and the physician may think that a neck mass is only a longstanding goiter. Other findings of Hashimoto's thyroiditis, including subnormal thyroid function or antithyroid antibodies, may add to the physician's confusion, rather than (as it should) trigger the suspicion of an associated lymphoma. Physicians must become more aware of the relationship between lymphoma and Hashimoto's thyroiditis, because early diagnosis, before extrathyroidal extension or involvement of adjacent lymph nodes, may be crucial in improving survival.[8,9]

Clinical Features Suggestive of Lymphoma of the Thyroid

The clinical features which have been associated with lymphoma of the thyroid include rapidly growing neck masses, often painful, associated with hoarseness, occurring usually in elderly women, many of whom have or have had evidence of Hashimoto's thyroiditis. Unfortunately this description, although valid, is the description of the late stage of the disease, a stage in which it is usually no longer possible to achieve a cure. Earlier diagnosis is needed. For this purpose perhaps the most important clinical feature is the association of Hashimoto's thyroiditis. Lymphoma should be suspected whenever the goiter of Hashimoto's thyroiditis is asymmetric with a localized prominence or nodularity. The nodular area may not feel much different from the rest of the goiter, for the goiter of Hashimoto's thyroiditis tends to be quite firm. Thyroid imaging will reveal reduced tracer concentration in the area of the mass. The difference in the functional activity of the tumor and the adjacent goiter of Hashimoto's thyroiditis may be more sharply outlined when ^{99m}Tc pertechnetate is used as the tracer, rather than isotopes of iodine. It should be emphasized that we do not refer to the patchy or small focal areas of reduced function seen on thyroid images of most patients with Hashimoto's thyroiditis, patients who do not have palpable nodules which correspond to these areas of reduced function. The defects to which we refer are sizable, 2–3 cm in diameter, and are associated with palpable masses. Even so, most of these lesions will prove to be part of the Hashimoto's thyroiditis, rather than lymphomas. Therefore it is important to make a differential diagnosis.

Needle Biopsy Is an Important Tool for Early Diagnosis of Lymphoma of the Thyroid

If surgical excision is employed for diagnostic purposes the number of operations which will be required for the detection of each lymphoma would be staggering. Since many suspect patients are elderly, surgical treatment would be risky. For these reasons the diagnosis is often delayed until there are clear-cut findings of malignant disease. However, this is too late for many patients. Also, operation is not needed for the treatment of most of these patients.[20]

Needle biopsy would seem to be the logical solution to early diagnosis. The procedure is simple and safe. Unfortunately, it also has a history of unreliability.[9,12] Diagnostic failures with needle biopsy have been emphasized, however, without attention to the circumstances in which they occurred. Many errors can be attributed to inexperience and, perhaps more important, to failure to consider the possibility of lymphoma. An abundance of cells resembling lymphocytes in a thyroid biopsy specimen may evoke a prompt diagnosis of Hashimoto's thyroiditis by many pathologists, especially if the clinician has provided compatible clinical data and particularly if the pathologist has seen many needle biopsy specimens from patients with Hashimoto's thyroiditis. Pathologists should consider lymphoma whenever the picture of Hashimoto's thyroiditis seems to be present. Sometimes smears prepared for FNAB specimens will provide cytologic evidence adequate to make the diagnosis if an experienced cytopathologist is available.[21] We, and others,[20] have had greater success with the LNB specimens which provide tissue cores for histologic evaluation. More does seem to be better in this instance. Whichever method is employed, we advise that multiple samples be taken, i.e., at least six grossly promising FNAB aspirates or three LNB tissue cores from different parts of the tumor. Since these tumors are usually 3 cm or larger, obtaining this much tissue is not difficult.

The pathologist, alert to the possibility of a lymphoma, will appreciate that he is dealing only with Hashimoto's thyroiditis if he sees the pattern of a polymorphous admixture of lymphocytes in various stages of transformation, but with an obvious predominance of mature well-differentiated small cells, a variable number of plasma cells, and the presence of germinal centers; rather than the monotonous monomorphic pattern of the lymphoma in which mature lymphocytes, if present at all, are always clearly in the minority.

Even after considerable experience it may not always be possible to make a specific diagnosis of lymphoma even from satisfactory needle biopsy specimens. Nevertheless most of the time it is, and for the remaining patients at least there should be an appreciation that malignant disease is probable. Therefore, greater use of needle biopsy for the diagnosis of nodular lesions of the thyroid, especially in association with Hashimoto's thyroiditis, will serve to eliminate unnecessary operations, as well as a possibly fatal delay in diagnosis.

COMMENTARY

William A. Hawk, M.D.

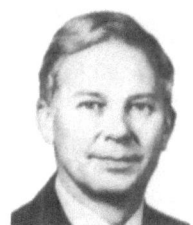

Frequency of Lymphoma of the Thyroid

The contention that primary lymphoma of the thyroid is increasing in frequency is probably valid. Primary lymphoma of the thyroid constitutes 4% or less of primary thyroidal malignancies. A recent report by Cumpagno and Ortell doubled the number of cases reported in the world literature.[8,22,23] Because of the rarity of the disorder, the addition of even small numbers of primary lymphomas of the thyroid can be appreciated as an absolute increase in the instance of the disease. The authors have experienced such an increase in their highly specialized medical practice and this has been the experience in other large centers. The true incidence of primary lymphoma of the thyroid is mercifully small. The authors have presented convincing evidence that an increasing awareness of primary lymphoma cannot account for this increasing incidence entirely, and other explanations must be invoked.

Relationship of Lymphoma of the Thyroid to Hashimoto's Thyroiditis

Inasmuch as primary lymphoma of the thyroid is principally non-Hodgkin's lymphoma, it is attractive to explore the relationship of this lymphoma to struma lymphomatosa. The origin of primary lymphoma of the thyroid gland in struma lymphomatosa was suggested as early as 1932, and sporadic reports have appeared since then.[24,25] The magnitude of the association of struma lymphomatosa with non-Hodgkin's lymphoma is attested by the finding of the association in nine of 14 patients reported by Miller et al. The majority of patients with non-Hodgkin's lymphoma primary in the thyroid seen at the Cleveland Clinic likewise demonstrate this strong association.[25] That struma lymphomatosa is increasing in incidence is generally accepted. The reasons for this extend beyond the purview of this commentary. The increased incidence of struma lymphomatosa correlates very well, therefore, with the increased incidence of primary lymphoma of non-Hodgkin's type.

In characterizing the relationship of struma lymphomatosa to non-Hodgkin's lymphoma of the thyroid, it is important that the diagnosis of struma lymphomatosa be made according to accepted and specific criteria. The use of antibody titers can be quite misleading since focal lymphocytic thyroiditis can produce antithyroid antibody titers of significance. In our experience focal lymphocytic thyroiditis has not been identified in association with lymphoma. The very nature of focal lymphocytic thyroiditis is such that it is very doubtful if the lesion could be recognized in the setting of an established primary lymphoma without resort to immunoperoxidase techniques that demonstrate the polyclonal nature of the thyroiditis as evidenced by the presence of kappa and lambda light chains. Miller et al. point out that an occasional primary lymphoma can give rise to antithyroid antibody titers without identifiable struma lymphomatosa. The diagnosis of struma lymphomatosa as an associated lesion must therefore be established on the basis of multiple parameters, i.e., an appropriate clinical history, evidence of reduced thyroidal function with associated elevated antithyroid antibody titers, and a consistent histologic appearance on biopsy.

The infrequency of lymphoma in struma lymphomatosa remains unexplained. Lymphomas occur in the elderly so that struma lymphomatosa may preexist for many years before the onset of lymphomatous disease. A breakdown in immune surveillance, the addition of an unknown etiologic agent, or both may be operative, but are currently unproven. The role of prior radiation therapy in the evolution of lymphoma of the thyroid has been well stated by Miller et al. The strength of this association is weak compared to the strength of the relationship between irradiation and carcinoma of the thyroid.

Clinical Findings Suggesting Lymphoma of the Thyroid

Little can be added to the discussion of the clinical features useful in suspecting lymphoma of the thyroid. The vast majority of primary thyroidal lymphomas will be of non-Hodgkin's type. In our experience with 35 cases, only three were primary Hodgkin's disease of the thyroid established on histologic grounds. These three patients had no clinical evidence of Hodgkin's disease elsewhere, but none had a staging laparotomy to exclude retroperitoneal disease. Of 35 cases of primary lymphoma of the thyroid, 30 were of histiocytic or lymphocytic type, and therefore of the type associated with struma lymphomatosa.

Needle Biopsy Diagnosis of Lymphoma of the Thyroid

The admonition that fine needle aspiration biopsy or large needle biopsy of the thyroid must be interpreted with knowledge of the clinical situation is well taken. Our experience indicates that needle biopsy of the thyroid is an accurate, safe, and rapid method to make a tissue diagnosis of thyroid disease.[26] Where the diagnosis does not appear to explain the clinical presentation, additional biopsy material, reinterpretation of the surgical biopsy, or open biopsy must be considered. With struma lymphomatosa and most lymphomas adequate large needle biopsy cores can be obtained readily, and these are usually sufficient for diagnostic purposes. If the suspicion of lymphoma is unusually strong a second core of tissue for immunoperoxidase studies may be beneficial, especially in subtyping the lymphoma. Experience with this is rudimentary, but the frozen section immunoperoxidase techniques have been invaluable in the classification of lymphomatous disease as diagnosed from open lymph node biopsy. The greatest diagnostic pitfall resides in failure to obtain a representative sample. This points up a need for close correlation of the needle biopsy interpretation with the clinical features. Communication among the endocrinologists or internists, the surgeon, and the pathologist will, in the majority of cases, obviate against an error in diagnosis.

Prognosis of Lymphoma of the Thyroid Is Related to Extent of Disease

It has been our experience, and that of others, that patients with lymphoma confined to the thyroid have a more favorable prognosis than those in whom the lymphomatous process has spread to extrathyroidal sites. Woolner et al. reported only four deaths attributable to lymphoma when the disease was confined to the thyroid, compared to 16 deaths in 20 patients in whom the disease had spread to extrathyroidal sites at the time treatment was begun.[2] The number of patients available in any series for study is small, and little can be reported concerning the effectiveness of modern chemotherapeutic protocols used for lymphomas in general. Clearly, there is an advantage to instituting therapy before extrathyroidal involvement has occurred.

Treatment of Lymphoma of the Thyroid

Irradiation has been the principal treatment in the past. The application of chemotherapy either as a primary modality, in combination with irradiation, or as adjuvant treatment is not definitely established. The accrual of small numbers of patients over long intervals of time complicates the determination of optimal treatment protocols.

Crile has also noted that patients treated with suppressive doses of thyroxine in addition to the therapy for their lymphomas have fared better than those who have not received thyroxine.[20] Again, the numbers are too small for accurate statistical evaluation, and the mechanism by which the benefit is achieved is unknown.

There is considerable merit in subtyping primary lymphoma of the thyroid. Plasmacytoma of the thyroid has an excellent prognosis with late appearance of extrathyroidal manifestations.[27] In the series of Cumpagno and Ortell[22] only one of 13 patients died of the disease. The outlook for patients with histiocytic lymphoma and lymphocytic lymphoma, poorly differentiated type, is approximately the same, with about half the patients succumbing to their disease. For patients with lymphocytic lymphoma with plasmacytoid features the outlook is considerably better, although it does not approach the survival achieved in plasmacytoma. The greater sophistication in chemotherapy warrants subclassifying lymphomas and it is quite possible that survival will be materially improved compared to patients treated with more traditional means.

COMMENTARY

C. Stratton Hill, Jr., M.D.

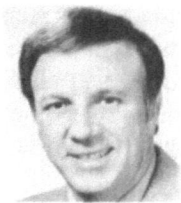

Miller et al. pose several important questions relative to lymphoma of the thyroid, but the most practical one seems to be, "What place does needle biopsy of the thyroid gland have in distinguishing virulent malignant disease from a relatively benign process?" As a corollary one might ask, "Is there a relationship between the relatively benign process and the virulent malignant disease?" The authors discuss the corollary question adequately, and probably answer it as well as possible at this time.

Needle Biopsy in the Diagnosis of Lymphoma of the Thyroid

Most malignant thyroid tumors are of the differentiated type and pursue a relatively indolent course over many years. This is the image most physicians have of thyroid cancer. There are three so-called primary malignant tumors that are more aggressive: medullary carcinoma of the thyroid, small cell carcinoma of the thyroid, and the highly virulent anaplastic carcinoma. There are also tumors of other-than-thyroid-follicular epithelium which occur in the thyroid, including lymphoma, that also usually pursue a more aggressive course. (Medullary carcinoma of the thyroid is of "other-than-follicular epithelium" (C cell), but by tradition it is classified as a "primary" thyroid tumor.) In experienced hands the needle biopsy can identify all these tumors.

For the more aggressive tumors it is necessary to obtain adequate specimens from several areas of the tumor. When these tumors are large and bulky they usually have grown rapidly. Such growth often outstrips growth of the blood supply, necrosis occurs, and if tissue specimens are taken from these areas they are uninterpretable. Another problem with anaplastic carcinoma, which makes multiple sampling necessary, is its frequent contiguous association with differentiated thyroid carcinoma. A sample obtained from the differentiated portion of the tumor mass will give a false impression of the patient's prognosis. When these two components occur in the same tumor mass the clinical course is almost always that of anaplastic carcinoma.

Lymphoma of the thyroid can usually be distinguished easily from the aggressive primary thyroid malignant tumors, excepting the small cell thyroid carcinoma. Small cell thyroid carcinoma is extremely rare and some authorities doubt its existence.[28] At the M. D. Anderson Hospital only three cases have been identified in over 1200 cases of thyroid cancer. It is most frequently confused with lymphoma of the thyroid. When this occurs it is a serious error because the treatment of lymphoma is different from that for small cell carcinoma. Prognosis in lymphoma therapy is related to the extent of disease when treatment is started. Misdiagnosis may delay therapy until the disease progresses to a more advanced stage, thus decreasing the chance of a favorable outcome. It is recommended that extreme caution be exercised in accepting a diagnosis of small cell carcinoma, based either upon a needle biopsy or surgical specimen.

Another difficult problem is distinguishing lymphoma from Hashimoto's thyroiditis. Miller et al. state this can only be done with experience, but that once experience is gained a high degree of accuracy is possible. But is merely making the diagnosis enough? One must remember that lymphoma of the thyroid is not a primary endocrine disease. The group of neoplastic diseases designated as lymphoma usually occur in nodal lymphoid tissue. Extranodal lymphoma may occur in almost any portion of almost any organ in the body. Lymphoma of the thyroid represents an extranodal lymphoma whose initial presentation happens to be in the thyroid gland. One must suspect any lymphoma, whether nodal or extranodal, of being "systemic," i.e., involving other portions of the lymphatic system in the case of nodal lymphoma, or involving the nodal portion of the lymphatic system in the case of extranodal lymphoma. For this reason it is necessary to determine the extent of involvement (stage) in all cases of both nodal and extranodal lymphoma. It has been shown that lymphoma when confined within the capsule of the thyroid gland has a better prognosis than that which has local soft tissue extension and regional lymph node involvement.[8] Patients with local soft tissue extension and regional lymph node involvement should be treated more vigorously than those patients whose disease is confined to the gland. Although needle biopsy of the thyroid in experienced hands can make an early diagnosis of lymphoma, it will likely not be adequate for staging purposes. (This is also true for needle biopsy of the liver and spleen for staging nodal lymphoma.) Therefore, it may not be possible to avoid a surgical procedure if one tailors therapy for lymphoma to the extent of disease (stage). Of course, a surgical procedure for staging is not necessary if clinical examination establishes fixation of the thyroid to surrounding structures, indicating extension of the disease beyond the capsule of the gland.

Frequency of Lymphoma of the Thyroid

The question of an increase in frequency of lymphoma is a difficult one. The evidence presented to support the notion that the NTL increase in frequency of making the diagnosis of lymphoma of the thyroid is tantamount to an increase in the frequency of the disease per se is not very convincing. To establish that there has been a real increase in the frequency of lymphoma of the thyroid would require data on the number of cases of lymphoma of the thyroid prior to 1976 possibly misdiagnosed as Hashimoto's thyroiditis. Additionally, there are many other factors that could account for the increase in the diagnosis of lymphoma. Accuracy of diagnosis can be increased by the interest of the group doing the biopsy. Attention to details of specimen collection is no doubt a factor. Experience of the operator in collecting the specimen and the pathologist in interpreting the results is extremely important. Knowledge by referring physicians of a special interest in any problem usually results in an increase of referrals and probably in selectivity.

It is impossible to analyze all the factors which may have been related to the increase in frequency of diagnosis of lymphoma of the thyroid. In the final analysis whether there is an actual increase in frequency of the disease is probably not critical. The fact that there has been an increase in frequency of diagnosis is significant in itself. The evidence presented indicates that a useful tool is available for early diagnosis of lymphoma of the thyroid and can probably be used successfully to differentiate between other malignant tumors of the thyroid. This will allow physicians to make appropriate therapy decisions. Unfortunately, needle biopsy of the thyroid will probably not prevent a surgical procedure because of the necessity of staging the disease. Should therapy for all lymphoma regardless of stage ever become uniform, the surgical procedure could be avoided.

COMMENTARY

Robert D. Leeper, M.D.

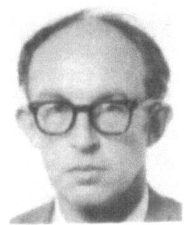

Frequency of Lymphoma of the Thyroid

Primary lymphomas of the thyroid are uncommon but important thyroid neoplasms, which were often not recognized as lymphomas by pathologists in past decades. These neoplasms constituted 1.7% of thyroid cancer at Memorial Hospital up to 1960.[29] In the past many lymphomas were classified as small cell carcinomas of the thyroid,[28] hence their lymphomatous nature went unrecognized. A few lymphomas were also categorized as anaplastic carcinomas, a diagnosis no doubt suggested by rapid growth rate.

It is important to determine whether the lymphoma is primary in the thyroid or whether the thyroid neoplasm is a secondary expression of a generalized process. It has been shown that 20% of generalized lymphomas will involve the thyroid.[30] The usual methods of diagnosis (lymphangiogram, chest radiograph, etc.) should be employed before a lymphoma is classified as a primary thyroid neoplasm. Case 3 in the series reported here may well have been a generalized process. Statistics on the prevalence of primary lymphoma of the thyroid can be heavily weighted by inclusion of secondary lymphomas.

Miller et al. have used their own data and cited published reports to suggest that the incidence of primary lymphoma of the thyroid is increasing. However, neither the author's data nor the data quoted in the cited reports include the total number of thyroid cancers diagnosed during the same time periods. These data are necessary to arrive at valid conclusions concerning changes of incidence in thyroid lymphomas. It is possible in the series of Miller et al. that in the period prior to 1976 more benign thyroid disease such as hyperthyroidism was being seen, and that referral patterns changed after 1976 and more thyroid cancers were seen. In the Memorial Hospital series, 705 cases of thyroid cancer were seen from 1930 to 1954 and 433 cases seen from 1955 to 1960.[29] Assuming a constant 1.7% incidence of lymphomas, the apparent rate per year for these neoplasms would seem to have increased from 0.48 to 1.47/year, a three-fold increase. When better pathologic recognition is taken into account the increase in the incidence of lymphoma may be more apparent than real. The increased use of cell surface marker studies in the future, specifically the identification of monoclonal immunoglobulin antigens for B-cell type tumors, will be helpful in identifying some thyroid lymphomas with more precision.

Association of Lymphoma of the Thyroid with Hashimoto's Thyroiditis

There is no doubt that lymphomas and Hashimoto's thyroiditis are not uncommonly associated in the same pathologic specimen. In fact this has been a cause of confusion in the past as recognized by the authors and others.[29,31] Whether Hashimoto's thyroiditis is a precursor lesion is purely speculative at this time. Areas of Hashimoto's thyroiditis are also found in the presence of other thyroid cancers and it may be that the Hashimoto's thyroiditis is a response to the presence of the neoplasm rather than being a precursor lesion. If lymphomas in general are the result of a prior existing autoimmune diathesis, then the transformation of autoimmune lymphocytes to lymphomatous cells must be a rare event, since it was estimated that only 28,800 cases of lymphoma would be diagnosed in 1975, in the United States.[32]

Diagnosis of Lymphoma of the Thyroid

The authors' case reports in general outline the clinical features of thyroid lymphoma. The process clinically involves the entire thyroid gland more often than is the case for most other thyroid neoplasms. The thyroid mass or masses are usually larger at the time of presentation than is the average differentiated thyroid cancer, which now averages 2.5 cm.[33] Many lymphomas will present with significantly elevated serum titers of antithyroglobulin or antimicrosomal antibodies. These findings are uncommon in other forms of thyroid cancer. Most cases of true Hashimoto's thyroiditis present with smaller glands and gland size decreases promptly with thyroid hormone suppression. A large gland in association with positive thyroid antibodies which enlarges fairly rapidly over the course of a few weeks or months in spite of adequate thyroid hormone suppression should make one suspect lymphoma. Giant and spindle cell cancers also enlarge rapidly but are uncommonly associated with markedly elevated thyroid antibodies.

Miller et al. have outlined the pitfalls of diagnosis. Even in the hands of a skilled pathologist the differential between Hashimoto's thyroiditis and lymphoma is sometimes difficult whether the specimen is a needle biopsy or a full surgical specimen. Growth patterns are such that some lymphomas may be classed as small cell carcinomas. The differences are more than academic since multidrug chemotherapy combined with external beam radiotherapy are indicated in lymphomas. The usefulness of combined modality therapy in other thyroid cancers has not yet been adequately studied.

It is of course important to make the diagnosis of lymphoma of the thyroid as soon as possible by any means including needle biopsy. The correct diagnosis prevents more than reasonable surgery, ensures prompt recourse to other diagnostic methods such as lymphangiograms and cell surface marker studies, and allows for the rapid introduction of multidrug chemotherapy and radiotherapy into the treatment program. This is important since lymphoma of the thyroid was the next most malignant neoplasm after giant and spindle cell cancer in the Memorial Hospital series.[29]

SUMMARY—CHAPTER 10

Our hypothesis that the incidence of lymphoma of the thyroid is increasing was also suggested by Cumpagno and Ortell,[22] who added 254 cases from the Armed Forces Institute of Pathology. This report was published after our paper was written and unfortunately makes no reference to the frequency of diagnoses for each year. Dr. Hawk also agreed with us, while Drs. Hill and Leeper had reservations about the possible error of equating numbers of cases diagnosed with incidence. We have made the assumption that errors in diagnosing lymphoma as Hashimoto's thyroiditis or missing a diagnosis of lymphoma altogether would be exposed in time. Our finding of increased numbers of papillary carcinomas of the thyroid was related partly (75%) to an increase in patient referrals and partly (25%) to the diagnosis of indolent tumors that might well have escaped clinical recognition.[34] Our experience with lymphoma during the same period would seem to be quite different.

The discussants are in agreement with us that the diagnosis of lymphoma of the thyroid can be made by needle biopsy. The previously accepted picture of this disease as an obvious malignancy in elderly females was appropriate for advanced disease. Our experience suggests that the diagnosis can be made earlier. For at least four patients, lymphoma was not on our original list of differential diagnoses.

Dr. Hill questions whether the diagnosis of lymphoma of the thyroid by needle biopsy serves any greater function than the identification of a candidate for thyroidectomy. If staging the disease in the neck by observation at surgery is necessary for selection of proper therapy, he is right. Some oncologists believe that if extracervical staging reveals no disease, and there is no evidence of extrathyroidal neck involvement on physical examination, cervical radiotherapy alone is reasonable treatment. Although the above position is controversial, if needle biopsy diagnosis of lymphoma of the thyroid leads to identification of extrathyroidal disease (perhaps with something as simple as a chest radiograph), then thyroidectomy would be unnecessary. The need for chemotherapy with or without radiotherapy would already be established.

Practically speaking, if one performs thyroid needle biopsies one will make earlier and possibly more frequent diagnoses of lymphoma. It is customary to biopsy enlarging thyroid masses with or without evidence of Hashimoto's thyroiditis. It is our current practice to biopsy all asymmetric or localized enlargements in glands with Hashimoto's thyroiditis that do not regress with TSH suppression by thyroid hormone. The physician who performs biopsies on such glands must be aware of the need for careful sampling and even more careful interpretation of the biopsy specimen.

J. Martin Miller, M.D.

REFERENCES

1. Lindsay S, Dailey ME: Malignant lymphoma of the thyroid gland and its relation to Hashimoto's disease: A clinical and pathologic study of 8 patients. J Clin Endocrinol Metab 15:1332, 1955
2. Woolner LB, McConahey WM, Beahrs OH, Black BM: Primary malignant lymphoma of the thyroid. Am J Surg 111:502, 1966
3. Crile G Jr.: Lymphosarcoma and reticulum cell sarcoma of the thyroid. Surg Gynecol Obstet 116:449, 1963
4. Cox MT: Malignant lymphoma of the thyroid. J Clin Path 17:591, 1964
5. Mikal S: Primary lymphoma of the thyroid gland. Surgery 55:233, 1964
6. Shimkin PM, Sagerman RH: Lymphoma of the thyroid gland. Radiology 92:812, 1969
7. Taylor I: Malignant lymphoma of the thyroid. Br J Surg 63:932, 1976
8. Burke JS, Butler JJ, Fuller LM: Malignant lymphomas of the thyroid. Cancer 39:1587, 1977
9. Sirota DK, Segal RL: Primary lymphomas of the thyroid gland. JAMA 242:1743, 1979
10. Gibson JM, Prinn MG: Hodgkin's disease involving the thyroid gland. Br J Surg 55:236, 1968
11. Hamburger JI, Miller JM, Kini SR: Clinical-Pathological Evaluation of Thyroid Nodules. Handbook and Atlas. Private publication, Southfield, 1979, p 65
12. Wang C, Vickery AL Jr, Maloof F: Needle biopsy of the thyroid. Surg Gynecol Obstet 143:365, 1976
13. Hamburger JI, Miller JM, Kini SR: Clinical-Pathological Evaluation of Thyroid Nodules. Handbook and Atlas. Private publication, Southfield, 1979, pp 10–19
14. Bisbee AC, Thoeny RH: Malignant lymphoma of the thyroid following irradiation. Cancer 35:1296, 1975
15. Cureton RJR, Harland DHC, Hosford J, Pike C: Reticulosarcoma in Hashimoto's disease. Br J Surg 44:561, 1957
16. Kenyon R, Ackerman LV: Malignant lymphoma of the thyroid apparently arising in struma lymphomatosa. Cancer 3:964, 1955
17. Smithers D: Malignant lymphomas of the thyroid gland. In Smithers D (ed): Monographs on Neoplastic Disease, Vol. VI. Tumors of the Thyroid Gland. Edinburgh, Livingstone, 1970, pp 141–154
18. Fujimoto V, Suzuki H, Abe K, Brook JR: Autoantibodies in malignant lymphoma of the thyroid gland. N Engl J Med 276:380, 1967
19. McConahey WM: Hashimoto's thyroiditis. Med Clin North Am 56:885, 1972
20. Crile G Jr: Struma lymphomatosa and carcinoma of the thyroid. Surg Gynecol Obstet 147:350, 1978

21. Einhorn J, Franzen S: Thin-needle biopsy in the diagnosis of thyroid disease. Acta Radiol 58:321, 1962
22. Cumpagno J, Ortell JE: Malignant lymphoma and other lymphoproliferative disorders of the thyroid gland. Am J Clin Pathol 74:1, 1980
23. Dinsmore RS, Dempsey WS, Hazard JB: Lymphosarcoma of thyroid. J Clin Endocrinol 9:1043, 1949
24. Graham A: Riedel's struma in contrast to struma lymphomatosa (Hashimoto). West J Surg 39:681, 1931
25. Crosby EH, Graham A: Mediastinal dermoid cyst containing pancreatic tissue simulating intrathoracic goiter. Cleve Clin Q 1:68, 1932
26. Hawk WA, Crile G Jr, Hazard JB, Barrett DL: Needle biopsy of the thyroid: an assessment of 625 biopsies. Surg Gynecol Obstet 122:1053, 1966
27. Hazard JM, Schildecker WW: Plasmacytoma of the thyroid. Am J Pathol 25:819, 1949
28. Rayfield EJ, Nishiyama RH, Sisson JC: Small cell tumors of the thyroid. A clinicopathologic study. Cancer 28:1023, 1971
29. Lieberman PH, Foote FW, Schottenfeld D: A study of the pathology of thyroid cancer, 1930–1960. MSKCC Clin Bull 2:7, 1972
30. Meissner WH: Pathology of the thyroid. In Werner SC, Ingbar SH (eds): The Thyroid. New York, Harper & Row, 1971, pp 343–363
31. Benua RS, Cicale NR, Sonenberg M, Rawson RW: The relation of radioiodine dosimetry to results and complications in the treatment of metastatic thyroid cancer. Am J Roentgenol Radium Ther Nucl Med 87:171, 1962
32. CA 25:8, 1975
33. Cady B, et al.: Changing clinical, pathologic, therapeutic, and survival patterns in differentiated thyroid carcinoma. Ann Surg 184:541, 1976
34. Miller JM, Hamburger JI, Kini SR: The needle biopsy diagnosis of papillary thyroid carcinoma. Cancer (in press)

Index

Physicians who wish to submit material for consideration for publication in the next edition of Controversies in Clinical Thyroidology should use the following format:

1. A title which states the major question to be addressed.

2. An introduction reviewing past and present attitudes on this matter which highlights the controversial issues which relate to the subject.

3. A listing of these issues.

4. A report of the author's experience including:
   a. Illustrative case reports
   b. Data
   c. Discussion
   d. References

5. A list of suggested authorities who might offer commentary on the subject, especially controversial commentary.

All submissions will be reviewed by the editors, and the authors will be advised promptly as to the suitability of the material.

Address all communications to: *Joel I. Hamburger, M.D.* and *J. Martin Miller, M.D.*, 4400 Prudential Town Center—Suite 275, Southfield, Michigan 48075, U.S.A.

* * *

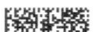